Aptasensors for Point-of-Care Diagnostics

The design and fabrication of aptamer-based biosensors for point-of-care testing of disease diagnostic and prognostic is an upthrust and interdisciplinary area of research. This book covers the design and development of novel cost-effective aptamer-based biosensors for disease diagnostic and prognostic including an understanding of health care management in terms of timely updates of disease situations in a particular geographical area. It also discusses the scaling up and market trend of aptamer-based devices for extension of research from lab to market, and end users.

Features:

- Explains the design and fabrication of aptasensors-based diagnostic devices.
- Includes novel approaches and comprehensive technology overview for diagnosis management towards early-stage detection of various biomarkers associated with several health conditions.
- Demonstrates possible benefits of combined diagnostics and therapeutic possibilities using aptamer-based point-of-care technologies devices.
- Discusses emerging implications and recent advances of biosensing platforms for designing and developing aptamer-based point-of-care testing (POCT) devices.
- Explores aptamer-based approach to develop advanced platforms for medical applications and open arena for state-of-the-art future research.

This book is aimed at researchers and graduate students in biomedical engineering, diagnostics, nanobiotechnology, and materials science.

Aptasensors for Point-of-Care Diagnostics

Fundamentals and Biomedical Applications

Edited by
Arpana Parihar and Raju Khan

CRC Press
Taylor & Francis Group
Boca Raton London New York

CRC Press is an imprint of the
Taylor & Francis Group, an **informa** business

Designed cover image: © Shutterstock

First edition published 2024
by CRC Press
2385 NW Executive Center Drive, Suite 320, Boca Raton FL 33431

and by CRC Press
4 Park Square, Milton Park, Abingdon, Oxon, OX14 4RN

CRC Press is an imprint of Taylor & Francis Group, LLC

ISBN: 9781032302621 (hbk)
ISBN: 9781032302645 (pbk)
ISBN: 9781003304227 (ebk)

DOI: 10.1201/9781003304227

Typeset in Times
by codeMantra

*Dedicated to Almighty, who gave us the strength
to complete this work*

Contents

Preface xv
About the Editors xvii
List of Contributors xix
Acknowledgements xxiii

Chapter 1   Overview of aptamer-based biosensors 1

Datta Maroti Pawde and Sankha Bhattacharya
1.1   Introduction 1
1.2   The brief history and market trend of aptamers 2
1.3   Benefits of aptamers over antibodies and enzymes 3
1.4   Applications of aptamer-based biosensors in diagnosis/
      analysis 4
      1.4.1   Small-molecule biomarkers 4
      1.4.2   Protein biomarkers 4
      1.4.3   Intact pathogens 6
      1.4.4   Circulating tumour cells 7
      1.4.5   Extracellular vesicles detection 11
      1.4.6   Tissue samples 13
1.5   Conclusions and future perspectives 14
References 15

Chapter 2   Biomarkers for aptamer-based diagnostic applications 21

*Sangeeta Ballav, Veda Joshi, Swarangi Tambat, Urwashi
Kumar, Shine Devarajan, Soumya Basu, and Jyotirmoi Aich*
2.1   Introduction 21
2.2   Aptamers as novel biomarkers 23
      2.2.1   What are aptamers? 23
      2.2.2   Types of aptamers 24
2.3   Distinctive attributes of aptamers 25
2.4   Aptamer designing 25
2.5   Aptamers in diagnostics 27
      2.5.1   Nanoparticles 27
      2.5.2   Aptamers in bioimaging 28
      2.5.3   How do aptamers detect the target? 30
      2.5.4   Aptamers in western blot 30
      2.5.5   Aptamers in PCR 31
      2.5.6   Aptamers in IHC 32
      2.5.7   Aptamers in emerging diagnostic applications 33

2.6   Aptamers as therapeutics..36
        2.6.1   Microbial or infectious diseases.......................36
        2.6.2   Oncology 37
        2.6.3   Metabolic disorders 38
        2.6.4   Anti-inflammation, anticoagulation and
                 anti-angiogenesis...38
        2.6.5   Neurological diseases.......................................39
2.7   Modifications for targeted drug delivery.......................39
2.8   Limitations and future prospective.................................40
2.9   Conclusion 41
References 43

Chapter 3   Designing and synthesis of aptamer via various approaches
                 (SELEX and ExSELEX)...49

                 Arpana Parihar, Kritika Gaur, Ayushi Singhal and Raju Khan
3.1   Introduction 49
3.2   Aptamer: potential and advantages 50
3.3   Aptamer synthesis methods...51
        3.3.1   SELEX 51
        3.3.2   Conventional SELEX 51
        3.3.3   Capillary electrophoresis SELEX 52
        3.3.4   Magnetic-bead-based SELEX..........................53
        3.3.5   Cell SELEX...53
        3.3.6   Microfluidic SELEX 55
        3.3.7   In vivo SELEX 55
        3.3.8   EX SELEX 55
3.4   Advanced methods 56
3.5   Application of aptamer..57
        3.5.1   Diagnostic approach..57
        3.5.2   Therapeutic approach 61
3.6   Challenges in aptamer synthesis 63
3.7   Conclusion and future outlook 65
References 66

Chapter 4   A comparative study of aptasensor versus immunosensor for
                 biomarker detection..72

                 Priya Chauhan, Annu Pandey, Ayushi Singhal and Raju Khan
4.1   Introduction 72
4.2   Aptasensors and immunosensors 75
4.3   Fundamentals of electrochemical detection of biomarker 79
4.4   Electrochemical behaviour of aptasensor and
        immunosensor 79
4.5   Role of biosensor as diagnostic tool 81
        4.5.1   Optical biosensors 82

4.5.2   Mechanical biosensors 82
4.5.3   Electrochemical biosensors....................................... 82
4.6   Detection of biological analytes using aptasensors................. 83
4.7   Application of aptasensors to detect several biomarkers 86
4.8   Application of aptasensors to detect cancer biomarkers 86
4.9   Voltammetric immunosensors to detect cancer biomarkers ...90
4.10   Future directions.. 90
References 91

Chapter 5   Aptamer-based point-of-care diagnostic devices for infectious
diseases... 99

Kalpesh V. Bhavsar, Hardik S. Churi, and Uday P. Jagtap

5.1   Introduction 99
5.2   Aptamer-based technologies.. 101
5.3   Introduction to POC technology...................................... 103
       5.3.1   Discovery of POCT...................................... 103
       5.3.2   Need for POC diagnostic technologies 104
5.4   POC diagnostics tools and devices.................................. 106
       5.4.1   Types of POC devices 106
       5.4.2   POC devices in the medical industry...................... 107
5.5   POC devices for infectious diseases................................ 109
       5.5.1   Bacterial infections.................................... 109
       5.5.2   Parasitic infection..................................... 112
       5.5.3   Viral infections.. 113
5.6   Additional aptamer-based detection methods 116
       5.6.1   Aptamer chemiluminescence immunosorbent assay..... 116
       5.6.2   Nanoarray aptamer-based chip assay 117
       5.6.3   Aptamer technique based on fluorescence energy
                transfer.. 117
5.7   Nanotechnology in diagnosis 118
5.8   Conclusion and future scope 119
References 120

Chapter 6   Aptamer-based colorimetric biosensor................................ 127

Yasmin Bano and Sadhana Chaturvedi

6.1   Introduction 127
6.2   Trends in aptamers-based techniques................................ 128
6.3   Aptamer-target configurations.. 129
6.4   Construction of aptamer-based biosensors 130
       6.4.1   Target-induced structure switching (TISS) mode 130
       6.4.2   Sandwich or sandwich-like mode........................ 132
       6.4.3   Target-induced dissociation/displacement (TID)
                mode.. 133
       6.4.4   Competitive replacement (CR) mode 133
       6.4.5   Target-induced reassembly (TIR) mode................. 134

6.5   Material-based colorimetric biosensors 135
        6.5.1   Gold nanomaterials-based colorimetric biosensors 135
        6.5.2   Graphene (Gr) based colorimetric biosensors 149
        6.5.3   Carbon dots (CDs) and nanotubes-based
                 colorimetric biosensors 150
        6.5.4   2D metal nanoplates 151
        6.5.5   Silica beads and silica nanoparticles (SiNPs) 152
        6.5.6   Magnetic beads (MBs) 152
        6.5.7   MOFs (metal-organic framework) 152
        6.5.8   Enzymes 153
6.6   Colorimetric biosensing assay as POC testing 154
6.7   Conclusion and future remarks 156
References 158

Chapter 7   Aptamer beacon probes for the detection and visualization of
             miRNA 171

             Jayavigneeswari Suresh Babu, Sailaja V. Eluchuri, and
             Janakiraman Narayanan
             7.1   Introduction 171
                     7.1.1   Aptamer and beacon probes 172
             7.2   Synthesis of nucleic acid aptamers 173
                     7.2.1   Variants of SELEX based on target types ... 173
                     7.2.2   SELEX variants with immobilized targets ... 174
                     7.2.3   SELEX variants involving cells or tissues ... 174
                     7.2.4   SELEX variants with immobilized aptamers ... 175
                     7.2.5   SELEX in solution 175
             7.3   Characterization of aptamers 177
                     7.3.1   Surface plasmon resonance (SPR) 177
                     7.3.2   Fluorescence polarization or fluorescence
                              anisotropy (FP or FA) 177
                     7.3.3   Isothermal titration calorimetry (ITC) 177
                     7.3.4   Flow cytometry 178
             7.4   Applications of aptamers 179
                     7.4.1   Aptasensors 179
                     7.4.2   Chemical toxins detection 180
                     7.4.3   Pathogen detection 180
                     7.4.4   Detection of biologically relevant molecules ... 182
                     7.4.5   Detection of different classes of cells 182
                     7.4.6   Nanovescicles secreted from human tissues
                              and cells detection by aptamer 184
                     7.4.7   Aptamers as drug delivery systems 185
             7.5   Peptide aptamers 185
                     7.5.1   Selection of peptide aptamers 185
                     7.5.2   Characterization of peptide aptamers 187
                     7.5.3   Applications of peptide aptamers 187
             7.6   Molecular aptamer beacon probes 188

7.6.1   Basic principle of molecular beacon probes............ 188
7.6.2   Beacon probes with aptamer engineering for
        biomolecule detection... 189
7.6.3   Aptamer-based beacon probes for pathogen
        detections... 189
7.6.4   Detection of RNA in living cells using molecular
        beacon probes.. 190
7.6.5   miRNA detection methods....................................... 190
7.6.6   Hybridization of the mature beacon to the mature
        miRNA target... 191
7.6.7   Aptamers beacon probes for the detection of
        miRNAs in different diseases 192
7.7   Therapeutic advances 194
7.7.1   Small RNA as therapy molecules 194
7.7.2   Chemical modifications of miRNA-based
        therapeutics... 195
7.7.3   Combination of miRNA and aptamers for therapy.... 195
7.7.4   Aptamer-modified exosomes as therapy 196
7.8   Future prospective 198
References 200

Chapter 8   Microfluidics-enabled aptamer-based sensing devices – the
             aptafluidics microdevices 211

*Vishal K. Sahu, Amit Ranjan, A.S.M. Shailaja, Jyotirmoi Aich,
and Soumya Basu*

8.1   Introduction 211
8.2   Microfluidic platforms patterning methods........................... 212
8.2.1   Wax printing.. 212
8.2.2   Inkjet printing.. 213
8.2.3   Digital light processing (DLP) printing 213
8.2.4   Plasma printing.. 213
8.2.5   Lithography 213
8.3   Detection and analytical methods 214
8.3.1   Electrochemical method... 214
8.3.2   Transistor-based method 214
8.3.3   Optical method... 214
8.3.4   Gravimetric method 215
8.4   The diverse microfluidics platforms..................................... 215
8.4.1   Paper microchips.. 215
8.4.2   Glass or plastic-based microchips............................ 215
8.5   Advantages 216
8.5.1   Rapid detection.. 216
8.5.2   High sensitivity and selectivity 216
8.5.3   Multiplexing of multiple signals.............................. 216
8.5.4   Miniaturized devices – LOC.................................... 216
8.5.5   Quantitative and qualitative detection...................... 218

        8.5.6   Multiple analyte detection 218

        8.5.7   Reusability and disposability 218

   8.6   Applications of aptafluidics microdevices (MeAS) 218

        8.6.1   Whole-cell detection and separation 218

        8.6.2   Detection and extraction of molecules 219

        8.6.3   Aptafluidics microdevices for cancer 220

        8.6.4   Detection and characterization of other diseases 221

        8.6.5   Screening and discovery of new potential agents
                 for diagnostics and treatment 222

   8.7   Challenges in the fabrication of MeAS devices
        and prospects 222

   8.8   MeAS patents 223

   8.9   Conclusion 224

   References 225

Chapter 9   Fabrication of aptamer-based electrochemical biosensor for
             health care monitoring 232

             Ayushi Singhal, Apoorva Shrivastava, Arpana Parihar, and
             Raju Khan

   9.1   Introduction 232

   9.2   Aptamers-based biosensors for point-of-care testing 234

   9.3   Application of aptasensors for the health care
        monitoring 236

   9.4   Conclusion and future perspective 243

   References 244

Chapter 10 Challenges and advances in aptamer-based biosensing
             approaches 248

             Srikanth Ponnada, Sarita Yadav, Demudu Babu Gorle, Meghali
             Devi, Anjali Palariya, Rapaka S. Chandra Bose, Rakesh K. Sharma

   10.1   Introduction 248

   10.2   Aptamer synthesis 250

   10.3   Aptamer-based POC diagnostic devices 251

        10.3.1 Aptamer-based optical biosensors 252

        10.3.2 Aptamer-based colorimetric biosensors 252

        10.3.3 Aptamer-based fluorescence biosensors 254

        10.3.4 SERS-based aptamers 255

        10.3.5 Aptamer-based electrochemical biosensors 257

        10.3.6 Aptamer-based microfluidic biosensors 258

        10.3.7 3D printing-based aptamers 260

   10.4   POC diagnostic applications of aptamer-based
        biosensor 261

        10.4.1 Protein biomarker identification 261

        10.4.2 Small-molecule biomarker detection 261

10.4.3   Intact pathogens detection.......................................263
10.4.4   Circulating tumour cells..263
10.5   Drawbacks of aptamer-based biosensors............................264
10.6   Future prospects and conclusions.......................................265
References 266

Chapter 11 Current perspectives of aptasensors as diagnostic tools for
oncological diseases 271

Suman Kumar Ray and Sukhes Mukherjee
11.1   Introduction 271
11.2   Aptasensor transduction mechanisms 273
11.2.1   Electrochemical aptasensors 273
11.2.2   Optical aptasensors 274
11.3   Aptasensors and detection of cancer biomarkers 275
11.3.1   Protein biomarkers for cancer 276
11.3.2   Biomarkers for antigens 276
11.3.3   Circulating tumor cells...276
11.3.4   Exosomes...276
11.4   Aptasensors for detection of the PSA in
prostate cancer...278
11.5   Aptasensors for detection of MCF-7 cells, Ramos cells,
and tumor necrosis factor-α...278
11.6   Aptasensors for detection of leukemia cells..........................278
11.7   Aptasensors for detection of MUC1 cells and CEA..............279
11.8   Application of aptasensors in clinical
diagnosis of cancer 280
11.9   Applications of aptasensors in the cancer
follow-up...280
11.10 Aptasensor and point-of-care diagnosis in cancer.................282
11.11 Conclusion and future outlook 282
References 284

Index..289

Preface

The aptamer-based biosensors also known as aptasensors have gained considerable interest in the development of diagnostic devices for various diseases. Aptamers are single-stranded DNA or RNA oligonucleotides that have a high affinity to bind with a diverse range of target molecules, like nucleic acids, proteins, and other small molecules. The higher affinity, target selectivity, and ultra-high sensitivity offered by aptasensors have been exploited for the design and development of several POCT devices. The target analyte-specific aptamers can be identified and purified using a process called Systematic Evolution of Ligands by Exponential Enrichment (SELEX). Further, aptamers can be produced at low cost and be easily modified with signal moieties when compared to other bioreceptors such as antibodies and enzymes. Due to these added advantages over other bioreceptors, the aptamer-based biosensors evolved rapidly and several aptamer-based biosensors (recognition and detection) for different target analytes have been successfully developed. Moreover, similar to the classical immunosorbent-based detection assays, aptasensors can be designed and fabricated in a single-site binding format, as a dual-site (sandwich) binding format, or one can use an aptamer and an antibody in a sandwich binding format. Besides, Aptasensors can be integrated with different transducers such as mass-, optical, or electrochemical for the sensitive detection of biomarkers. The aptasensor-based point-of-care diagnostics at near patients' settings holds great promise to deal with critical situations in terms of decision-making and specific therapy prescription. Aptasensors-based diagnostic technologies have emerged as a boon to society for POCT of disease diagnostics as they are cost-effective, easily accessible, and scalable. Several studies revealed that aptamer-based biosensors exhibit great potential for disease diagnosis as they offer high sensitivity and selectivity for the detection of target biomarkers associated with particular disease conditions. Several Aptasensors are commercially available for the diagnosis of various diseases and are routinely used in clinical, industrial, environmental, and agricultural applications. In the present scenario, due to lifestyle changes and emerging pathogens, there is a need of a novel highly sensitive cost-effective biosensing platform for point-of-care diagnostics of diseases in mass population. The advantages such as rapid and precise response, portability, low cost, and requirement of simple equipment made aptasensor-based POCT a valuable tool for disease diagnostics at low resource settings. This book describes the fundamental process of designing and fabricating aptamer-based biosensors for various infectious and oncological diseases. Besides, types of aptasensors based on various transducers and biomarkers have been discussed. Apart from this, an insight into scaling up of devices using various approaches along with the current market trend for the detection of the disease has been included in this book. It is expected that this book would help researchers and clinicians to design and develop novel aptasensors for point-of-care disease diagnostics. Moreover, in this book, we highlight the fabrication strategies along with biomedical applications of advanced aptamer-based biosensors which would not only provide a greater understanding of disease diagnostics but also be helpful in terms of technology adoption by the end users in resource-limited settings.

The book comprises 11 chapters. Chapter 1 deals with an overview and basic information of aptamer used for the development of biosensors. Chapter 2 provides brief details of aptamer-based biomarkers and highlights the emerging biomarkers in several diseases which can be explored for the development of sensing devices. Chapter 3 discusses the approaches of aptamer designing and synthesis. Further, it would also enable readers the screening process of biomarker-specific aptamer. Chapter 4 provides a comparative study of aptasensors and immunosensors for biomarker detection. Different types of bioreceptors such as enzymes, antibodies and aptamers along with their associated biosensing applications, chemical linking procedures, and transduction mechanisms. Chapter 5 deals with the point-of-care aptasensors for rapid monitoring of viral and bacterial-born infectious diseases. Chapter 6 attempts to cover basic principle and fabrication strategy of aptamer-based colorimetric biosensors for the detection of biomarkers for health care monitoring. Chapter 7 discusses miniaturization strategies and overview details of surface-based miniaturized platforms for biomarker detection. Chapter 8 would enable the reader to understand the importance of microfluidics-based aptasensors, their performance, sensitivity, and specificity for detection of biomarkers. Chapter 9 discusses various types of electrochemical aptasensors such as field-effect transistors, DPV, EIS, etc. Besides, sensing strategies based on the unique properties of aptamers will be summarized for biomedical devices. Chapter 10 covers current progress, advances and challenges in the development of aptamer-based next-generation biosensors. Chapter 11 deals with current aptamer-based diagnostics devices for monitoring oncological diseases. The required references are cited in each chapter for further study on the respective topic.

About the Editors

Dr. Arpana Parihar is currently working as a Women Scientist B at CSIR-Advanced Materials and Processes Research Institute (AMPRI), Bhopal, MP, India, under the scheme of DST-WoS-B awarded from the Department of Science and Technology, Government of India. She did her Ph.D. at Raja Rammana Centre for Advanced Technology, Indore, and postdoctoral research work at the Centre for Biomedical Engineering (CBME), Indian Institute of Technology (IIT) Delhi. Dr. Parihar has been awarded with prestigious GATE, CSIR-NET, DST-WoS A, and WoS B fellowships. She has more than 8 years of research and teaching experience in the field of disease therapeutics and diagnostics. Her current research activity includes the fabrication of biosensors for early diagnosis of cancer, molecular docking and simulation for drug designing, tissue engineering, targeted cancer therapy, and 3D cell culture. She has published 45 articles and edited 7 books with renowned publishers.

Dr. Raju Khan is currently working as a Principal Scientist and Associate Professor at CSIR-AMPRI Bhopal, Madhya Pradesh, India. He has more than 15 years of experience in electrochemistry, and the development of biosensors-based diagnostics. He is a member of the International Advisory Committee, World Academy of Science, Engineering and Technology, and a Fellow of the Royal Society of Chemistry. He published more than 90 research articles with high citation scores. He has edited 20 books with various reputed publishers. He has several ongoing/completed projects including National/International scientific collaborations with the USA, Czech Republic, and Russia.

Contributors

Jyotirmoi Aich
School of Biotechnology and
  Bioinformatics, DY Patil Deemed-
  to-Be University, CBD
  Belapur, Navi Mumbai,
  Maharashtra, India

Sangeeta Ballav
Cancer and Translational Research
  Centre, Dr. D.Y. Patil Biotechnology
  & Bioinformatics Institute, Dr. D. Y.
  Patil Vidyapeeth, Pune, Maharashtra,
  India

Yasmin Bano
Molecular and Human Genetics, Jiwaji
  University, Gwalior, India

Soumya Basu
Cancer and Translational Research
  Centre, Dr. D.Y. Patil Biotechnology
  & Bioinformatics Institute, Dr. D. Y.
  Patil Vidyapeeth, Pune, Maharashtra,
  India

Sankha Bhattacharya
Department of Pharmaceutics, School
  of Pharmacy & Technology
  Management, SVKM'S NMIMS
  Deemed-To-Be University, Shirpur,
  Maharashtra, India

Kalpesh V. Bhavsar
National Centre for Nanosciences
  and Nanotechnology, University of
  Mumbai, Kalina Campus.Kalina,
  Santacruz (E), Mumbai, India

Rapaka S. Chandra Bose
Centre for Materials for Electronics
  Technology, Thrissur, Kerala, India

Sadhana Chaturvedi
School of Sciences, ITM University,
  Gwalior, India

Priya Chauhan
SOS in Environmental Chemistry,
  Jiwaji University, Gwalior, India

Hardik S. Churi
Sonopant Dandekar Shikshan Mandali
  (SDSM) College, College Road,
  Tembhode, Palghar, Maharashtra,
  India

Shine Devarajan
School of Biotechnology and
  Bioinformatics, DY Patil Deemed-
  To-Be University, CBD Belapur,
  Navi Mumbai, Maharashtra, India

Meghali Devi
Department of Chemistry, National
  Institute of Technology, Silichar, India

Sailaja V. Eluchuri
Department of Nanobiotechnology,
  Vision Research Foundation,
  Kamalnayan Bajaj Institute
  for Research in Vision and
  Ophthalmology, Chennai, Tamil
  Nadu, India

Kritika Gaur
Central sheep and wool research
  institute. ICAR – Indian Council of
  Agricultural Research, Avikanagr,
  Malpura, Rajasthan, India

Demudu Babu Gorle
Materials Research Centre, Indian
  Institute of Science, Bangalore, India

Uday P. Jagtap
National Centre for Nanosciences
    and Nanotechnology, University of
    Mumbai, Kalina Campus.Kalina,
    Santacruz (E), Mumbai, India

Veda Joshi
School of Biotechnology and
    Bioinformatics, DY Patil Deemed-
    To-Be University, CBD Belapur,
    Navi Mumbai, Maharashtra, India

Raju Khan
Academy of Scientific and Innovative
    Research (AcSIR), Ghaziabad, India

Urwashi Kumar
School of Biotechnology and
    Bioinformatics, DY Patil Deemed-
    To-Be University, CBD Belapur,
    Navi Mumbai, Maharashtra, India

Sukhes Mukherjee
Department of Biochemistry, All
    India Institute of Medical Sciences,
    Bhopal, Madhya Pradesh, India

Janakiraman Narayanan
Department of Nanobiotechnology,
    Vision Research Foundation,
    Kamalnayan Bajaj Institute
    for Research in Vision and
    Ophthalmology, Chennai, Tamil
    Nadu, India

Anjali Palariya
Department of Chemistry, Jai Narayan
    Vyas University (New Campus),
    Jodhpur, Rajasthan, India

Annu Pandey
Department of Chemistry, Institute of
    Science, Chandigarh University,
    Chandigarh, India

Arpana Parihar
Industrial Waste Utilization, Nano and
    Biomaterials, CSIR-AMPRI, Bhopal,
    Madhya Pradesh, India

Datta Maroti Pawde
Department of Pharmaceutics, School
    of Pharmacy & Technology
    Management, SVKM'S NMIMS
    Deemed-To-Be University, Shirpur,
    Maharashtra, India

Srikanth Ponnada
Sustainable Materials and Catalysis
    Research Laboratory (SMCRL),
    Department of Chemistry, IIT
    Jodhpur, Karwad,
    Jodhpur, India

Amit Ranjan
Cancer and Translational Research
    Centre, Dr. D.Y. Patil Biotechnology
    & Bioinformatics Institute, Dr. D. Y.
    Patil Vidyapeeth, Pune, Maharashtra,
    India

Suman Kumar Ray
Independent Researcher, Bhopal,
    Madhya Pradesh, India

Vishal K. Sahu
Cancer and Translational Research
    Centre, Dr. D.Y. Patil Biotechnology
    & Bioinformatics Institute, Dr. D. Y.
    Patil Vidyapeeth, Pune, Maharashtra,
    India

A.S.M. Shailaja
Cancer and Translational Research
    Centre, Dr. D.Y. Patil Biotechnology
    & Bioinformatics Institute, Dr. D. Y.
    Patil Vidyapeeth, Pune, Maharashtra,
    India

Rakesh K. Sharma
SMCRL, Department of Chemistry,
    IIT Jodhpur, Karwad, Jodhpur,
    India

Apoorva Shrivastava
D. Y. Patil Biotechnology and
    Bioinformatics Institute, Dr. D. Y.
    Patil Vidyapeeth, Sr. No. 87-88,
    Mumbai-Bangalore Highway,
    Tathawade, Pune,
    Maharashtra, Ghaziabad, India

Ayushi Singhal
AcSIR, Ghaziabad, India

Jayavigneeswari Suresh Babu
Department of Nanobiotechnology, Vision
    Research Foundation, Kamalnayan
    Bajaj Institute for Research in Vision
    and Ophthalmology, Chennai, Tamil
    Nadu, India

Swarangi Tambat
School of Biotechnology and
    Bioinformatics, DY Patil Deemed-
    To-Be University, CBD Belapur,
    Navi Mumbai, Maharashtra, India

Sarita Yadav
Department of Chemistry, National
    Institute of Technology Warangal,
    Telangana, India

Acknowledgements

All contributors to the respective chapters in this book are thankfully acknowledged by the editors. Their honest efforts, hard work, and analytical approach have been well appreciated and recognized. The editors are thankful to the Director, CSIR-AMPRI, Bhopal, MP, India, for his invaluable advice and direction. Dr. Arpana Parihar is thankful to the Department of Science and Technology, Government of India, for providing her fellowship (DST/WOS-B/HN-4/2021) under the DST-WoS-B Scheme. Dr. Raju Khan acknowledges funding from SERB (IPA/2020/000130).

1 Overview of aptamer-based biosensors

Datta Maroti Pawde and Sankha Bhattacharya

1.1 INTRODUCTION

Aptamers are single-stranded nucleic acids that have been 3D-folded and have the capacity selectively bind to target molecules (Li & Champion 2022). Aptasensors are one of the most promising possibilities to help accelerate the transformation of old-style benchtop therapeutic diagnostics into point-of-care tests in the innovative era of cutting-edge medicine (Sharma et al. 2022). Throughout the history of our culture, health care has consistently been regarded as a top priority and given a high value. Even though there has been a significant increase in funding for healthcare in recent decades, there are still a number of significant obstacles to overcome. For instance, epidemic infectious diseases like the 2019 coronavirus disease as well as other diseases can be found in every region of the world. Global health is the study of interdisciplinary collaboration among medical practitioners, scientists, funding agencies, policymakers, and the common community to promote efficient ways to solve problems that arise globally and cross-national boundaries. These problems can range from people-based prevention to single person-level medical attention (Lee & Lee 2021).

Well-known large-scale problems like non-communicable diseases, infant health, HIV/AIDS, malnutrition, maternal and vaccination, also preferred scientific or technical developments that would improve the access to medical care and conquer socioeconomic obstacles for public incarnate in assets-limited areas, are among the magnificent tasks facing the arena of overall health (Jakovljevic et al. 2021).

Diagnostic technologies are essential for early detection of health disorders or diseases, treatment planning, and monitoring of the outcomes of medical interventions. Current diagnostic techniques, on the other hand, are frequently developed for laboratory usage and so are lacking to address the health necessities of developing countries (Pohanka 2021).

The development of point-of-care (POC) technologies to provide fast, self-assisted testing in outpatient or remote locations to accompany routine clinical diagnostics is a current trend in medical diagnostics. The widespread availability of these low-cost tests, as well as their amalgamation with digital strategies for inaccessible records broadcast and examination, are projected to create a primarily novel approach for

DOI: 10.1201/9781003304227-1

global, near-real-time public health interventions (Flahault et al. 2017; Steinhubl et al. 2015). This book chapter seeks to deliver a well-timed overview of the latest advancements in the use of aptamer-associated biosensors for POC diagnostics and public well-being.

1.2 THE BRIEF HISTORY AND MARKET TREND OF APTAMERS

The aptamers are presented for the first stint in 1990. Andy Ellington and Jack Szostak, in independent experiments that formulated a similar common scheme for the SELEX process, the subsequent agents were termed "aptamers" (derived from the Greek word aptus means "to fit") (Ellington & Szostak 1990; Green et al. 1990). In 1992, the development of NeXagen continued history; NeXagen turned into an industry named NeXstar. NeXagen and NeXstar were devoted to developing aptamers as medicaments, precisely equivalent to antibodies or antibody mimics. NX1838 (currently named Macugen) came to the market as the first aptamer. It is a modified RNA aptamer that has a vascular endothelial growth factor (VEGF) antagonist, and hence it works as an angiogenesis inhibitor (Ruckman et al. 1998).

The recently published research report provides a thorough analysis of the aptamers market's prospects, as well as the industry's drivers, restraints, and challenges, to aid in acquiring an in-depth understanding of the current and future market landscape. Moreover, the study offers in-depth data on a variety of factors, including product category, use case, technology, end user, and geographical location. Fact.MR is an Unbiased Source of Market Research and Business Intelligence. The global aptamers market is expected to increase at a compound annual growth rate (CAGR) of 21.6% from 2022 to 2030. By the year 2030, it is expected that market sales will have hit $11.5 billion US dollars. Growth over the assessment period is expected to be fuelled by a number of factors, including the rising global use of aptamers in R&D and the high prevalence of chronic diseases (2022–2030). Several nations are boosting their financial and funding commitments to the study of novel vaccinations for the treatment of a wide variety of diseases, including cancer. Numerous illnesses have been eradicated because of vaccines and other medical advancements. Aptamer industry participants stand to benefit from the spotlight being shone on chronic disease therapy and other upbeat endeavours. One reason contributing to the increased need for aptamers is the rising cost of providing healthcare for an ever-increasing elderly population. Census estimates put the number of Americans 65 and up at more than 54 million. The prevalence of chronic diseases is rising alongside the senior population, driving up the need for specialized medical treatment. Aptamers are used extensively in the pursuit of novel therapies, therefore it stands to reason that demand for aptamers will rise during the course of the horizon of analysis. In addition, North America is considered the largest market for aptamers, and this area is expected to continue leading the pack during the course of the forecast. The United States is expected to dominate the North American market, surpassing Canada's current market share. Aptamers are predicted to maintain brisk sales across the globe, particularly in the Americas, Europe, and Asia (Di Ruscio & de Franciscis 2022). The market trends of aptamers are summarized in Figure 1.1.

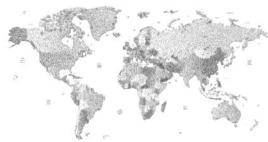

Aptamers Market Trends

151 USD
Million in 2021

342 USD
Million in 2026

The expansion of research and development efforts focused on aptamers, as well as the manufacturing of products based on these aptamers, can be credited with driving growth in the Asia-Pacific region market.

CAGR
17.7%

The global market for aptamers is projected to reach $342 million by 2026, representing a compound annual growth rate (CAGR) of 17.7% throughout the period covered by this projection.

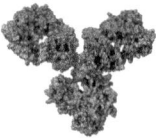

The increasing number of clinical studies being conducted to develop aptamer-based medicines as well as the increasing expenditure in pharmaceutical R&D are the primary factors driving the growth of the market.

This market has an opportunity for growth thanks to an increase in investment from venture capitalists for research on aptamers.

According to certain estimates, the market in Asia and the Pacific would see the highest CAGR during the first period.

It is possible that the market expansion may be affected by the shortage of experienced and trained individuals.

FIGURE 1.1 Market trends of aptamers (Di Ruscio & de Franciscis 2022).

1.3 BENEFITS OF APTAMERS OVER ANTIBODIES AND ENZYMES

Aptamers are now incredibly significant diagnostic and therapeutic molecular tools. Aptamer-associated biosensors, in particular, have unrivalled benefits over biosensors grounded on regular receptors such as antibodies and enzymes. Following are the benefits of aptamers over antibodies and enzymes (Candia et al. 2017; Di Ruscio & de Franciscis 2022).

- Aptamers with great specificity and affinity can feasibly be chosen in vitro for any goal, extending from minor molecules to bulky proteins and the level of cells, allowing for the development of a diverse spectrum of aptamer-associated biosensors.
- Aptamers are able to be manufactured with extraordinary purity and reproducibility from marketable sources once they've been chosen. DNA aptamers are also usually chemically stable, unlike protein-associated antibodies or enzymes.
- When aptamers attach to a target, they frequently undergo considerable conformational changes. This provides a lot of leeway when it comes to creating novel biosensors with excellent detection sensitivity and selectivity.

Additionally, aptamers have several advantages over alternative methods, and as drug transport, purification, and the development of drugs for killing target cells continue to advance, more and more researchers will be compelled to use them. Several benefits distinguish aptamers from antibodies, including reduced production costs, smaller molecular size, less side effects, and less immunogenicity (Li & Champion 2022). These benefits should help propel the global aptamers market forward throughout the next decade.

1.4 APPLICATIONS OF APTAMER-BASED BIOSENSORS IN DIAGNOSIS/ANALYSIS

1.4.1 Small-Molecule Biomarkers

Small molecules consist of an enormous number of compounds which are biologically active. These small molecules have a vital role in human health. Because of their small size, they have limitations in the accessibility for the targeting ligand (e.g., aptamer) to bind on the binding site. Aptamers have been extensively used in the diagnosis/analysis of antibiotics, drug molecules, heavy metals, pesticide residues, and toxins. Table 1.1 shows the non-comprehensive reports of aptasensors that are particularly cast-off in the diagnosis of small molecules, along with their LOD and aptasensing strategy.

1.4.2 Protein Biomarkers

The presence of many protein biomarkers in the biological fluid such as serum, sweat, etc. can be done with the aid of aptasensors. For the detection of main inflammatory markers like cytokine tumour necrosis factor-α (TNF-α), aptasensors have been developed. The assay was linear from 6 nM and able to detect 58 pM of TNF-α. The blood plasma samples can be analysed for the detection of the protein related to lung cancer with the help of EC aptasensors. The detection limit of the aptasensors was enhanced by employing silica-coated iron oxide MBs (Zamay et al. 2016). An assay was developed by applying the same principles as that of EC aptasensing for the detection of C-reactive protein (Jarczewska et al. 2018; Wang et al. 2017), interleukin-6 (Kumar et al. 2016), lysozyme (Rodríguez & Rivas 2009), prostate-specific antigen (Crulhas et al. 2017) and vascular endothelial growth factor (Crulhas et al. 2017). Mycobacterium tuberculosis secretes protein MPT64. This protein is utilized as a biomarker of tuberculosis. An assay was developed in a recent study employing aptasensors for the detection of MPT64 in serum in 30 min time and 81 pM of sensitivity (Sypabekova et al. 2019). The subtyping of the influenza A H1N1 virus was successfully done by Bhardwaj et al. (2019) with the application of a DNA aptamer that targets the hemagglutinin's stem region. The thrombin detection was enhanced successfully by Ren et al. (2020) to 0.57 fM with the development of an aptamer derived from a porous carbon nanocontainer that has a framework with zeolitic imidazolate. The mucin 16 protein was detected with the help of a newly developed aptamer-antibody sandwich assay. This assay has 0.02 units/mL of LOD (Lu et al. 2020). The insulin-like growth

TABLE 1.1

Small molecules detection employing developed aptasensors in the last 10 years

Target compound	Aptasensing strategy	LOD	References
• Acetamiprid	• Electrochemical	• 0.33 pM	• Jiang et al. (2015)
• Atrazine	• Electrochemical	• 40 pM	• Madianos et al. (2018)
• Carbofuran	• Chemiluminescent	• 88 pM	• Li et al. (2016)
• Chloramphenicol	• Colorimetric	• 18.3 pM	• Javidi et al. (2018)
• Chlorpyrifos	• Electrochemical	• 0.35 fM	• Roushani et al. (2018)
• Isocarbophos	• Electrochemical	• 0.01 nM	• Bala et al. (2016a)
• Malathion	• Colorimetric	• 0.06 pM	• Fu et al. (2019)
• Omethoate	• Electrochemical	• 0.1 nM	• Fu et al. (2020)
• Phorate	• Colorimetric	• 0.01 nM	• Bala et al. (2016b)
• Profenofos	• Electrochemical	• 0.003 nM	• Fu et al. (2019)
• Aminoglycoside antibiotics	• Colorimetric	• 1–100 nM	• Derbyshire et al. (2012)
• Chloramphenicol	• Photoelectrochemical	• 3.1 nM	• Liu et al. (2015)
• Kanamycin	• Electrochemical	• 5.8 nM	• Sun et al. (2014)
• Lincomycin	• Chemiluminescent	• 1.6×10^{-13} mol/L	• Li et al. (2017)
• Tetracycline	• Colorimetric	• 45.8 nM	• He et al. (2013)
• As^{3+}	• Colorimetric	• 5.3 ppb	• Wu et al. (2012a, 2012b)
• Cu^{2+}	• Electrochemical	• 0.1 pM	• Chen et al. (2011)
• Hg^{2+}	• Surface plasmon resonance spectroscopy	• 10 fM	• Pelossof et al. (2011)
• Aflatoxin B1	• Spectrophotometry	• 0.1 ng/mL	• Seok et al. (2015)
• Fumonisin B1	• Fluorescence resonance energy transfer	• 0.1 ng/mL	• Yang et al. (2011)
• Ochratoxin A	• Colorimetric	• 20 nM	• Rivas et al. (2015)
	• Impedimetric	• 14 pM	• Temur et al. (2012)
• Staphylococcal enterotoxin B	• Surface-enhanced Raman spectroscopy	• 224 aM	• Ramezani et al. (2015)
• ATP	• Electrochemical	• 0.1 pM	• Wang et al. (2018)
• BPA	• Electrochemical	• 5 nM	• Zhou et al. (2014)
	• Surface-enhanced Raman spectroscopy	• 3 nM	• Marks et al. (2014)
• Cocaine	• Molecular beacons	• 0.48 nM	• Taghdisi et al. (2015)
	• Electrochemical	• 105 pM	• Ma et al. (2011)
• Mat lysozyme	• Colorimetric	• 1×10^{-4} µg/mL	• Wang et al. (2011)

ATP, adenosine 5¢-triphosphate; BPA, bisphenol A.

factor 2 receptor protein was detected through a SERS assay reported by Liu et al. (2020). The detection limit of the developed assay is 141.2 fM.

1.4.3 INTACT PATHOGENS

The intact pathogens like whole bacteria and viruses can be detected with the help of aptamers. The application of aptamers in this field is directed to progress for various pathogen detection with quick and highly sensitive diagnostics technologies. These aptasensors have benefits such as ease of use, high throughput, low cost, minimum batch-to-batch variability, and stability over the traditional antibody-based assays (Li & Champion 2022). In the future, diagnostics development using aptasensors will increase due to the above-stated advantages. The topic is huge. The published literature is extensive and due to space constraints, we have only listed a selected recent report on aptasensors for pathogen detection which is shown in Table 1.2.

At an extremely low level, even at a single-cell level, detection of the pathogen can be possible with the help of aptamers. Unfortunately, even after the accomplishment of the patent stage, there is no translation of the major part of the research, for the accomplishment of the substantial successes, necessary to improve the strategies for

TABLE 1.2

The non-exhaustive list of aptasensing assays used for pathogen detection

Aptasensing strategy	Limit of detection	Pathogen	References
• Impedimetric	• 3×10^3 CFU/mL	• *Bacillus anthracis*	• Mazzaracchio et al. (2019)
• Colorimetric paper chip	• 3×10^7 CFU/mL	• *Bacillus thuringiensis*	• Zhou et al. (2020)
• Fluorometric/ luminescence sensors coupled with magnetic separation	• 10–250 CFU	• *Campylobacter jejuni*	• Bruno et al. (2009)
• Fluorescence	• *100 CFU*	• *Escherichia coli* O157:H7	• Li et al. (2019)
• Electrochemical	• 0.0014 fg/mL	• Hepatitis B	• Mohsin et al. (2021)
• Aptamer qPCR	• 5 CFU/mL	• *Listeria monocytogenes*	• Suh et al. (2018)
• Colorimetric	• 200 virus particles/mL	• Norovirus	• Weerathunge et al. (2019)
• Colorimetric and electrochemical	• 60 CFU/mL	• *Pseudomonas aeruginosa*	• Das et al. (2019)
• Fluorescence	• 10^2 CFU/mL	• *Salmonella paratyphi A*	• Liang et al. (2019)
• Electrochemical graphene composite	• 5 CFU/mL	• *Salmonella typhimurium*	• Dai et al. (2019)
• Resonance Rayleigh scattering (single cell)	–	• *Staphylococcus aureus*	• Chang et al. (2013)
• Colorimetric	• 10 CFU/mL	• *Vibrio parahaemolyticus*	• Sun et al. (2019)

manufacturing and the innovation of translational technologies. In comparison to the antibodies, aptamers have high stability which creates a chance for the amalgamation of aptasensors into bulk production and fetching for detection of the whole-cell pathogen from the lab to the market (Sun et al. 2022).

1.4.4 CIRCULATING TUMOUR CELLS

The second leading reason for death revolves around cancer (Ayele et al. 2022). For the improvement in the therapeutic outcome and early diagnosis, there is always a high requisite to develop advanced tools. Molecular biomarkers such as cell-free DNA and circulating tumour cells (CTCs) out housed in the bloodstream by the solid tumours (Williams 2013). In the case of personalized treatment of cancer, non-invasive analysis of various cancers is done by liquid biopsy (Fang & Tan 2010). CTCs are the foundation of liquid biopsy. For CTC isolation, analysis, and detection with targeted imaging, there has been a lot of progress in diagnostic assays and aptamer-based biosensors.

1.4.4.1 Aptamers for CTC isolation as separation ligands

In the isolation and capturing of CTCs (Fang & Tan 2010) aptamers have been employed as recognition ligands by targeting various cell membrane proteins (Ferreira et al. 2006), epithelial cell adhesion molecules (EpCAM) (Song et al. 2013) and epidermal growth factor receptor (EGFR) (Wan et al. 2010). For the capturing of CTCs from the clinical or culture samples, the aptamer is functionalized to the surface with the help of microfluidic and nanomaterials. In 2018, Sun et al. aptamers were conjugated to the superficial of gold, which resulted in the formation of a DNA-based nanotetrahedron (NTH) bioscaffold. This increases the binding capability to human hepatocellular carcinoma (HepG2) CTC by conforming aptamers to higher availability in the CTCs targeting. With a LOD of 3 cells/mL, this means wedged few quantities of HepG2 cells. Shen et al. (2016) added an additional 19-nucleotide segment to the particular aptamer. The aptamer was partially mongrelized with a complimentary probe linked to the gold exterior that leads the capturing of CTCs with an LOD of 10 cells/mL.

Rapid testing with aptamers produced from cell-SELEX for CTC isolation on microchips is also widespread. For the capture cells like human Burkitt's lymphoma cells (Ramos) and lymphocytes, Xu et al. (2009) used aptamer-based microfluidic chips. The capture effectiveness of this technology was comparable to that of cell-affinity chromatography (Nagrath et al. 2007). Several other researchers used sgc8 aptamers for the isolation of acute lymphocytic leukaemia cells from persons' bloodstreams using a micropillar device (Sheng et al. 2012), a gold NP-herringbone microchip (Sheng et al. 2013), or a 3D DNA network-based microchip (Zhao et al. 2012). The multivalent interactions and rough surfaces introduction into microchip devices have become a typical method to enhance CTC capture efficiency. A micropillar array, for example, was put into a microchip device to boost the likelihood of tumour cells interacting with the sgc8 aptamer, resulting in roughly 95% capture efficiency and 81% purity (Sheng et al. 2012). The usage of a gold NP-herringbone microchip, on the other hand, enabled scaffolding for the formation of multivalent aptamer nanospheres, which increased binding affinity and consequently CTC capture effectiveness by up to 93% (Sheng et al. 2012). Rolling circle amplification (RCA) was used to create a 3D DNA network-based microchip with a multivalent binding network for improved capture efficiency (Zhao et al. 2012). A NanoVelcro Chip with an integrated aptamer-silicon nanowire substrate (SiNS) was also produced for capturing non-small-cell lung cancer (NSCLC) cells from blood samples. The device had a capture efficiency of more than 80% (Shen et al. 2013). A customized microfluidic device with different aptamer combinations was also created to capture CTCs with varied phenotypes from patient samples. The aptamer cocktail improved capture efficiency, which is helpful in determining CTC heterogeneity quickly (Zhao et al. 2016).

1.4.4.2   Aptamers for CTC imaging as targeting ligands

For Targeted CTC imaging, aptamers have also been coupled to imaging contrast agents including fluorophores and NPs to serve as selective optical probes for CTC imaging. Aptamer-conjugated NPs (ACNPs) have been produced for cell targeting and imaging. In this study, aptamer-conjugated magnetic NPs (MNPs) were utilized to extract target cells from blood samples, and aptamer-conjugated fluorescent NPs (FNPs) were employed for sensitive and rapid detection via signal amplification (Smith et al. 2007). Moreover, ACNPs were used to capture and identify multiple CTCs from complex samples in a selective manner. MNPs and FNPs coupled with aptamers, for example, were used to capture and photograph cells from pseudocomplex samples concurrently (Smith et al. 2007).

1.4.4.3   CTC detection and analysis using aptamer-based biosensors or assays

For quick CTC detection and analysis, a plethora of aptamer-based technologies have been developed. Optoaptasensors are one of the most widely used detecting technologies. With a LOD of 10 cancer cells, Chiu et al. (2015) developed a gold nanofilm chip functionalized with an aptamer for the detection of CTCs from breast, gastric, and ovarian cancer cells. The employment of an aptamer in conjunction with a volumetric bar-chart chip (V-chip) allowed both visual and quantitative detection of Ramos (leukaemia) cells (Figure 1.2a). The enzymatic reaction between ACNPs and H_2O_2 was used in this chip to quantify the biomarkers in a way that a readily noticeable visual signal was generated from the number of CTCs (Abate et al. 2019). Using HB5 and SYL3C aptamers, Labib et al. (2016) created an aptamer-embedded 2D microfluidic chip to sort distinct types of CTCs in ratio to the expression levels of EpCAM (adenocarcinoma) and HER2 (breast, gastric) (Figure 1.2b). Zhang et al. (2018a) also designed aptamers for identifying CTC subpopulations by analyzing membrane proteins of several cell lines (Figure 1.2c). SERS was used to profile cell phenotypes after CTCs were sieved using a microfluidic chip (Zhang et al. 2018a). Using an NP-mediated 2D sorting apparatus, Green and colleagues (Green et al. 2017; Labib et al. 2016) showed the biochemical and functional characteristics of CTC subpopulations (Figure 1.2d). The EpCAM expression level was used to separate the cell subpopulations on the microfluidic device. A fluorescent collagen uptake assay and a metabolic NAD(P)H assay were used to evaluate the separated tumour cells (Green et al. 2017; Labib et al. 2016). A genetic mutation of the TP53 gene, which promotes to abnormal growth of the cells and thus the development of cancer, was also detected using aptamer-embedded microfluidic chips. The detection was accomplished by extracting genomic DNA from cancer cells (cervical and ovarian) and then Sanger sequencing the results, which was then compared to the sequence of the wildtype TP53 gene (Reinholt & Craighead 2018).

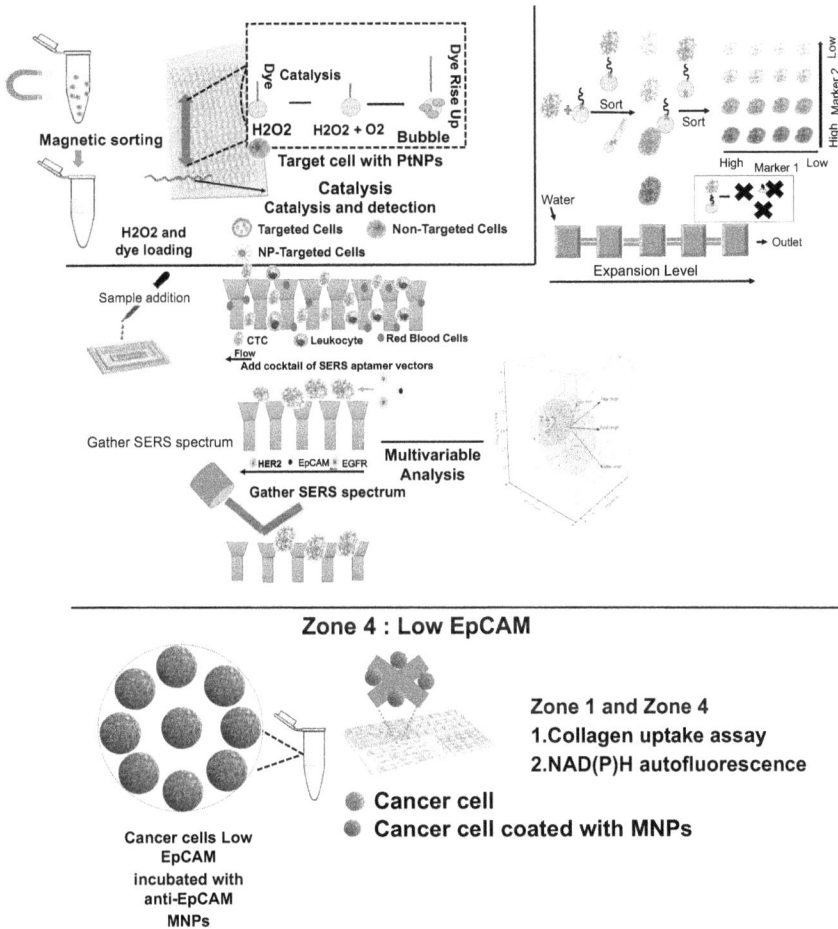

FIGURE 1.2 Aptamer-linked tools for CTC capture and detection. (a) The operational principle of the volumetric bar-chart chip (b) Depiction of a 2D categorization microfluidic tools to capture and separate cells stating EpCAM and HER2 diversely. (c) Illustration of a chip-linked tool for in situ capture and outlining of CTCs grounded on SERS finding. (d) Diagrammatic depiction of phenotypic profiling of CTC subpopulations as per the level of EpCAM manifestation (Stanciu et al. 2021).

1.4.4.4   Role of aptamers in cancer therapy

Today, there are a lot of chemical drugs that can kill cancer cells, but they can also kill normal cells and have serious side effects. Because of this, it is now important for the success of cancer treatment that drugs are given in a targeted way (Figure 1.3). Because of their unique mix of chemical and physical properties, aptamers have become a cutting-edge way to use drugs to target tumours and a great tool for use in therapeutic applications. Some of these therapies are aptamer-drug conjugates (AptDC), aptamer-functionalized nanoparticles, and therapeutic aptamers. As more aptamers are made from cell-SELEX, they can be used as medicines to treat diseases. For example, in 2004, the Food and Drug Administration (FDA) approved the first human VEGF-targeted aptamer to treat age-related macular degeneration. There is a non-SELEX aptamer that binds to nucleolin and has a G-quadruplex structure. AS1411 demonstrated during in vitro testing that it could halt the development of a variety of cancer cells. Additionally, AS1411 may interact with nuclear factor B (NF-B), which would reduce NF-activity and decrease the stability of BCL-2 mRNA. These two conditions would prevent cell division. Because they can intensify their affinity with the target, induce the receptor to produce more copies of itself, and initiate downstream signalling, multivalent aptamers are more effective at combating cancer than monovalent aptamers. The creation of a trivalent form of the HER2 aptamer was recently discovered. The trivalent HER2 aptamer was two times more effective than the HER2 antibody at preventing cancer, according to the findings. A greater chance exists for the trivalent CD30 aptamer to inhibit tumour growth.

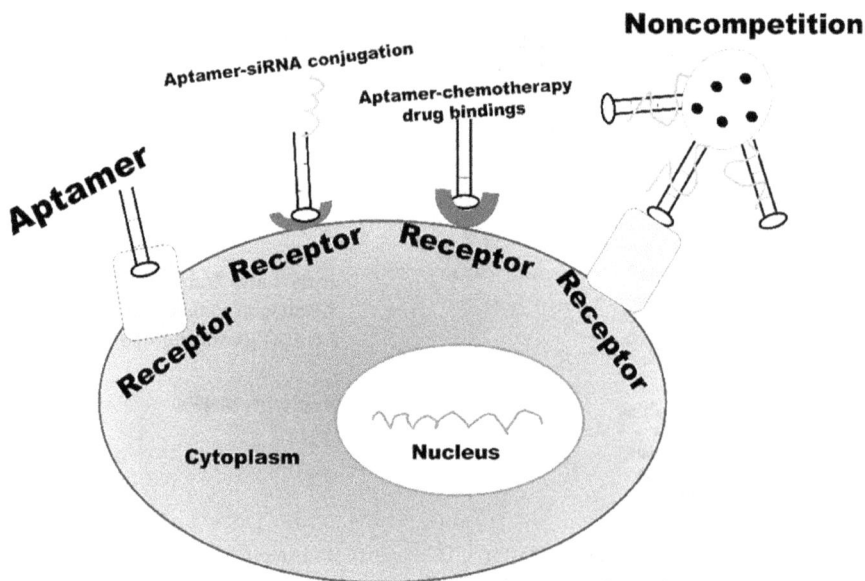

FIGURE 1.3   The diagram demonstrates that in addition to their use as a therapeutic drug, aptamers can also be combined with siRNA, chemotherapeutic agents, and nanoparticles in order to kill cancer cells.

1.4.5 EXTRACELLULAR VESICLES DETECTION

Exosomes, microvesicles, and apoptotic bodies are three forms of lipid-bound extracellular vesicles (EVs) present in the extracellular space that are released by cells (Yáñez-Mó et al. 2015; Zaborowski et al. 2015). Exosomes are found in a variety of biofluids, including synovial fluid, amniotic fluid, bile, breast milk, bronchial fluid, cerebral spinal fluid, gastric acid, plasma, lymph, sperm, saliva, serum, urine, and tears (Doyle & Wang 2019). Exosomes has a characteristic diameter of 30–150 nanometer (Bebelman et al. 2018). It is secreted by almost all kinds of cells.

Microvesicles, on the other hand, have a diameter of 0.1–1 μm. They are made by straight outward budding or pinching of the plasma cell membrane (Bebelman et al. 2018). Apoptotic bodies are larger (0.05–5 μm) than the two forms of EVs discussed above. Dead cells create apoptosis bodies, which contain intact organelles, chromatin, and modest amounts of glycosylated proteins and are discharged into the extracellular space. Exosomes, in particular, are carriers of a variety of biomarkers (e.g., surface proteins, microRNA) in extracellular space and have recently gained a lot of interest for diagnostic purposes (Doyle & Wang 2019).

1.4.5.1 EV isolation and capture by aptamers

The preanalytical separation and purification process is critical for clinical applications while investigating the function and diagnostic potential of EVs (Contreras-Naranjo et al. 2017). Aptamers have been shown to effectively bind EVs via exosomal proteins, which may then be evaluated using a variety of assay techniques, such as simple colorimetric profiling tests (Jiang et al. 2017). Several groups exploited complementary sequences to disrupt the DNA aptamer-exosomal protein complex structure (Zhao et al. 2012) before cleaving the aptamer structure and releasing the intact EVs with restriction enzymes (Zhang et al. 2018b). Downstream molecular analysis can be done on a single platform because of the captured Evs' nondestructive release manner. Huang et al. (2018) created a dual-signal amplification aptasensor for the detection of leukemia-derived exosomes. They successfully isolated exosomes using MBs coupled with anti-CD63 antibodies and subsequently detected them using a nucleolin-recognition DNA aptamer. For the initial stage of signal amplification, the identification aptamer was coupled to an RCA primer. The RCA products were then detected using a gold NP-quenched fluorescent probe (GNP-DNA-FAM), which magnified the fluorescence signals a second time in the vicinity of a nicking endonuclease (Nb.BbvCl). The LOD of this aptasensor was 105 particles/mL. Separation of EVs by size is another key issue. Liu et al. (2019) used HER2 and EpCAM aptamers in combination with λ-DNA-mediated viscoelastic microfluidics for sorting and evaluating EVs produced from breast cancer cells at the same time (Figure 1.4a). The addition of viscoelastic λ-DNA to the EV mixture and the lateral displacement of microvesicles and apoptotic bodies due to the elastic lift force resulted in particle size-dependent sorting (Fe). Targeting EV surface proteins and machine learning-based categorization were used to detect distinct EV kinds (Liu et al. 2019). For capturing LNCaP cell-derived exosomes, Dong et al. (2018) designed an aptamer–magnetic bead bioconjugate (Figure 1.4b). Three messenger DNAs were released by the bioconjugate after magnetic separation, which hybridized with probe DNAs linked to a gold electrode. Exonuclease III then broke the probe DNAs, releasing messenger DNAs that could subsequently spread and bind newer DNA probes. In differential pulse voltammetry, cyclic enzymatic amplification (repeated cleavage events) created a turn-off signal, which was connected to the initial exosome concentration. The LOD on this platform was 7×10^4 particles/mL (Dong et al. 2018). For the isolation of EVs employing DNA aptamers, Xu et al. (2018) developed a noninvasive ExoPCD microfluidic chip in which founded on the basis of a label-free and immobilization-free EC technique. With a LOD of 4.39×10^3 particles/mL, this diagnostic tool had a high detection sensitivity for CD63 proteins on exosomes (Xu et al. 2018). Zhang et al. (2019) created a DNA aptamer-based magnetic isolation method that captures MUC1-positive EVs in breast cancer plasma samples quickly and releases them non-destructively in 90 minutes with a release efficiency of about 78%, which is comparable to ultracentrifugation. Streptavidin MBs were combined with a biotin-labelled anti-CD63 aptamer to capture EVs. The EVs were then liberated in a nondestructive manner via magnetic separation (Zhang et al. 2019).

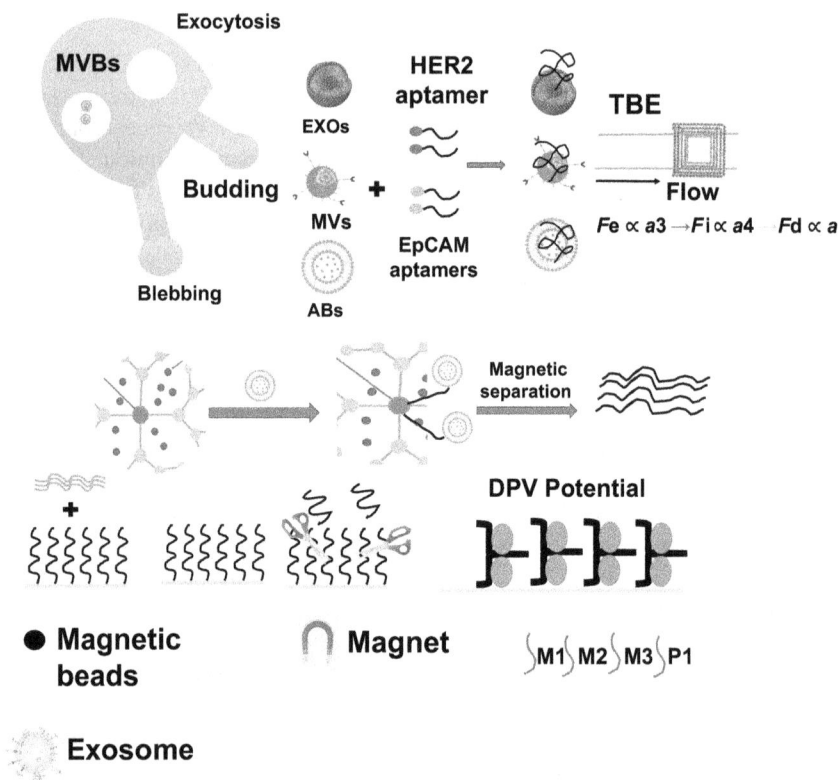

FIGURE 1.4 (a) Diagrammatic explanation of the aptamer-associated targeting agents. (b) Depiction of a cancerous tissue-derived exosome detection mechanism founded on differential pulse voltammetry (Stanciu et al. 2021).

1.4.5.2 EV detection by aptamers

Numerous aptamer-associated detection approaches for exosome analysis have been established and have shown significant potential as diagnostic instruments for studying EVs, particularly exosomes. Fluorescent aptasensors that use fluorescence signal amplification, fluorescence resonance energy transfer, or fluorescence polarization have a simple operation and great diagnostic sensitivity. An RCA aptasensor with an LOD of 4.27×10^4 particles/mL was recently created for the detection and amplification of captured exosomes by producing in situ double-stranded DNA products. Exosome capture was combined with a hairpin DNA cascade hybridization reaction (HD-CHR) in this method, for quantification it was turned the amount of exosomes captured into double-stranded DNA products (Huang et al. 2020). Li et al. (2019) developed magnetic isolation using aptamer-functionalized Fe_3O_4 beads to improve exosome purity. A urine exosome with a LOD of 10^5 particles/mL was found using this aptamer probe. Zhao et al. (2020) also combined a CD63 aptamer with a CRISPR/Cas12a system for improved signal amplification. The CD63 aptamer released a complementary DNA sequence termed a blocker upon capturing the exosomal surface protein. The CRISPR/Cas12a complex then identified the blocker and cleaved a reporter probe, amplifying the fluorescence signals.

1.4.6 TISSUE SAMPLES

In situ immunostaining of tumour tissues has also been used to obtain diagnostic information using aptamer-based ligands. Aptamer-aided staining of formalin-immobilized and paraffin-inserted tumour tissues is accomplishing admiration in comparison to antibody-based immunostaining because of its high penetration effectiveness and capacity to minimize nonspecific signals from the necrotic section (Zeng et al. 2010). A number of aptamers produced from cell/tissue SELEX have been created for staining breast, colorectal, gastric, and prostate cancer tissues. Pu et al. (2015) developed a SYL3C-CY3 aptamer for staining tissue samples of colorectal cancer patients. The immunofluorescence method was used to identify EpCAM-positive colorectal cells in frozen tissue components. For the imaging of metastatic colorectal cancer cells, Li et al. (2014) developed a recognition probe based on W3 aptamer–treated QDs. This probe was also employed for immunostaining tumour-bearing mouse tissues (Li et al. 2014). Yuan et al. (2017) created a J3 DNA aptamer tagged with Cy5 dye that bound to colorectal cancer cells selectively and specifically. This aptamer-aided probe produced favourable fluorescence pictures of colorectal cancer tissue slices, which gave useful immunostaining data for colorectal cancer metastasis clinical verdict.

Shao and colleagues (Li et al. 2009) created a BC-15 DNA aptamer that can selectively recognize cancerous breast tissue.

In summary, aptamer-associated tissue staining has developed as an encouraging substitute for monoclonal antibody linked immunostaining for histopathological diagnosis because of its wide temperature range stability, penetration efficacy, and ease of chemical alteration (Bukari et al. 2017).

1.5　CONCLUSIONS AND FUTURE PERSPECTIVES

Aptasensors gained popularity over the preceding few years. Their benefits over old-style antibody-aided identification have been thoroughly acknowledged in the literature. In the last few years, the prospective of aptamer-aided biosensors or assay approaches in the perspective of POC diagnostics for universal well-being has been speedily studied. Their distinctive characteristics, such as dry reagent stability, little products' specification fluctuation in the high scale production, great profit, and extraordinary detection sensitivity and specificity, make them particularly desirable for field deployment or adoption in low-resource environments.

This book chapter includes a few exemplary instances since a slew of current research on aptamer-aided sensing tools for the detection of small molecules, proteins, nucleic acids, etc. The following two instances are representative of several noteworthy patterns. First, most studies utilize aptamers as binding or targeting agents for the discriminating identification of specific components, though a few findings used the 3D architecture of aptamers as part of the signal transduction tool (e.g., arrangement change-influenced signalling). Next, aptamers are typically coupled with microfluidic devices or nanomaterials to enable high-throughput screening or novel signal-producing mechanisms, resulting in arena-deployable POC sensing or diagnostic tools.

Currently exhibited aptasensors confront a number of significant obstacles. First, more clinical trials are needed to confirm their ability to analyze actual patient samples. Several previous findings were based on small ideal provisions like isolated cell cultures. Various aptamer-associated approaches should be evaluated in additional complicated biological samples, like serum, saliva, urine, etc. To expedite convergent science and further boost sensing systems, stronger multi-disciplinary teamwork among sensor designers (engineers) and healthcare staffs (clinicians) would be required.

Second, because early disease detection is critical for better medical intervention, the new generation of aptasensors will be required to indicate changes in health status or disease development in real time. Aptamer-based biosensors with real-time and constant observing proficiencies are projected to lead forthcoming advancement in the area discoursed. This presents a substantial task in terms of developing an entirely new class of aptasensors that do not depend on permanent binding happenings and instead, emphasize on changeable chemical interactions to allow constant components sampling.

Regardless of the obstacles faced, the current advancement of POC-approachable aptamer-aided biosensors has shown great promise for enhancing tailored diagnostics and universal health on a wide-ranging scale. A combination of aptamer biosensors with developing wearable technology could bring a better approach to long-term ailment management and monitoring. Aptasensors could have a bigger influence in the approaching era of advanced treatment if they have greater clinical validation, scalability, and commercialization.

CREDIT AUTHORSHIP CONTRIBUTION STATEMENT

All the authors equally help in conceptualization; supervision; validation; visualization; writing – original draft; writing – review and editing.

ACKNOWLEDGEMENT

This initiative would not have been possible without the help and support of Dr. R.S. Gaud, Director of SVKM's NMIMS Deemed-to-be University, Shirpur.

DECLARATION OF COMPETING INTEREST

There is no conflict of interest reported.

REFERENCES

Abate MF, Jia S, Ahmed MG, Li X, Lin L, Chen X, Zhu Z, Yang C. 2019. Visual quantitative detection of circulating tumor cells with single-cell sensitivity using a portable microfluidic device. *Small*. 15(14):1804890.

Ayele W, Führer A, Braun GA, Formazin F, Wienke A, Taylor L, et al. 2022. Breast cancer morbidity and mortality in rural Ethiopia: data from 788 verbal autopsies. *BMC Women's Health*. 22(1):1–9.

Bala R, Kumar M, Bansal K, Sharma RK, Wangoo N. 2016a. Ultrasensitive aptamer biosensor for malathion detection based on cationic polymer and gold nanoparticles. *Biosens. Bioelectron*. 85:445–449.

Bala R, Sharma RK, Wangoo N. 2016b. Development of gold nanoparticles-based aptasensor for the colorimetric detection of organophosphorus pesticide phorate. *Anal. Bioanal. Chem*. 408(1):333–338.

Bebelman MP, Smit MJ, Pegtel DM, Baglio SR. 2018. Biogenesis and function of extracellular vesicles in cancer. *Pharmacol. Ther*. 188:1.

Bhardwaj J, Chaudhary N, Kim H, Jang J. 2019. Subtyping of influenza A H1N1 virus using a label-free electrochemical biosensor based on the DNA aptamer targeting the stem region of HA protein. *Anal. Chim. Acta*. 1064:94–103.

Bruno JG, Phillips T, Carrillo MP, Crowell R. 2009. Plastic-adherent DNA aptamer-magnetic bead and quantum dot sandwich assay for Campylobacter detection. *J. Fluoresc*. 19(3):427–435.

Bukari BA, Citartan M, Ch'ng ES, Bilibana MP, Rozhdestvensky T, Tang TH. 2017. Aptahistochemistry in diagnostic pathology: technical scrutiny and feasibility. *Histochem. Cell Biol*. 147(5):545.

Candia J, Cheung F, Kotliarov Y, Fantoni G, Sellers B, Griesman T, et al. 2017. Assessment of variability in the SOMAscan assay. *Sci. Rep*. 7(1):1–3.

Chang YC, Yang CY, Sun RL, Cheng YF, Kao WC, Yang PC. 2013. Rapid single cell detection of *Staphylococcus aureus* by aptamer-conjugated gold nanoparticles. *Sci. Rep*. 3(1):1–7.

Chen Z, Li L, Mu X, Zhao H, Guo L. 2011. Electrochemical aptasensor for detection of copper based on a reagentless signal-on architecture and amplification by gold nanoparticles. *Talanta*. 85(1):730–735.

Chiu WJ, Ling TK, Chiang HP, Lin HJ, Huang CC. 2015. Monitoring cluster ions derived from aptamer-modified gold nanofilms under laser desorption/ionization for the detection of circulating tumor cells. *ACS Appl. Mater. Interfaces*. 7(16):8622–8630.

Contreras-Naranjo JC, Wu HJ, Ugaz VM. 2017. Microfluidics for exosome isolation and analysis: enabling liquid biopsy for personalized medicine. *Lab Chip*. 17(21):3558–3577.

Crulhas BP, Karpik AE, Delella FK, Castro GR, Pedrosa VA. 2017. Electrochemical aptamer-based biosensor developed to monitor PSA and VEGF released by prostate cancer cells. *Anal. Bioanal. Chem*. 409(29):6771–6780.

Dai G, Li Z, Luo F, Ai S, Chen B, Wang Q. 2019. Electrochemical determination of Salmonella typhimurium by using aptamer-loaded gold nanoparticles and a composite prepared from a metal-organic framework (type UiO-67) and graphene. *MCA*. 186(9):1–9.

Das R, Dhiman A, Kapil A, Bansal V, Sharma TK. 2019. Aptamer-mediated colorimetric and electrochemical detection of Pseudomonas aeruginosa utilizing peroxidase-mimic activity of gold NanoZyme. *Anal. Bioanal. Chem.* 411(6):1229–1238.

Derbyshire N, White SJ, Bunka DH, Song L, Stead S, Tarbin J, et al. 2012. Toggled RNA aptamers against aminoglycosides allowing facile detection of antibiotics using gold nanoparticle assays. *Anal. Chem.* 84(15):6595–6602.

Di Ruscio A, de Franciscis V. 2022. Minding the gap: Unlocking the therapeutic potential of aptamers and making up for lost time. *Mol. Ther. Nucleic Acids.* 29:384–386.

Dong H, Chen H, Jiang J, Zhang H, Cai C, Shen Q. 2018. Highly sensitive electrochemical detection of tumor exosomes based on aptamer recognition-induced multi-DNA release and cyclic enzymatic amplification. *Anal. Chem.* 90(7):4507–4513.

Doyle LM, Wang MZ. 2019. Overview of extracellular vesicles, their origin, composition, purpose, and methods for exosome isolation and analysis. *Cells.* 8(7):727.

Ellington AD and Szostak JW. 1990. *In vitro* selection of RNA molecules that bind specific ligands. *Nature.* 346:818–822.

Fang X, Tan W. 2010. Aptamers generated from cell-SELEX for molecular medicine: a chemical biology approach. *Acc. Chem. Res.* 43(1):48–57.

Ferreira CS, Matthews CS, Missailidis S. 2006. DNA aptamers that bind to MUC1 tumour marker: design and characterization of MUC1-binding single-stranded DNA aptamers. *Tumor Biol.* 27(6):289–301.

Flahault A, Geissbuhler A, Guessous I, Guérin P, Bolon I, Salathé M, et al. 2017. Precision global health in the digital age. *Swiss Med. Wkly.* 147:w14423.

Fu J, An X, Yao Y, Guo Y, Sun X. 2019. Electrochemical aptasensor based on one step co-electrodeposition of aptamer and GO-CuNPs nanocomposite for organophosphorus pesticide detection. *Sens. Actuators B Chem.* 287:503–509.

Fu J, Yao Y, An X, Wang G, Guo Y, Sun X, et al. 2020. Voltammetric determination of organophosphorus pesticides using a hairpin aptamer immobilized in a graphene oxide-chitosan composite. *MCA.* 187(1):1–8.

Green BJ, Kermanshah L, Labib M, Ahmed SU, Silva PN, Mahmoudian L, et al. 2017. Isolation of phenotypically distinct cancer cells using nanoparticle-mediated sorting. *ACS Appl. Mater. Interfaces.* 9(24):20435–20443.

Green R, Ellington AD, Szostak JW. 1990. *In vitro* genetic analysis of the tetrahymena self-splicing intron. *Nature.* 347:406–408.

He L, Luo Y, Zhi W, Zhou P. 2013. Colorimetric sensing of tetracyclines in milk based on the assembly of cationic conjugated polymer-aggregated gold nanoparticles. *Food Anal. Methods.* 6(6):1704–1711.

Huang L, Wang DB, Singh N, Yang F, Gu N, Zhang XE. 2018. A dual-signal amplification platform for sensitive fluorescence biosensing of leukemia-derived exosomes. *Nanoscale.* 10(43):20289–20295.

Huang R, He L, Li S, Liu H, Jin L, Chen Z, et al. 2020. A simple fluorescence aptasensor for gastric cancer exosome detection based on branched rolling circle amplification. *Nanoscale.* 12(4):2445–2451.

Jakovljevic M, Liu Y, Cerda A, Simonyan M, Correia T, Mariita RM, et al. 2021. The global South political economy of health financing and spending landscape–history and presence. *J. Med. Econ.* 24:25–33.

Jarczewska M, Rębiś J, Górski Ł, Malinowska E. 2018. Development of DNA aptamer-based sensor for electrochemical detection of C-reactive protein. *Talanta.* 189:45–54.

Javidi M, Housaindokht MR, Verdian A, Razavizadeh BM. 2018. Detection of chloramphenicol using a novel apta-sensing platform based on aptamer terminal-lock in milk samples. *Anal. Chim. Acta.* 1039:116–123.

Jiang D, Du X, Liu Q, Zhou L, Dai L, Qian J, et al. 2015. Silver nanoparticles anchored on nitrogen-doped graphene as a novel electrochemical biosensing platform with enhanced sensitivity for aptamer-based pesticide assay. *Analyst.* 140(18):6404–6411.

Jiang Y, Shi M, Liu Y, Wan S, Cui C, Zhang L, et al. 2017. Aptamer/AuNP biosensor for colorimetric profiling of exosomal proteins. *Angew. Chem. Int. Ed. Engl.* 56(39):11916–11920.

Kumar LS, Wang X, Hagen J, Naik R, Papautsky I, Heikenfeld J. 2016. Label free nanoaptasensor for interleukin-6 in protein-dilute bio fluids such as sweat. *Anal. Methods.* 8(17):3440–3444.

Labib M, Green B, Mohamadi RM, Mepham A, Ahmed SU, Mahmoudian L, et al. 2016. Aptamer and antisense-mediated two-dimensional isolation of specific cancer cell subpopulations. *J. Am. Chem.* 138(8):2476–2479.

Lee SM, Lee D. 2021. Opportunities and challenges for contactless healthcare services in the post-COVID-19 era. *Technol. Forecast. Soc. Change.* 167:120712.

Li Y, Champion JA. 2022. Self-assembling nanocarriers from engineered proteins: design, functionalization, and application for drug delivery. *Adv. Drug Deliv. Rev.* 189:114462.

Li P, Yu X, Han W, Kong Y, Bao W, Zhang J, et al. 2019. Ultrasensitive and reversible nanoplatform of urinary exosomes for prostate cancer diagnosis. *ACS Sens.* 4(5):1433–1441.

Li S, Liu C, Yin G, Zhang Q, Luo J, Wu N. 2017. Aptamer-molecularly imprinted sensor base on electrogenerated chemiluminescence energy transfer for detection of lincomycin. *Biosens. Bioelectron.* 91:687–691.

Li S, Wu X, Liu C, Yin G, Luo J, Xu Z. 2016. Application of DNA aptamers as sensing layers for detection of carbofuran by electrogenerated chemiluminescence energy transfer. *Anal Chim Acta.* 941:94–100.

Li S, Xu H, Ding H, Huang Y, Cao X, Yang G, et al. 2009. Identification of an aptamer targeting hnRNP A1 by tissue slide-based SELEX. *J. Pathol.* 218(3):327–336.

Li WM, Bing T, Wei JY, Chen ZZ, Shangguan DH, Fang J. 2014. Cell-SELEX-based selection of aptamers that recognize distinct targets on metastatic colorectal cancer cells. *Biomaterials.* 35(25):6998–7007.

Liang J, Zhou J, Tan J, Wang Z, Deng L. 2019. Aptamer-based fluorescent determination of Salmonella paratyphi a using Phi29-DNA polymerase-assisted cyclic amplification. *Anal. Lett.* 52(6):919–931.

Liu C, Zhao J, Tian F, Chang J, Zhang W, Sun J. 2019. λ-DNA-and aptamer-mediated sorting and analysis of extracellular vesicles. *J. Am. Chem.* 141(9):3817–3821.

Liu Y, Tian H, Chen X, Liu W, Xia K, Huang J, et al. 2020. Indirect surface-enhanced Raman scattering assay of insulin-like growth factor 2 receptor protein by combining the aptamer modified gold substrate and silver nanoprobes. *MCA.* 187(3):1–9.

Liu Y, Yan K, Okoth OK, Zhang J. 2015. A label-free photoelectrochemical aptasensor based on nitrogen-doped graphene quantum dots for chloramphenicol determination. *Biosens. Bioelectron.* 74:1016–1021.

Lu L, Liu B, Leng J, Ma X, Peng H. 2020. Electrochemical mixed aptamer-antibody sandwich assay for mucin protein 16 detection through hybridization chain reaction amplification. *Anal. Bioanal. Chem.* 412(26):7169–7178.

Ma C, Wang W, Yang Q, Shi C, Cao L. 2011. Cocaine detection via rolling circle amplification of short DNA strand separated by magnetic beads. *Biosens. Bioelectron.* 26(7):3309–3312.

Madianos L, Skotadis E, Tsekenis G, Patsiouras L, Tsigkourakos M, Tsoukalas D. 2018. Impedimetric nanoparticle aptasensor for selective and label free pesticide detection. *Microelectron. Eng.* 189:39–45.

Marks HL, Pishko MV, Jackson GW, Coté GL. 2014. Rational design of a bisphenol A aptamer selective surface-enhanced Raman scattering nanoprobe. *Anal. Chem.* 86(23):11614–11619.

Mazzaracchio V, Neagu D, Porchetta A, Marcoccio E, Pomponi A, Faggioni G, et al. 2019. A label-free impedimetric aptasensor for the detection of Bacillus anthracis spore simulant. *Biosens. Bioelectron.* 126:640–646.

Mohsin DH, Mashkour MS, Fatemi F. 2021. Design of aptamer-based sensing platform using gold nanoparticles functionalized reduced graphene oxide for ultrasensitive detection of Hepatitis B virus. *Chem. Paper* 75(1):279–295.

Nagrath S, Sequist LV, Maheswaran S, Bell DW, Irimia D, Ulkus L, et al. 2007. Isolation of rare circulating tumour cells in cancer patients by microchip technology. *Nature*. 450(7173):1235–1239.

Pelossof G, Tel-Vered R, Liu XQ, Willner I. 2011. Amplified surface plasmon resonance based DNA biosensors, aptasensors, and Hg^{2+} sensors using hemin/G-quadruplexes and Au nanoparticles. *Eur. J. Chem.* 17(32):8904–8912.

Pohanka M. 2021. Current biomedical and diagnostic applications of gold micro and nanoparticles. *Mini Rev. Med. Chem.* 21(9):1085–1095.

Pu Y, Liu Z, Lu Y, Yuan P, Liu J, Yu B, et al. 2015. Using DNA aptamer probe for immunostaining of cancer frozen tissues. *Anal. Chem.* 87(3):1919–1924.

Ramezani M, Danesh NM, Lavaee P, Abnous K, Taghdisi SM. 2015. A novel colorimetric triple-helix molecular switch aptasensor for ultrasensitive detection of tetracycline. *Biosens. Bioelectron.* 70:181–187.

Reinholt SJ, Craighead HG. 2018. Microfluidic device for aptamer-based cancer cell capture and genetic mutation detection. *Anal. Chem.* 90(4):2601–2608.

Ren Q, Mou J, Guo Y, Wang H, Cao X, Zhang F, et al. 2020. Simple homogeneous electrochemical target-responsive aptasensor based on aptamer bio-gated and porous carbon nanocontainer derived from ZIF-8. *Biosens. Bioelectron.* 166:112448.

Rivas L, Mayorga-Martinez CC, Quesada-González D, Zamora-Gálvez A, De La Escosura-Muñiz A and Merkoçi A. 2015. Label-free impedimetric aptasensor for ochratoxin-A detection using iridium oxide nanoparticles. *Anal. Chem.* 87(10):5167–5172.

Rodríguez MC, Rivas GA. 2009. Label-free electrochemical aptasensor for the detection of lysozyme. *Talanta*. 78(1):212–216.

Roushani M, Nezhadali A, Jalilian Z. 2018. An electrochemical chlorpyrifos aptasensor based on the use of a glassy carbon electrode modified with an electropolymerized aptamer-imprinted polymer and gold nanorods. *MCA*. 185(12):1–8.

Ruckman J, Green LS, Beeson J, Waugh S, Gillette WL, Henninger DD, et al. 1998. 2′-Fluoropyrimidine RNA-based aptamers to the 165-amino acid form of vascular endothelial growth factor (VEGF165). Inhibition of receptor binding and VEGF-induced vascular permeability through interactions requiring the exon 7-encoded domain. *JBC*. 273:20556–20567.

Seok Y, Byun JY, Shim WB, Kim MG. 2015. A structure-switchable aptasensor for aflatoxin B1 detection based on assembly of an aptamer/split DNAzyme. *Anal. Chim. Acta*. 886:182–187.

Sharma A, Dulta K, Nagraik R, Dua K, Singh SK, Chellappan DK, et al. 2022. Potentialities of aptasensors in cancer diagnosis. *Mater. Lett.* 308:131240.

Shen H, Yang J, Chen Z, Chen X, Wang L, Hu J, et al. 2016. A novel label-free and reusable electrochemical cytosensor for highly sensitive detection and specific collection of CTCs. *Biosens. Bioelectron.* 81:495–502.

Shen Q, Xu L, Zhao L, Wu D, Fan Y, Zhou Y, et al. 2013. Specific capture and release of circulating tumor cells using aptamer-modified nanosubstrates. *Adv. Mater. Lett.* 25(16):2368–2373.

Sheng W, Chen T, Kamath R, Xiong X, Tan W, Fan ZH. 2012. Aptamer-enabled efficient isolation of cancer cells from whole blood using a microfluidic device. *Anal. Chem.* 84(9):4199–4206.

Sheng W, Chen T, Tan W, Fan ZH. 2013. Multivalent DNA nanospheres for enhanced capture of cancer cells in microfluidic devices. *ACS Nano*. 7(8):7067–7076.

Smith JE, Medley CD, Tang Z, Shangguan D, Lofton C, Tan W. 2007. Aptamer-conjugated nanoparticles for the collection and detection of multiple cancer cells. *Anal. Chem.* 79(8):3075–3082.

Song Y, Zhu Z, An Y, Zhang W, Zhang H, Liu D, et al. 2013. Selection of DNA aptamers against epithelial cell adhesion molecule for cancer cell imaging and circulating tumor cell capture. *Anal. Chem.* 85(8):4141–4149.

Stanciu LA, Wei Q, Barui AK, Mohammad N. 2021. Recent advances in aptamer-based biosensors for global health applications. *Annu. Rev. Biomed. Eng.* 23:433–459.

Steinhubl SR, Muse ED, Topol EJ. 2015. The emerging field of mobile health. *Sci. Transl. Med.* 7(283):283rv3.

Suh SH, Choi SJ, Dwivedi HP, Moore MD, Escudero-Abarca BI, Jaykus LA. 2018. Use of DNA aptamer for sandwich type detection of Listeria monocytogenes. *Anal. Biochem.* 557:27–33.

Sun D, Lu J, Luo Z, Zhang L, Liu P, Chen Z. 2018. Competitive electrochemical platform for ultrasensitive cytosensing of liver cancer cells by using nanotetrahedra structure with rolling circle amplification. *Biosens. Bioelectron.* 120:8–14.

Sun M, Ma N, Shi H, Cheong LZ, Yang W, Qiao Z. 2022. A HCR based multivalent aptamer amplifier for ultrasensitive detection of Salmonella. *Sens. Actuators B Chem.* 17:132860.

Sun X, Li F, Shen G, Huang J, Wang X. 2014. Aptasensor based on the synergistic contributions of chitosan–gold nanoparticles, graphene–gold nanoparticles and multi-walled carbon nanotubes-cobalt phthalocyanine nanocomposites for kanamycin detection. *Analyst.* 139(1):299–308.

Sun Y, Duan N, Ma P, Liang Y, Zhu X, Wang Z. 2019. Colorimetric aptasensor based on truncated aptamer and trivalent DNAzyme for Vibrio parahemolyticus determination. *J. Agric. Food Chem.* 67(8):2313–2320.

Sypabekova M, Jolly P, Estrela P, Kanayeva D. 2019. Electrochemical aptasensor using optimized surface chemistry for the detection of Mycobacterium tuberculosis secreted protein MPT64 in human serum. *Biosens. Bioelectron.* 123:141–151.

Taghdisi SM, Danesh NM, Emrani AS, Ramezani M, Abnous K. 2015. A novel electrochemical aptasensor based on single-walled carbon nanotubes, gold electrode and complimentary strand of aptamer for ultrasensitive detection of cocaine. *Biosens. Bioelectron.* 73:245–250.

Temur E, Zengin A, Boyacı IH, Dudak FC, Torul H, Tamer U. 2012. Attomole sensitivity of staphylococcal enterotoxin B detection using an aptamer-modified surface-enhanced Raman scattering probe. *Anal. Chem.* 84(24):10600–10606.

Wan Y, Kim YT, Li N, Cho SK, Bachoo R, Ellington AD, et al. 2010. Surface-immobilized aptamers for cancer cell isolation and microscopic cytology. *Cancer Res.* 70(22):9371–9380.

Wang G, Su X, Xu Q, Xu G, Lin J, Luo X. 2018. Antifouling aptasensor for the detection of adenosine triphosphate in biological media based on mixed self-assembled aptamer and zwitterionic peptide. *Biosens. Bioelectron.* 101:129–134.

Wang J, Guo J, Zhang J, Zhang W, Zhang Y. 2017. RNA aptamer-based electrochemical aptasensor for C-reactive protein detection using functionalized silica microspheres as immunoprobes. *Biosens. Bioelectron.* 95:100–105.

Wang W, Wu WY, Zhong X, Miao Q, Zhu JJ. 2011. Aptamer-based PDMS–gold nanoparticle composite as a platform for visual detection of biomolecules with silver enhancement. *Biosens. Bioelectron.* 26(7):3110–3114.

Weerathunge P, Ramanathan R, Torok VA, Hodgson K, Xu Y, Goodacre R, et al. 2019. Ultrasensitive colorimetric detection of murine norovirus using NanoZyme aptasensor. *Anal. Chem.* 91(5):3270–3276.

Williams SC. 2013. Circulating tumor cells. *PNAS.* 110(13):4861.

Wu S, Duan N, Ma X, Xia Y, Wang H, Wang Z, et al. 2012a. Multiplexed fluorescence resonance energy transfer aptasensor between upconversion nanoparticles and graphene oxide for the simultaneous determination of mycotoxins. *Anal. Chem.* 84(14):6263–6270.

Wu Y, Zhan S, Wang F, He L, Zhi W, Zhou P. 2012b. Cationic polymers and aptamers mediated aggregation of gold nanoparticles for the colorimetric detection of arsenic (III) in aqueous solution. *Chem. Commun.* 48(37):4459–4461.

Xu H, Liao C, Zuo P, Liu Z, Ye BC. 2018. Magnetic-based microfluidic device for on-chip isolation and detection of tumor-derived exosomes. *Anal. Chem.* 90(22):13451–13458.

Xu Y, Phillips JA, Yan J, Li Q, Fan ZH, Tan W. 2009. Aptamer-based microfluidic device for enrichment, sorting, and detection of multiple cancer cells. *Anal. Chem.* 81(17):7436–7442.

Yáñez-Mó M, Siljander PR, Andreu Z, Bedina Zavec A, Borràs FE, Buzas EI, et al. 2015. Biological properties of extracellular vesicles and their physiological functions. *J. Extracell.* 4(1):27066.

Yang C, Wang Y, Marty JL, Yang X. 2011. Aptamer-based colorimetric biosensing of Ochratoxin A using unmodified gold nanoparticles indicator. *Biosens. Bioelectron.* 26(5):2724–2727.

Yuan B, Jiang X, Chen Y, Guo Q, Wang K, Meng X, et al. 2017. Metastatic cancer cell and tissue-specific fluorescence imaging using a new DNA aptamer developed by Cell-SELEX. *Talanta.* 170:56–62.

Zaborowski MP, Balaj L, Breakefield XO, Lai CP. 2015. Extracellular vesicles: composition, biological relevance, and methods of study. *Bioscience.* 65(8):783–797.

Zamay GS, Zamay TN, Kolovskii VA, Shabanov AV, Glazyrin YE, Veprintsev DV, et al. 2016. Electrochemical aptasensor for lung cancer-related protein detection in crude blood plasma samples. *Sci. Rep.* 6(1):1–8.

Zeng Z, Zhang P, Zhao N, Sheehan AM, Tung CH, Chang CC, et al. 2010. Using oligonucleotide aptamer probes for immunostaining of formalin-fixed and paraffin-embedded tissues. *Mod. Pathol.* 23(12):1553–1558.

Zhang K, Deng R, Teng X, Li Y, Sun Y, Ren X, et al. 2018a. Direct visualization of single-nucleotide variation in mtDNA using a CRISPR/Cas9-mediated proximity ligation assay. *J. Am. Chem.* 140(36):11293–11301.

Zhang K, Yue Y, Wu S, Liu W, Shi J, Zhang Z. 2019. Rapid capture and nondestructive release of extracellular vesicles using aptamer-based magnetic isolation. *ACS Sens.* 4(5):1245–1251.

Zhang Y, Wang Z, Wu L, Zong S, Yun B, Cui Y. 2018b. Combining multiplex SERS nanovectors and multivariate analysis for in situ profiling of circulating tumor cell phenotype using a microfluidic chip. *Small.* 14(20):1704433.

Zhao L, Tang C, Xu L, Zhang Z, Li X, Hu H, et al. 2016. Enhanced and differential capture of circulating tumor cells from lung cancer patients by microfluidic assays using aptamer cocktail. *Small.* 12(8):1072–1081.

Zhao W, Cui CH, Bose S, Guo D, Shen C, Wong WP, et al. 2012. Bioinspired multivalent DNA network for capture and release of cells. *PNAS.* 109(48):19626–19631.

Zhao X, Zhang W, Qiu X, Mei Q, Luo Y, Fu W. 2020. Rapid and sensitive exosome detection with CRISPR/Cas12a. *Anal. Bioanal. Chem.* 412(3):601–609.

Zhou C, You T, Jang H, Ryu H, Lee ES, Oh MH, et al. 2020. Aptamer-conjugated polydiacetylene colorimetric paper chip for the detection of *Bacillus thuringiensis* spores. *Sensors.* 20(11):3124.

Zhou L, Wang J, Li D and Li Y. 2014. An electrochemical aptasensor based on gold nanoparticles dotted graphene modified glassy carbon electrode for label-free detection of bisphenol A in milk samples. *Food Chem.* 162:34–40.

2 Biomarkers for aptamer-based diagnostic applications

Sangeeta Ballav, Veda Joshi, Swarangi Tambat, Urwashi Kumar, Shine Devarajan, Soumya Basu, and Jyotirmoi Aich

2.1 INTRODUCTION

The present Aeon of scientific research has always aimed to seek up-gradation in the realm of prognostics and diagnostics to enhance the survival chances by looking at the level of the insurgence of human health hazards being on a constant rise. The urgency in establishing a strong prognosis for any given disease has become a mandate to deal with the disease as soon as possible to mitigate the further repercussions of disease pathogenesis. For this, the need to search for compounds that can validate the presence or absence of a certain health condition right at the early stage leads to the discovery of biomarkers. Biomarkers can be defined as any molecular or cellular components located in tissue or body fluids that can act as an indicator of the normal or transmuted physiological state of the body and can be measured via analytical tools on tissue or liquid biopsy (Strimbu and Tavel 2010). These biomarkers are very specific to a particular health condition, directly correlate to the disease, and provide a very helpful means of detection at its early onset. For example, blood pressure acts as a biomarker for cardiovascular functioning, swelling, and rashes indicate inflammation, and fever indicates infection. Early medical practices were hugely dependent on such biomarkers. But with the advent of genomics, transcriptomics, and advances in molecular biology have garnered the attention of medical practitioners to look out for more biomarkers of high precision that can have a positive impact on current therapeutics, especially in cancers (McDermott et al. 2012). The earliest cancer biomarker identified as the light chain of immunoglobulin in urine was found in 75% of myeloma patients in 1848 (Jones 1848). Thereafter, several hormones, peptides, and proteins were identified that had altered concentrations in the serum of cancer patients. The heyday of hybridoma technology in the 1980s prompted the discovery of the ovarian epithelial carcinoma marker carbohydrate antigen CA25 (Bast et al. 1981).

The biomarkers can be classified depending on the clinical requirements. The first class includes "biomarkers of exposure". The biomarkers for exposure are used

DOI: 10.1201/9781003304227-2

for risk prediction for an individual when exposed to environmental toxins. These biomarkers generally reflect the degree of exposure a person has to that toxin and correlate it with the chances of disease occurrence (Mayeux 2004). Appraising the biomarkers of exposure is far better than analyzing the history of exposure as it gives the accurate "internal dosage" of exposure and improves the precision in the measurement of toxins in body tissue or fluids. Lead exposure is a type of biomarker for assessing the risk factor associated with an individual's contact with lead. Likewise, organophosphate pesticides account for toxicity and are measured in blood and urine (Mayeux 2004).

Another class of biomarkers is "biomarkers of disease". These biomarkers can be subcategorized depending on the clinical requirement. Different biomarkers are available for screening, prognosis, and disease staging (Tong and Li 2016). These are the markers that are already present in the body and have undergone aberrant changes due to certain health conditions. By detecting and quantifying these biomarkers the disease progression can be understood and aid in the manifestation of treatment. Based on this classification, biomarkers can be proteins, missing genes, extra gene copies, gene mutations, gene rearrangements, enzymes, serum proteins, hormones, peptides, nucleic acid, and other molecules (Coppedè 2014).

The characteristic properties required for a molecule or compound to be a biomarker are as follows:

> A biomarker should be able to showcase and relate the differences at the molecular as well as the physiological level at the time of disease occurrence and then disease progression, it should be able to generate dose-response statistical data, and it should be unique to every type of disease be it cancer or any other health condition like cardiovascular ailment, diabetes, etc. and it should be a quantifiable entity.
>
> *(Spitz and Bondy 2009)*

The recent applied sciences and methodologies adopted for biomarker discovery are genomics, proteomics, and epigenomics (Scaros and Fisler 2005). In genomics, the molecular diagnostics approach is applied in techniques like polymerase chain reaction (PCR), microarrays, serial analysis of gene expression (SAGE), tangerine expression profiling, gene expression profiling, and expressed sequence tag (ESTs) analysis (Jain 2010) that locates the aberrant gene expressions as the biomarker of health conditions. In the proteomics approach, electrophoresis, Matrix-assisted laser desorption/ionization (MALDI-MS), and immunohistochemistry (IHC) are the most followed techniques that recognize tissue-specific proteins or protein sequence as the biomarker or molecular marker of disease (Wu et al. 2010). the epigenetics approach like pyrosequencing, MALDI-TOF, and bisulphite genome sequencing (Sandoval et al. 2013) was adopted to locate heritable changes in gene expressions like gene mutations that can be considered as biomarkers by DNA or RNA sequencing (Sandoval et al. 2013).

Despite having a wide range of biomarkers specific for each cell type that can help diagnose even a fatal health condition in its early stages and present a reliable cure, the target-specific remedies have not yet grasped the roots in medical fields due to major setbacks in the identification of biomarkers. The most commonly used techniques are the application of antibodies as recognition elements. However, their high production cost and variability in batch-to-batch production limit their usage (Bauer et al. 2016). The quest for finding an alternative to antibodies led to the discovery of aptamers – oligonucleotide or peptide sequences which contains unique to specific cell surface markers that mimic antibodies with respect to their binding affinity and specificity and nullify all the discrepancies raised due to antibodies (Briones 2011). These aptamers are artificially synthesized by systematic evolution of ligands by exponential enrichment (SELEX) and SoMER methods. They are designed for specific binding to the biomarkers and can be detected even at low concentrations. This leads to an increased sensitivity and reliability of the technique (Adachi and Nakamura 2019). The advent of aptamers in clinical research has boosted biomarker discovery to design and develop more aptamers which can be tested in different diseases. Their use in diagnostics and molecular techniques like western blotting, PCR, and IHC have aided in the manifestation of early detection of diseases. The use of aptamers is just not limited to diagnostic purposes but has widened to therapeutic applications and has made a remarkable impact in current cancer therapeutics and ventures a promising role in the future of personalized medicine and in the field of oncology.

2.2 APTAMERS AS NOVEL BIOMARKERS

2.2.1 What are aptamers?

The word "aptamer" derives its roots from the Latin word "aptus" which means "to fit" and the Greek word "meros" which means "part" (Gold et al. 2012). Literally, aptamers refer to the high-affinity binding molecules, precisely, oligonucleotides or peptide residues that bind to a variety of specific targets like microorganisms, cells and cellular proteins, carbohydrates, toxins, metals, compounds of diverse nature, small molecules, etc. (Wang et al. 2019). Aptamers, although different in their biomolecular origin as a peptide or an oligonucleotide molecule, bind with very high specificity and affinity to their respective targets. This specificity and binding ability are in turn, due to their three-dimensionally folded structures (Song et al. 2012). The use and significance of aptamers as potential biomarkers in diagnostics and therapeutics can be accredited to the efforts of Craig Tuerk and Larry Gold (1990) who generated specifically binding ligands with the help of SELEX and Andy Ellington and Jack Szostak (1990) who coined the generated ligands as now scientifically acclaimed "aptamers" in an independent work to select the high-affinity RNA molecules in vitro (Gold et al. 2012; Wang et al. 2019).

As mentioned in the previous section, the diagnostic and therapeutic implications of novel biomarkers have broadened the chances of correct and quick detection as well as proper treatment of multiple diseases in recent years. The chief reasons for the novelty of aptamers are rooted at the molecular level, disclosing its small size (5–15 kDa) and the convenience of chemical modification. The small size allows easy aptamer diffusion into the binding sites and lowers the chances of steric restrictions (Li et al. 2021). The focus on aptamers as potent biomarkers has gained worldwide due to their superior characteristics over other biomarkers and even antibiotics with cost-efficient synthesis, ease of chemical modification, structural flexibility, and low immunogenicity (Huang et al. 2021). The oligonucleotide aptamers i.e., either DNA or RNA molecules can form tertiary structures which in turn, are responsible for their specific binding to their targets (Ni et al. 2011). This specificity and high affinity have interested scientists globally as both properties are of utmost importance for an optimum diagnosis and prevention of any disease.

2.2.2 TYPES OF APTAMERS

Based on their occurrence, aptamers can be naturally occurring (unmodified) or synthetically modified. Naturally occurring aptamers can be broadly classified as nucleic acid aptamers and peptide aptamers. Nucleic acid aptamers further consist of single-stranded DNA (ssDNA) and RNA (ssRNA) aptamers (Huang et al. 2021). These short DNA or RNA sequences can stabilize as secondary and tertiary systems capable of especially binding proteins or different targets in the cell. Due to their closeness to antibodies as far as the specificity and binding are concerned, they may be regarded as equivalents of antibodies chemically (Ni et al. 2011). This concept of utilization of short ssDNA or ssRNA as affinity molecules for diverse targets relies on their property to form characteristic tertiary structures, allowing specific interactions with their target compounds (Adachi and Nakamura 2019).

ssRNA molecules fold into a colossal set of tertiary structures according to their varying primary structures. This validates their high capability to function as molecular mimics of proteins (Adachi and Nakamura 2019). RNA aptamers, thus, can be defined as ssRNA oligonucleotides which are capable of binding to their targets with high specificity and binding affinity (Germer et al. 2013). The selection of RNA aptamers over other macromolecules is advantageous due to the following reasons – (1) RNA aptamers have comparatively very low or negligible immunogenicity. (2) They are relatively easier to synthesize in bulk and under controlled conditions. (3) They easily attain the desired configuration and conformation. (4) They are thermodynamically much more stable than antibodies, peptides, or proteins (Germer et al. 2013).

Both the DNA and RNA aptamers function similarly but they differ in their degree of stability and utility. As compared to DNA aptamers, RNA aptamers are chemically unstable due to the presence of a free, reactive hydroxyl group at the 2′ position of the ribose sugar in RNA molecules. This hydroxyl group can get deprotonated in solution very easily, specifically, in alkaline solutions. The phosphorus atom involved in the phosphodiester linkage of the nucleotide may get nucleophilically attacked by the resulting anionic 2′-O, causing the hydrolysis of RNA molecules (Zhu et al. 2015). DNA aptamers have been explicitly researched for their applications in diverse fields such as diagnostics and therapeutics. Although the working of DNA and RNA aptamers is in a similar way, DNA aptamers bear few advantages over RNA aptamers because - (1) RNA aptamers formation needs reverse transcription in vitro for each round of selection, as well as an initial transcription for the generation of the RNA library from a DNA library. (2) The production cost for DNA aptamers is less than the cost of producing RNA aptamers (Zhu et al. 2015).

Peptide aptamers are short conjugational proteins that can bind to specific sites on their targets (New et al. 2020). They are composed of approximately 5–20 amino acid residues, generally embedded as a loop within a stable protein scaffold (Reverdatto et al. 2015). They are extremely small and compact molecules with high solubility, high stability, feasible kinetics for quick folding, and high availability through the possible chemical mechanisms and bacterial expressions (Reverdatto et al. 2015). The chemically modified aptamer examples include the SELEX-based aptamer called "Spiegelmer" developed for its nuclease resistance (Adachi and Nakamura 2019). It can be defined as an aptamer whose all sugar moieties in the oligonucleotides enantiomers or mirror images of those found naturally (Keefe et al. 2010). They consist of L-nucleotides rather than D-nucleotides which are naturally found in the nucleic acids (Ni et al. 2021). Yet another modification strategy has been developed slow off-rate modified aptamers (SOMAmers) that can target a huge number of proteins with a high binding affinity and specificity (Duo et al. 2018; Jankowski et al. 2020).

2.3 DISTINCTIVE ATTRIBUTES OF APTAMERS

Aptamers have an edge over other macromolecules due to their small size and negligible immunogenicity (Ni et al. 2011). In contrast to antibodies, aptamers have many advantages including easy chemical synthesis and modification and flexible design (Huang et al. 2021). Aptamers have a great scope in the near future as alternatives to antibodies as they overcome their drawbacks. The various advantages of aptamers over antibodies include – (1) High stability of aptamers as oligonucleotides are thermodynamically stable whereas the peptide or proteins can easily get denatured at higher temperatures and lose their tertiary or quaternary structures. (2) Ease and cost-efficient commercial production and chemical modification of aptamers. (3) Antibodies are significantly immunogenic which necessitates repeated dose administration whereas aptamers are low or negligibly immunogenic. (4) Aptamers can target a wide range of molecules even those which are often not recognized by antibodies (Keefe et al. 2010; Song et al. 2012). In addition, aptamers can also be used as binding domains for more complex regulatory RNA modules like ribozymes and natural riboswitches (regulatory elements within mRNA) thus, regulating the gene expression (Weigand and Suess 2009).

2.4 APTAMER DESIGNING

At present, there are different aptamer-based technologies for designing and synthesizing biomarkers, namely, Cell-SELEX and SOMAScan technology. Cell-SELEX technology is utilized for the identification of the surface biomarkers on the cell membrane of various cells whereas SOMAScan technology is utilized for the detection of enormous amounts of proteins of different kinds in the biological samples at the same time (Huang et al. 2021). The traditional and most common method for aptamer designing or engineering i.e., SELEX can be segregated into two alternating stages – In the first stage, PCR is used to amplify the original oligonucleotides. In the case of RNA aptamers selection, the in vitro transcription of dsDNA with the enzyme T7 RNA-polymerase generates a large pool of single-stranded oligoribonucleotides. In the case of DNA aptamers, the strands of the double-stranded products obtained after PCR are separated to produce single-stranded oligodeoxyribonucleotides.

In the second stage, the binding oligonucleotides are identified by incubating the pool of amplified oligonucleotides with the target molecules. These interacting ssDNA or ssRNA molecules are then used for the first stage of the subsequent SELEX round (Lakhin et al. 2013).

Thus, the general or conventional type of SELEX is composed of three, iterative steps in order to find the best binding nucleotides. The first step of the general SELEX strategy starts with the generation of combinatorial libraries (Song et al. 2012). The second step of binding and elution or separation involves the isolation of specifically binding components by repeated ligand binding and elution process (Song et al. 2012). The third step of amplification involves the PCR-based amplification of the target-bound nucleotides to generate a new library to be used in the subsequent round of SELEX (Lakhin et al. 2013). Aptamers are unceasingly being developed through this technology, and their properties are studied with the help of numerous biological assays (Song et al. 2012).

In recent years, many variations and modifications in the SELEX technology are observed like Cell-SELEX, Capillary electrophoresis-based SELEX, microfluidic-based SELEX, affinity chromatography, and magnetic bead-based SELEX, nitrocellulose membrane filtration-based SELEX, etc. (Song et al. 2012). As opposed to the other types of SELEX technologies, Cell-SELEX aims at the entire direct screening of aptamers from the entire cell (Huang et al. 2021). The process consists of iterative cycles of (1) the positive selection of oligonucleotides by incubating the initial oligonucleotides with the target cells. (2) The negative selection of the oligonucleotides by incubation of target-bound oligonucleotides with non-target cells. (3) Amplification of the unbound oligonucleotides (to the non-target cells) to create a new library of oligonucleotides for the subsequent oligonucleotide selection round (Lakhin et al. 2013). After around 20 cycles, the different aptamers can be selected. The desired candidate aptamers are selected with the help of cloning and sequencing of the generated aptamer pool. Cell-SELEX technology has been successfully utilized for the diagnostic and therapeutic applications of aptamers as biomarkers, reportedly, in cancers like leukaemia, glioblastoma, pancreatic cancers, and carcinomas (Huang et al. 2021).

Cell-SELEX bears many advantages over other SELEX types – (1) This generation is capable of picking out aptamers that may differentiate ordinary cells from diseased cells without understanding the distinction among the cells in advance. (2) Cell-SELEX is a solution to the limitation that the aptamers engineered can bind only to purified proteins and not to impurified proteins that are in their native state. (3) This area is under research to discover new biomarkers in different types of diseased cells. (4) The aptamers obtained are also able to differentiate between various cell lines like cancer cells, benign tumour cells, or other cell lines of a known or unknown disease, and also various subtypes of cells (Huang et al. 2021; Meyer et al. 2011). The illustration of steps involved in SELEX and Cell-SELEX are described in Figure 2.1.

SOMAScan is used to generate synthetically a different type of aptamers called the SOMAmers. As compared to conventional aptamers, SOMAmers are advantageous because of the increment in the binding force between the oligonucleotides and the target proteins as a result of chemical modification. The SOMAScan

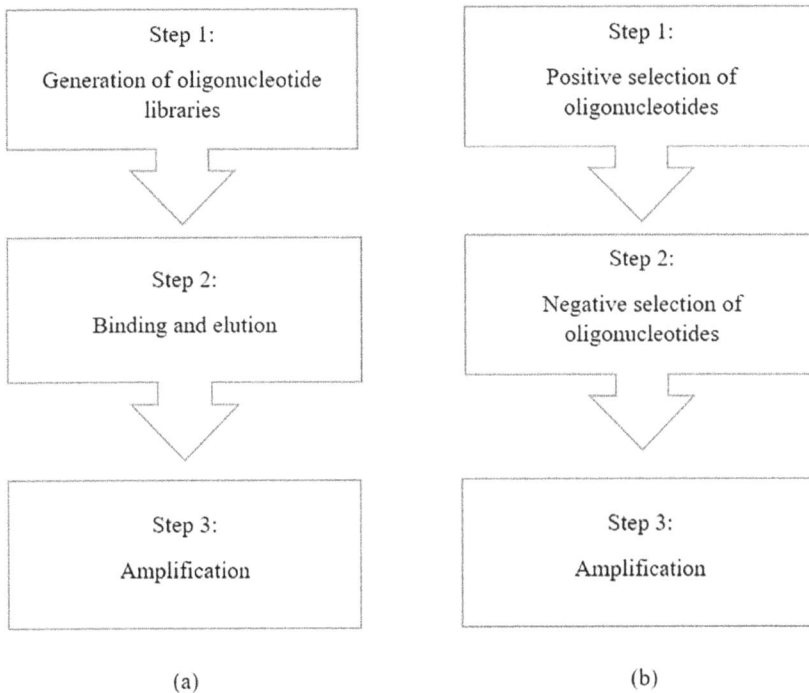

FIGURE 2.1 Schematic representation of steps involved in general (a) SELEX and (b) Cell-SELEX.

strategy involves – (1) Mixing of the SOMAmers with the target molecules forming SOMAmer-protein complexes. (2) Tagging of the complexes with fluorescent tags and with biotin. (3) These complexes are immobilized on avidin beads with the help of streptavidin. (4) The captured proteins are then labelled with biotin. (5) The complexes are separated from the beads with the help of UV light. (6) Polyanionic competitors are then added to facilitate the separation of proteins bound to non-specific SOMAmers. (7) The bound complexes are then immobilized onto the primer beads. (8) The obtained complexes are detached with the help of sodium hydroxide solution (20 mM) (Huang et al. 2021). SOMAScan technology has been used in the diagnosis and therapy of various cancers namely lung, colon, ovarian, breast, and liver as well as neurodegenerative disorders such as Parkinson's disease and multiple sclerosis, rheumatoid arthritis, infectious diseases (Huang et al. 2021).

2.5 APTAMERS IN DIAGNOSTICS

2.5.1 NANOPARTICLES

Chemotherapy and radiotherapy are the current cancer therapeutics in practice and has alarmed many concerns regarding side effect due to their non-specificity for cancer cells thereby killing normal cells (Pearce et al. 2017). Hence, the recent endeavours to establish a targeted drug delivery system have potentiated an exorbitant class of compounds that can accomplish target-based therapeutic approaches. One such is the use of nanotechnology wherein a fixed amount of anti-cancer drug is delivered to cancer cells over an extended period of time and ensures that the nearby cells are not affected (Farokhzad et al. 2006). The major hindrance to this is directing the drug conjugated with nanoparticles to a proper site. This requires the identification of a biomarker highly specific to that particular cancer. Aptamers which are short oligonucleotide sequences of proteins or DNA or RNA have helped to overcome this problem and are a widely accepted new field in oncology antidotes (Chang et al. 2013). In this technique, the aptamers are designed complementary to the biomarkers that are generally available as cell receptors unique to the cancer cell. Such aptamers are conjugated to the nanoparticles and administered to the patients where the drug is directed towards the tumour which is released slowly from the nanoparticle in the solid tumour (Figure 2.2). Aptamer-guided nanoparticles are profoundly studied in prostate cancer (Dhar et al. 2008). Cisplatin a well-known anti-cancer drug was constructed as Pt(IV) encasing nanoparticles of poly(d,l-lactic-co-glycolic acid) (PLGA)-poly(ethylene glycol) (PEG)-functionalized controlled release polymers conjugated with prostate-specific membrane antigen (PSMA) targeting aptamer (Dhar et al. 2008) where PSMA is cancer biomarker for prostate cancer (Srikantan et al. 2000).

Yu et al. 2011 proposed the use of mucin short variant S1 (MUC1) antigen aptamer in adenocarcinoma treatment (Yu et al. 2011). MUC1 – a large transmembrane glycoprotein was observed to manifest a 10-fold increase in its expression in adenocarcinomas and hence was considered to be a suitable target (Taylor-Papadimitriou et al. 1999). The MUC1 aptamer S2.2 – a 25 bases long oligonucleotide complementary to MUC1 receptors was conjugated with nanoparticles by carboxyl (–COOH) and amine (–NH$_2$) cross-linkage to deliver paclitaxel at the target site in the MCF-7 breast cancer cell line positive for MUC1 receptors (Yu et al. 2011).

The cellular binding of aptamers and the release of the paclitaxel (PTX) from aptamer-conjugated nanoparticles (Apt-NPs) conjugates were determined by flow cytometry and membrane diffusion technique respectively (Yu et al. 2011) and the cumulative PTX release was calculated. The two cancer cell lines chosen for the study were MCF-7, a MUC1 positive breast cancer cell line (Ren et al. 1997) as a test group, and HepG, a MUC1 negative hepatic cancer cell line as a control group (Yu et al. 2011). The results displayed the binding of MUC1 aptamers only to the MCF-7 cancer cells and showed no binding affinity towards the HepG2 cells (Yu et al. 2011). These results assured that the aptamer-guided nanoparticle therapy targeted the cancer biomarkers accurately and has a great scope in future cancer therapeutics.

2.5.2 APTAMERS IN BIOIMAGING

Bioimaging refers to the non-invasive procedure carried out to visualize the ongoing metabolic activities in living cells without causing any kind of hindrance or obstacle in the biological processes (Malik et al. 2019). It is quite possible to observe cellular movements under a light microscope but when it comes to the identification of any intracellular metabolism or pathways happening live, observations under the

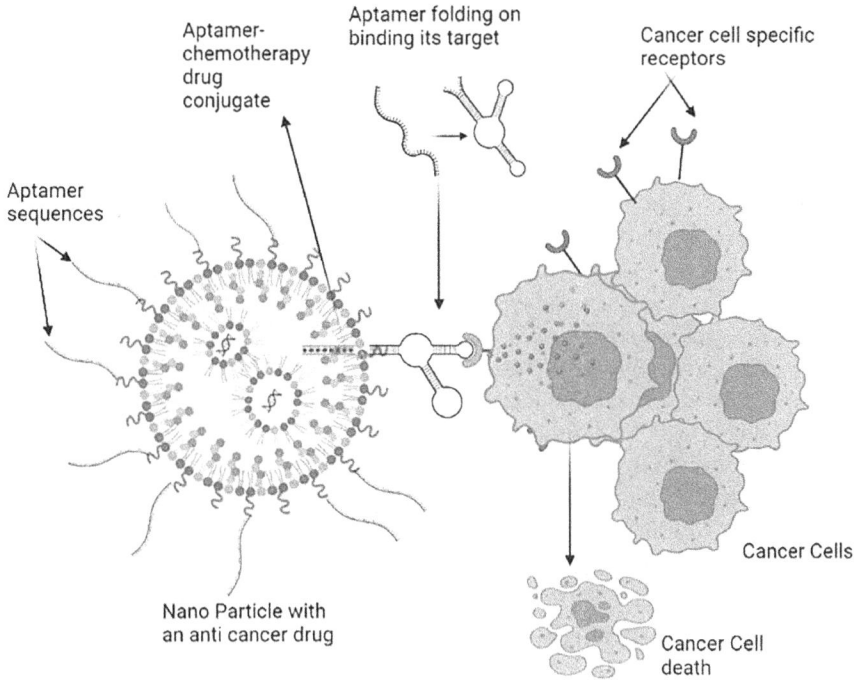

FIGURE 2.2 Cancer cell-specific binding of aptamer-conjugated nanoparticles for target-specific drug delivery.

microscope become difficult. For this, when small molecules or compounds are to be identified that are actively taking part in a metabolic process biosensors are required. Biosensors are the tools utilized to quantify the molecular analytes produced inside a live cell during a metabolic process that plays a major role in disease target validation, diagnostics, and drug delivery (Bhalla et al. 2016). Biological elements like enzymes, DNA probes, proteins, and antibodies are used as the recognition elements that infer appreciable target specificity (Guan et al. 2020). However, with the recent advancements in aptamer-based diagnostics biosensors termed aptasensors, are emerging as the most suitable molecular biology tool for sensing small molecules even at a very low concentration due to their high precision target identification (Wang and Ray 2012).

Aptasensors have two basic modules, the first one is the aptamer probe that is synthesized according to the required molecule that must be quantified and another is the imaging modality (Wang and Ray 2012). The aptamer probe has a sensing domain that deploys the aptamer as a recognition element (ideal probe reagents) that recognizes the target molecule and upon binding with the help of the signalling domain, the signal is transduced further through a reporter that can be radionuclides, microbubbles or fluorophore that result in fluorescence (Wang and Ray 2012). The effects of such reporter elements are analyzed on imaging modalities, mainly fluorescence microscopy, radiography, computed tomography, or magnetic resonance imaging

(MRI) (Song et al. 2008). The aptamer probes used are selected by considering the parameters like having high affinity and specificity, and good pharmacokinetic properties. When the target is a small molecule or a protein, direct aptamer target interaction is considered ideal (Chen and Chen 2010). Sometimes, rational designing is done wherein the aptamers are linked to an aptamer ligand which is then enriched on the target and produces readable results (Wang and Ray 2012).

The advancements in molecular biology have unleashed the importance of different types of RNAs like mRNA, tRNA, rRNA, siRNA, and microRNA each one having different roles like RNA translation, localization, splicing, gene silencing, etc. in cellular dynamics. The most probable technologies suited for such analysis make use of hybridization-based probes like fluorescence in situ hybridization (FISH) or molecular beacons (Bao et al. 2009; Itzkovitz and van Oudenaarden 2011). These techniques involve invasive procedures of prob delivery to the target for the detection of endogenous RNAs without tagging them. To avoid these invasive procedures, aptamer-based RNA imaging has been devised. Here, aptamers are designed for RNA imaging where the multiple copies of aptamer tags are linked to their target RNA in untranslated regions via physical linkage or hybridization to detect the presence of different RNAs by binding a fluorescent ligand to it and elucidate their expressions levels in an individual and interpret their health conditions (Wang and Ray 2012).

2.5.3 How do aptamers detect the target?

To take an example, for detection and quantification of potassium ion (K^+) in a live cell, a thrombin aptamer that is a G-quartet by structure was used as a recognition element owing to its structural sensitivity to potassium ion (K^+) (Wang and Ray 2012). At the 5′ end, a biotinylated neutral peptide (PSO 5) was linked to carboxytetramethylrhodamine (TAMRA) fluorophore, and at the 3′ end, fluorescein amidites (FAM) was linked. A nuclear export signal was synthesized namely B-NES. Streptavidin (four sites for biotin attachment) has the unique feature of capturing both PSO 5 and B– NES signals and a ternary complex was formed that included streptavidin, PSO5, and B– NES in the ratio 1:3:1 (Wang and Ray 2012). For K^+ imaging, this ternary complex was retained in the cytoplasm rather than in the nucleus. When the K+ is absent, the thrombin aptamer undergoes structural unfolding such that the two fluorophores, TAMRA and FAM are far away from each other. On the other hand, when potassium ions are present, the thrombin aptamer forms the G-quartet structure such that the two fluorophores TAMRA and FAM are close to each other to be able to generate a fluorescence resonance energy transfer (FRET) signal for K^+ imaging (Figure 2.3; Wang and Ray 2012). When the ternary complex was incorporated into HeLa cells, it recorded cytosolic K+ levels and dynamics in real time. Likewise, many other aptasensors are contrived for the detection of specific biomarkers, thus improvising the currently used diagnostic methodologies.

2.5.4 Aptamers in western blot

Western blotting is a predominant molecular biology technique for detecting sensitive and specific proteins with the help of antibodies or probes (Kim 2017; Nybo 2012).

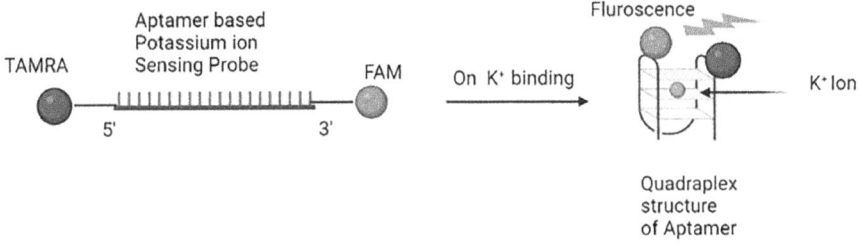

FIGURE 2.3 Aptamer sensing based on FRET.

This technique involves electrophoretic separation of proteins proceeded by transfer to nitrocellulose membrane thereby blocking non-specific adsorption. The desired proteins are identified by conjugation with primary and secondary antibodies and, in turn, conjugated with fluorophores or horseradish peroxidase (Han et al. 2019; Mishra et al. 2019). Although being an effective method, tedious protocols, colossal time consumption, high antibodies production cost that can have irreversible denaturation and variations from batch-to-batch production, and long incubation time for ensuring proper protein antibody binding, limit the use of this technique (Wang and Ray 2012). The recent findings have shown how aptamers can be used as a protein recognition substitute for antibodies and overcome all of the disadvantages associated with the use of antibodies. This technique is also referred to as apt blotting or southwestern blotting where the primary antibody is replaced with an aptamer. Conversely, aptamers might be intrinsically linked to a reporter moiety such as fluorophore and quantum dot, which would make protein recognition more convenient and speedier (Li et al. 2011; Shin et al. 2010). In a study presented by Wang and Ray (2012), the binding affinity of three aptamers namely G1, M1, and H1 for their respective target proteins glutathione S-transferase (GST), maltose binding protein (MPB), and polyhistidine tag (His-tag) protein were determined by western blotting and compared with the western blotting performed with the help of antibodies. The results depicted that aptamer-based western blotting produced better results in terms of being able to reduce non-specific binding being less time-consuming and cost-effective, and can be sensitive to detecting proteins in nanomolar concentrations. The only drawback this method suffers is that the denaturation of target protein due to sodium dodecyl-sulfate polyacrylamide gel electrophoresis (SDS page) decreases the binding affinity of the DNA aptamers as they require their protein targets to be in the same condition as retrieved from natural isolates (Wang et al. 2020). But surely, they embark on a promising role to be played in future diagnostics.

2.5.5 APTAMERS IN PCR

PCR is a widely used analytical tool for amplifying double-stranded DNA fragments and infers many clinical applications. Many subtypes of PCR have been developed in different medical fields such as fast-cycling PCR for gene cloning, reverse transcriptase PCR for detecting the presence of any viral infection, and real-time PCR for evaluating the actual viral load in a given sample (Lakhin et al. 2013). The scope of these techniques has expanded hugely in almost every clinical research field and has imparted many promising roles in the establishment of therapeutics. The advancements in target-specific therapeutics have increased the demand for disease-specific target protein discoveries and for this several methods and techniques are emerging (Song et al. 2012). One such novel approach of using PCR in target protein discovery with the help of aptamers has gained much attention in the discipline of diagnostics and therapeutics. The PCR amplification of specific DNA sequence aptamers procured from the SELEX or SoMER methods has shown the efficacy of detecting target proteins even at the lowest concentration of 10^{-14} mol/L (Lin and McNatty 2009).

Another type of PCR developed by aptamer technology is the aptamer-based regionally protected PCR (ARP-PCR). In ARP-PCR, ssDNA segments are obtained from dot plotting or western blotting by performing an SDS page. In this pool of ssDNA, the aptamers designed specifically for the target proteins are incorporated. DNase I (DNA denaturing enzyme) is administered to this solution. The target sequences to which the aptamers are bound to remain intact, whereas the rest free unbound ssDNA gets degraded by DNase I. Thereafter the remaining ssDNA-aptamer conjugate is subjected to PCR to further amplify the desired ssDNA sequence (Lin and McNatty 2009). This unique approach of filtering out required target protein sequences and amplifying them lends an easy and cost-effective way for developing aptamer-based therapeutics, especially in cancers where cancer-specific biomarkers are the prerequisites for desirable treatment outcomes (Lakhin et al. 2013). A study by Lin and McNatty (2009) described the accuracy and sensitivity of ARP-PCR by incorporating the Ovine follicle-stimulating hormone (oFSH-α) model protein for generating Ofsh-α receptor-specific DNA aptamers. It revealed that ARP-PCR can detect native Ofsh-α at the lowest concentration of 10^{-14} mol/L (Lin and McNatty 2009).

2.5.6 APTAMERS IN IHC

IHC can be considered the paradigm for the current tumour diagnosis practices across the globe. Previously, the surgical procedures followed to diagnose cancer which involved staining a tumour susceptible tissue section with eosin and haematoxylin and studied using contrast microscopy (Jaffer and Bleiweiss 2004). The results revealed frail molecular features that were inadequate for a conclusive diagnosis like deciphering stage and grade of cancer (Wu et al. 2010). The use is limited due to poor contrast between the cellular components and a complete lack of knowledge of biomarkers especially when the tumour in its early stage is undifferentiated (Bauer et al. 2016). On the other hand, IHC works on the idea that each cell type does have a molecular marker and can aid in differential diagnosis with respect to cancer cells and normal cells (Hofman and Taylor 2013)

IHC can be defined as an immunological technique that renders monoclonal or polyclonal antibodies of specific types to bind to their corresponding cell surface markers or antigens located in tissues and selectively identify those tissue antigens (Ramos-Vara and Miller 2013). However, along with the precision in the selectivity of antibodies, there are a few drawbacks that raise concerns about the validity of antibodies. In general, IHC is performed by vaccinating a mouse model with the desired target protein epitope which forms the primary antibodies. This is followed by surgical removal of the spleen from the mouse model, and the plasma cells collected from here are fused with myeloma tumour cells to form a hybridoma cell lineage that would ensure continuous production of monoclonal antibodies. Such antibodies are collected and used in IHC (Jaffer and Bleiweiss 2004). Similarly, for secondary antibodies, an antigen complementary to the Fc region of the primary antibody is injected, and via hybridoma technology secondary antibodies are produced. Every time, the antibodies are produced in a new modal organism by new immune cells with slightly different genetic makeup. This can add up to the variability in the antibodies, thus, questioning the validity of the antibody as the recognition element. Also, the antibody production cost makes them unsuitable for procuring consistent results where a repetitive experimental setup is required (Bauer et al. 2016). According to one analysis, 42% of diagnostic discrepancies were attributed to improper antibody selection and antibody cross-reactivity (De Matos et al. 2010; Leong 2004). Therefore, to enhance the processivity of IHC, aptamers that bestow thermal stability, low production cost, and ease in discovery and quantification are currently well researched for developing robust target-specific therapeutics.

Recently, a study on atherosclerosis revealed the involvement of the matrix metalloproteinase-2 (MMP2) enzyme in the development of atherosclerotic plaque leading to coronary heart diseases (Han et al. 2014). In order to visualize the MMP2 activity in pathological tissues, aptamer named MMP2, was designed by performing eight rounds of SELEX with an affinity of (K_d = 5.59 nM). This aptamer was able to precipitate MMP2 and detect it in tissue samples of atherosclerotic plaques and gastric cancer. When this MMP2 aptamer was conjugated with a fluorophore to develop a nanoprobe, it was able to successfully visualize the atherosclerotic plaques in Apolipoprotein E knockout mice (Han et al. 2014).

The epithelial cell adhesion molecules (EpCAM) are well-known biomarkers that are generally found to be overexpressed in cancers of epithelial origin (Pu et al. 2015). In a recent study, a DNA-based aptamer SYL3C was designed for the EpCAM biomarker expressed in colorectal cancer. This aptamer was tested for its binding specificity in frozen and paraffin-embedded sections of colorectal cancer tissue samples against commercialized antibodies for EpCAM standard control. The aptamer displayed specific recognition of cancer nests within the tissue section and stained exactly those regions by excluding the background cells benign lesions and inflammation of colorectal cancer tissue. SYL3C showed no cross-linkage to EpCAM-negative malignant tissue samples (Pu et al. 2015). These results supported the high specificity of DNA aptamers and their further applications in clinical research.

2.5.7 APTAMERS IN EMERGING DIAGNOSTIC APPLICATIONS

Flow cytometry is one of the most extensively used techniques for cell characterization that hydrodynamically focuses them in a fluid streamlet where they pass through intersecting laser beams that result in scattering of light and generate fluorescent signals that tell us about the cell size, intracellular and granularity (Meyer et al. 2013). The pressing need for biomarker discovery has impelled researchers to consider aptamer application in flow cytometry. These aptamers are used as fluorescent probes that detect only those cells in the cell subpopulation that carry a molecular marker specific for that cell type – a cancer cell or a normal cell (Meyer et al. 2013). Recently, Aptamer Science Inc. (AptSciSci, Inc.) located in South Korea was successful in synthesizing aptamers against CD31, hepatocyte growth factor receptor (HGFR), vascular endothelial growth factor receptor 2 (VEGFR2), intercellular adhesion molecule 1 (ICAM-2), human epidermal growth factor receptor 2 (HER-2), and epidermal growth factor receptor (EGFR) biomarkers and developed magnetic bead-based cell isolation kits that expeditiously detected and isolated the above-mentioned biomarker-positive cells using flow cytometry (Kaur et al. 2018). These aptamers are dually labelled as in from one end it is linked to biotin for capturing the biomarker-positive cells with streptavidin that is coated with magnetic beads. The other end is labelled with fluorescein isothiocyanate (FITC) for monitoring the captured cells and recording the fluorescence produced by them (Kaur et al. 2018). The aptamer used in diagnostics applications is enlisted in Table 2.1.

Another implication of aptamers is being studied in immunoprecipitation techniques. When the quantity of biomarkers in a sample is below the detectable levels in enzyme-linked immunosorbent assay (ELISA) or western blotting assays, aptamers can be a suitable substitute for antibodies. Also, the use of antibodies infers sometimes cross-reactivity and protein contamination thus causing hindrance in downstreaming processes. For this, Aptoprep kits are developed that contain conjugates of the aptamers complementary to the biomarkers like CD31, HER2, HGFR, ICAM-2, etc., and magnetic beads that pull down the biomarkers from the serum and aid in their precipitation. This technique is also termed aptoprecipitation. This technique yields biomarkers of the highest purity (Kaur et al. 2018).

TABLE 2.1
Aptamers in diagnostic applications

Aptamer	Detection mode	Diagnostic application	Mode of signal transduction	References
DNA streptavidin labelled	ELISA-Like array	To quantify IgE antibodies	SPR	Wang et al. (2008)
DNA labelled with quantum dot	Fluorescence techniques: FRET	Detection of MUC1 Cancer-specific biomarker	Fluorescence	Cheng et al. (2009)
MB-conjugated DNA aptamer	Quartz crystal microbalance system	Leukaemia cells	QCM	Pan et al. (2010)
Biotin-conjugated RNA aptamer	Biosensor	HIV-Tat	SPR, QCM	Tombelli et al. (2005)
RNA aptamer	Chip-based	Hepatitis C Core antigen	Fluorescence	Lee et al. (2007)

Another commercially available aptamer-based sensing technology used is Ochratoxin A (OTA)-Sense. This was developed by the Neoventures of Biotechnology Inc. under the guidance of Dr. Gregory Penner (Penner 2012). The purpose of OTA-sense is to detect the OTA mycotoxins produced by fungi like Aspergillus, penicillin, etc. in food products like cereals, wines, fruits, grapes, etc. Even the low levels of OTA toxin are highly hazardous to health and are considered carcinogenic, therefore the European Union has set a bar for the maximum allowed level of this toxin in foods like cereals, wines, and baby food to be 5, 2, and 0.5 ppb (Kaur et al. 2018). The OTA-sense fluorescent diagnostic kit does the detection of the toxin in the sample in a high-throughput manner that deploys high sensitivity, and its application is broadened in alcohol industries for detecting toxins (Penner 2012).

2.5.7.1   Aptamers in SARS-CoV-2 virus detection

The recent application of aptamers in severe acute respiratory syndrome Coronavirus 2 (SARS-CoV-2) detection can be studied by Chen et al. (2021). In this research article, the authors have proposed that a spike in protein DNA aptamer having high sensitivity for the protein of the SARS-CoV-2 virus can be utilized for diagnosis of COVID-19 infection. The detection of the same is based on surface-enhanced Raman scattering (SERS). Here, the DNA aptamers conjugated with cy3-Raman receptor molecules were immobilized on the gold Nano popcorn surface that would act as a sensor surface and would measure the deflection in the electromagnetic field. When the sample solution containing the protein of interest to be detected is added, the DNA aptamer specific for that protein binds to it causing it to move slightly away from the cy3-Raman receptor. This results in the localized surface plasmon resonance and is recorded as the deflection in the electromagnetic field leading to a change in Raman peak intensity. This method not only gives the qualitative data i.e., tells about the presence or absence of the protein but also relays the quantitative data as the change in the Raman peak intensity is inversely proportional to the concentration of SARS-CoV-2 spike protein in the test solution with threshold less than 10 PFU/mL (Chen et al. 2021). The selectivity of this aptamer-based biosensor exclusively for SARS-CoV-2 viral particles was cross-verified by having different viral particles e.g., influenza viral particles where no changes were observed in the reading. By this, the selectivity and specificity of this biosensor were confirmed. This new technique of detection poses several advantages over the conventional methods of viral infection diagnostics (Song et al. 2020). Unlike the other conventional methods that rely on antibody production for the detection of viral infection, aptamers-based biosensors with their high specificity for the viral antigens themselves, enable one to detect the viral infection in its very early stage. One need not wait for the window period to be completed for accurate diagnostics. This would help the medicos to administer a suitable treatment in early stages only which would aid in reducing the fatality rate. This technique is comparatively inexpensive, reliable, robust, and short-time stipulated method to detect SARS-CoV-2 infection would potentiate the efficacy of handling the pandemic, the world is apparently seeing (Song et al. 2020). The illustration of the same is mentioned in Figure 2.4.

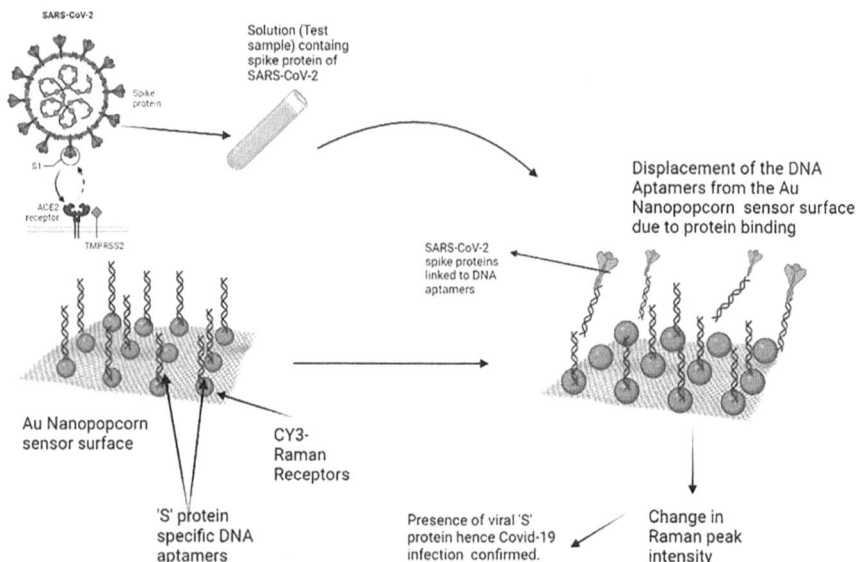

FIGURE 2.4   Aptamer-based biosensor for detection of SARS-CoV-2 viral infection.

2.6   APTAMERS AS THERAPEUTICS

The consistently increasing disease burden on the world has led to the emergence of newer possibilities in the field of therapeutics. The hunt for better medicinal alternatives has taken into consideration novel biomolecules like aptamers for the treatment of various diseases. Aptamers, as well, have been showing promising therapeutic results in a diverse set of diseases. A few of its therapeutic effects are discussed below:

2.6.1 MICROBIAL OR INFECTIOUS DISEASES

The recent efforts in the field of therapeutics have reported the production and validation of aptamers against many microbial pathogens, their toxins, and diseases (Table 2.2). RNA aptamer has been produced using the Cell-SELEX method to target the blood-borne organism *Trypanosama cruzi* which is the causative parasitic agent of Chagas disease in the blood (Nagarkatti et al. 2012). Yet another example includes the treatment of food poisoning and other food-borne diseases caused by *Salmonella* sp. The design of a twenty-seven nucleotide aptamer (LA 27) targeted the Lipopolysaccharides (LPS) of *Salmonella typhimurium* (Srivastava et al. 2021). A few examples of DNA aptamers targeting bacterial species include Lyd-3 aptamer targeting *Streptococcus pneumoniae*, SAL26 aptamer targeting *S. typhimurium,* and BB16-11f targeting *Bifidobacterium breve* (Afrasiabi et al. 2020). The notable DNA aptamers acting against bacterial toxins include CT916 targeting cholera toxin and ML12 targeting anthrax toxin (Afrasiabi et al. 2020).

Most viruses escape through the effects of medications due to their mutative behaviour and ability to hide from the host's immune system. The most notorious viral diseases remain hepatitis C, SARS, human immunodeficiency virus (HIV-1), and Middle East respiratory syndrome (MERS) (Song et al. 2020). Additionally, many antiviral medications increase the risk of health due to their untreated side effects. Studies have been undertaken to confirm the action of aptamers not just as therapeutic but also as preventive at any diagnosed stage of the disease. Researchers have been focusing upon the inhibition of attachment and penetration into the host and the blocking of the virus' replication machinery (main replication enzymes) as the prime antiviral mechanisms (Fesseha et al. 2020). The DNA aptamers targeting the hepatitis B virus target its core protein and prevent the replication of the virus, those targeting the influenza A virus prevent its host cell invasion by targeting its haemagglutinin protein, and many others are witnessed to be targeting vaccinia and rabies virus. Several RNA aptamers have also been under extensive research for targeting viruses like Ebola, SCV, HSV-1, Influenza B virus, and HIV-1 (Afrasiabi et al. 2020).

The recent COVID-19 pandemic has forced the medical community to search for the most affirmative alternatives for the correct detection and treatment of the virus. As the current tests and medications lack the optimum specificity and are extremely time-consuming for any observable results, aptamer-based biomarkers are emerging as one of the substitutes for the present-day detection kits and curatives (Byun 2021). Studies have further confirmed the therapeutic effects of aptamers against parasites. The RNA aptamers targeting *Entamoeba histolytica* cease its proliferation and thus kill it. *Trypanosoma cruzi* and *Trypanosoma brucei* are also known to be targeted by RNA aptamers. The DNA aptamer targeting *Leishmania infantum* ceases its transcription process by disturbing the normal functioning of the Poly(A)-binding protein (PABP) (Afrasiabi et al. 2020).

2.6.2 Oncology

The diverse types based on the tissue origin and tumour progression, cancer treatment, and management are of great concern. Antisoma or AS1411 is a guanine-rich aptamer which targets the nucleolar phosphoprotein of eukaryotes called nucleolin. This inhibition blocks the normal ribosomal synthesis and maturation which is a target for many anti-cancer therapies. The different cancers that have shown effects in favour of AS1411 therapy are acute myeloid leukaemia, breast cancer, and metastatic renal cell carcinoma as evident from the clinical trial reports of each one of them (Ni et al. 2011; Zhu et al. 2015). Another important target of anti-cancer therapy for breast cancer is the HER-2which is significantly overexpressed in a large number of breast cancers as well as other tumours of the epithelium. A DNA aptamer is produced which has been shown to interact and bind HER-2 causing the cessation of growth of gastric cancer cells in vitro. Attempts have been made to develop an RNA aptamer that can bind and internalize into HER-2-expressing cells with the help of Cell-SELEX (Nimjee et al. 2017). Another example includes a nuclease-resistant aptamer against the AXL tyrosine kinase receptor which is recognised as a transforming gene in myeloid leukaemia and its expression is amplified in several solid tumours (Nimjee et al. 2017). One of the foremost crucial aptamers was created to target the protein tyrosine kinase 7 (PTK7), which is a cell surface receptor, in T-cell acute leukaemia (Nimjee et al. 2017).

2.6.3 METABOLIC DISORDERS

A spiegelmer (L-RNA aptamer) named NOX-E36 has been under study for the treatment of type 2 diabetes. The 40-nucleotide long aptamer binds with C–C chemokine ligand 2 (CCL2) which is a human chemokine. Also known as monocyte chemoattractant protein 1 (MCP-1). Many inflammatory diseases have been reported to involve the overexpression of CCL2 and C–C chemokine receptor 2 (CCR2) which is its receptor. Clinical trials have been carried out for type 2 diabetes (Kaur et al. 2018). Research is being carried out to confirm the aptamer's involvement in the treatment of the disease and its exact therapeutic mechanism.

2.6.4 ANTI-INFLAMMATION, ANTICOAGULATION AND ANTI-ANGIOGENESIS

A 44-nucleotide long speigelmer named NOX-H94 is an L-RNA aptamer reported to have a high binding affinity with hepcidin. The aptamer is modified to bear forty kilodaltons of polyethylene glycol (PEG) tail and it is the third speigelmer to have successfully entered the clinical trials. The aptamer is being studied for its effect on anti-inflammatory diseases. As hepcidin is one of the prime regulators of normal iron levels in the body, the blocking of the regulator is studied to be involved in the treatment of anaemia of chronic inflammation (ACI) (Kaur et al. 2018). Achemix or ARC1779 is a PEGylated DNA aptamer which is used to identify the platelet ligand-receptor von Willebrand factor that is responsible for the recruitment of platelets. ARC1779 is responsible for producing an antithrombotic effect as it inhibits the binding between von Willebrand factor and the platelets (Ni et al. 2011; Nimjee et al. 2017; Zhu et al. 2015). Another example of an anti-coagulating aptamer is NU172 which is an unmodified DNA aptamer targeting thrombin. This interaction delays blood clotting (Ni et al. 2011; Zhu et al. 2015).

The anti-angiogenic aptamers include E10030 and pegaptanib or macugen. E10030 is a PEGylated DNA aptamer that is antagonistic to platelet-derived growth factor. E10030 along with correct concentrations of anti-VEGF drugs can evidently prevent angiogenesis or blood vessel formation. The anti-angiogenic effect of E10030 in wet age-related macular degeneration is at present under study (Zhu et al. 2015). Pegaptanib is an anti-VEGF RNA aptamer. Reportedly, the U.S. Food and Drug Administration (FDA) had approved pegaptanib as the first nucleic acid aptamer. Pegaptanib targets VEGF165, which is a homodimeric protein and the most profuse isoform of VEGF, responsible for blood vessel formation and regulating the permeability of the blood vessels. Pegaptanib blocks normal blood vessel formation by blocking the interaction between VEGF and its receptor. Also, its ability to lower the permeability of blood vessels is being explored in the treatment of neovascular age-related macular degeneration which involves vision loss due to increased vascular permeability in the eyes (Ni et al. 2011; Nimjee et al. 2017).

2.6.5 NEUROLOGICAL DISEASES

The diagnosis and treatment of neurological diseases is difficult and the options for permanent treatment are still under research. Aptamers prove to be promising therapeutics in nervous system disorders due to their high affinity which lowers the chances of side effects and loss of drug. Their relatively smaller size aids in crossing the blood-brain barrier and deeply penetrating the nervous tissue. Two aptamers against multiple sclerosis are under study in mice i.e., the IL-17 and the midkine aptamer. Both aptamers were reported to lower the level of inflammation (Zhou et al. 2012). Studies of the effects of aptamers as therapeutics in other neurological disorders like Alzheimer's disease, Parkinson's disease, ischemic stroke, etc. are in progress (Zhou et al. 2012).

2.7 MODIFICATIONS FOR TARGETED DRUG DELIVERY

Aptamer degradation is one of the major limitations to their optimum utilisation in biological systems. Aptamers, specifically RNA aptamers, get readily degraded by nucleases and there arises a need for modifications for the protection of aptamers from the action of nucleases. One of the traditional methods used to produce nuclease-resistant aptamers is by using SELEX with oligonucleotides with modified nucleotide structures. Characteristic DNA and RNA polymerases which can use chemically modified nucleoside triphosphate substrates are used in the production of such oligonucleotides (Lakhin et al. 2013; Ni et al. 2021). Examples include modified oligonucleotides with a 2′ sugar position. The sole modified aptamer which is validated and approved as a therapeutic is pegaptanib or macugen. Another major limitation to efficient aptamer-based drug delivery is renal excretion and quick removal from the bloodstream. The modification by conjugating aptamers with PEG of the appropriate molecular weight has been found to resolve the problem (Lakhin et al. 2013; Ni et al. 2021). Many long-length aptamers undergo truncation as their long length limits their therapeutic effects. Truncation, in addition to increasing the therapeutic effects of aptamers, also lessens the cost of components required for aptamer production and lessens the number of unexpected and unnecessary interactions of aptamers (Adachi and Nakamura 2019).

Various aptamer conjugates are being studied, designed, and explored for their possible benefits as drug delivery systems. Aptamer–drug conjugates (ApDCs) are devised in order to overcome the individual limitations of the aptamer as well as the drug. Aptamer–RNA conjugated complexes are under study for target-specific delivery of bioactive RNA molecules, like small hairpin RNA (shRNA), microRNA (miRNA), and small interfering RNA (siRNA) to the target location (Ni et al. 2021). Bi-specific aptamers or bivalent aptamers are generated by the interaction or linking of two aptamers. Because of their dual targeting nature, bi-specific aptamers can regulate the immune response between the physiological molecules and the target cells. Bi-specific aptamers may be composed of two different aptamers which can target two drug sites, or one therapeutic aptamer with the opposite acting as a targeting moiety. Other aptamer-conjugated systems include aptamer–peptide conjugated systems, aptamer–liposome delivery systems, and aptamer-gold nanoparticle conjugated systems (Ni et al. 2021). A summary of different types of aptamers along with their reported targets is enlisted in Table 2.1.

2.8   LIMITATIONS AND FUTURE PROSPECTIVE

Although bestowed with numerous advantages over conventional biomarkers, there are still many challenges to be fully resolved related to its feasible and economical usage. As discussed in the earlier section, the main limitations of aptamers include their enzymatic degradation, quick removal from the body through the excretory system, cross-reactivity, relatively high production cost at present, its interconnection with intracellular components (Lakhin et al. 2013). To overcome all the pre-found and yet unfound drawbacks, a high cost and a lot of effort need to be put into the process. The most reliable and promising techniques involve the chemical modification of aptamers for their effective therapeutic action and undisturbed targeted drug delivery. Moreover, it has been found that the unmodified aptamer candidates are at an extreme risk of serum degradation (Keefe et al. 2010). This intensifies the necessity of appropriate techniques and novel approaches to ensure the safeguarded delivery of aptamers.

Simultaneously dealing with the drawbacks, scientists are keen on uncovering newer possibilities revolving around the applications of aptamers. Recent efforts have been emphasizing the discovery of not just the cellular but also the intracellular targets for aptamers. Examples of the same include nanoparticle utilization for the delivery of nucleic acids, the use of conjugated systems like cholesterol to increase the intracellular delivery of siRNA, decoy oligonucleotides (ssRNA molecules with the ribose molecule modified at the 2'-O position with a methyl group) that can target the splicing factors and novel antiviral delivery systems that can enter organs in vivo (Adachi and Nakamura 2019).

It has been believed that successive generations of aptamers are going to be notably helpful for diagnostic purposes, together with aptamer-based magnetic cell sorting, molecular probes, biosensors, and immunoassays. Also, there is an analogous level of enthusiasm for its therapeutic applications in many domains, including microbial diseases and their manifestations, cancer, neurological disorders, and cardiovascular diseases (Nimjee et al. 2017). Not just the chemical modifications that permit increased bioavailability and other beneficial corollaries, but also the introduction of different aptamer formulations (conjugated and unconjugated) welcomes an arena of opportunities as therapeutic compounds. A few examples include the inhibition of proinflammatory factors, coagulation factors, etc. (Nimjee et al. 2017). Due to the ascension of population, and totally different forms of viruses that are often impervious to customary treatment, there is constant pressure to develop novel diagnostic procedures with high specificity and sensitivity, allowing for early and rapid detection of infectious agents (Fesseha et al. 2020). Therefore, it can be concluded that aptamers are an emerging group of molecules that can be trusted upon for favourable target identification and targeted therapy. They are a class of designer drugs that can be modified and selected based upon our requirements. This property in addition to their high binding affinity, specificity for several target macromolecules like proteins, and their advantageous behaviour over antibodies secures them

TABLE 2.2
Therapeutic targets of different types of aptamers

Name of drug	Type of aptamer	Target	Disease	References
Pegaptanib (Macugen)	RNA	VEGF165	Age-related Macular degeneration	Byun (2021), Ni et al. (2021), Kaur et al. (2018)
E10030	DNA	PDGF	Age-related Macular degeneration	Byun (2021), Ni et al. (2021), Kaur et al. (2018)
AS1411 (Antisoma)	DNA	Nucleolin	Acute Myeloid leukaemia, metastatic renal cell carcinoma	Byun (2021), Meyer et al. (2011), Ni et al. (2021), Kaur et al. (2018)
NOX- E36	RNA	CCL2	Type II diabetes melitus	Byun (2021), Ni et al. (2021), Kaur et al. (2018)
NU172	DNA	Thrombin	Heart diseases	Byun (2021)
SAL 26	DNA	Salmonella typhimurium	Food-borne diseases	Afrasiabi et al. (2020)

as candidates of interest. Furthermore, with the knowledge of the human genome and proteome, the development of aptamers as inhibitors of cellular components deregulated in diseased conditions will become irreplaceable for the entire medical field (White et al. 2000).

2.9 CONCLUSION

The above book chapter focusses upon the potential of aptamers in the field of diagnostics and therapeutics. The increasing frequencies of diseases, mostly fatal, going undiagnosed and untreated at the early stages make it even more crucial to search for and validate the use of novel biomarkers. Aptamers, which are small-size biomolecules like oligonucleotides and peptides, harbour many advantages over conventional diagnostic biomarkers and antibiotics. Their small size favours their easy chemical modification and their high target-binding abilities. Also, their low immunogenicity and cost-efficient production enhance their chances of potential diagnostic and therapeutic elements. There are various ways by which we can target different diseased conditions by exploiting the diverse types of aptamers. Aptamers can be natural or artificial and their origins and modifications can be utilized for high specificity and high affinity binding with the targets. Many techniques and approaches for the synthesis and modification of aptamers have been developed and many are still under way. The two most common artificial synthesis technologies are the SELEX and SOMAScan technologies utilized for the production of Spiegelmers and SOMAmers respectively.

Aptamers have been explored in recent years for their possible actions as therapeutics. The various experimentations have opened a wide arena for the field of curatives due to the positive outcomes of aptamer-based treatments. Many studies have formulated the therapeutic effects of aptamers against microbes including bacteria and viruses; few even show significant results for the detection and treatment of the novel Coronavirus. Different cancers, and metabolic conditions like diabetes, neurological diseases, and inflammatory diseases are also employing the use of aptamers as their potential drug candidates in the future. The anti-coagulatory and anti-angiogenic aptamers are also under study for their use in diseases involving abnormal coagulation or increased vascular formation and permeability.

Though possessing a lot of possible advantages, some limitations of aptamers have kept them at bay. Their enzymatic digestion, quick elimination from the body, cross-reactivity, etc. need to be looked upon for their emergence as reliable and feasible diagnostic and therapeutic applications. Through the various modifications of aptamers for their targeted and efficient drug delivery, these limitations might as well dissolve in the near future.

CONFLICT OF INTEREST

The authors have declared no conflict of interest.

ACKNOWLEDGEMENTS

The authors are thankful to the School of Biotechnology and Bioinformatics, D Y Patil Deemed to be University, Maharashtra, India for providing research facilities. Sangeeta Ballav is thankful to Dr. D. Y. Patil Vidyapeeth, Pune for Junior Research Fellowship (DPU/291/2021).

ABBREVIATIONS

ACI	anaemia of chronic inflammation
ApDCs	aptamer–drug conjugates
Apt-NPs	aptamer-conjugated nanoparticles
ARP-PCR	aptamer-based regionally protected PCR
CCL2	C-C chemokine ligand 2
CCR2	C-C chemokine receptor 2
EGFR	epidermal growth factor receptor
ELISA	enzyme-linked immunosorbent assay
EpCAM	epithelial cell adhesion molecules
ESTs	expressed sequence tags
FAM	fluorescein amidites
FDA	food and drug administration
FISH	fluorescence in situ hybridization
FITC	fluorescein isothiocyanate
FRET	fluorescence resonance energy transfer
GST	glutathione S-transferase
HER-2	human epidermal growth factor receptor 2
HGFR	hepatocyte growth factor receptor

His-tag	poly histidine tag
HIV	human immunodeficiency virus
ICAM	2-intercellular adhesion molecule 1
IHC	immunohistochemistry
K+	potassium ion
LA 27	twenty-seven nucleotide aptamer
LPS	lipopolysaccharides
MALDI-MS	matrix-assisted laser desorption/ionization
MCP-1	monocyte chemoattractant protein 1
MERS	middle east respiratory syndrome
MMP2	matrix metalloproteinase-2
MPB	maltose binding protein
MRI	magnetic resonance imaging
MUC1	mucin short variant S1
oFSH-α	ovine follicle-stimulating hormone
OTA	ochratoxin A
PABP	Poly(A)-binding protein
PCR	polymerase chain reaction
PEG	polyethylene glycol
PSMA	prostate-specific membrane antigen
PTX	paclitaxel
SAGE	serial analysis of gene expression
SARS-CoV-2	severe acute respiratory syndrome Coronavirus 2
SELEX	systematic evolution of ligands by exponential enrichment
SERS	surface-enhanced Raman scattering
SOMAmers	slow off-rate modified aptamers
ssDNA	single-stranded DNA
ssRNA	single-stranded RNA
TAMRA	carboxytetramethylrhodamine
VEGFR2	vascular endothelial growth factor receptor

REFERENCES

Adachi, Tatsuo, and Yoshikazu Nakamura. 2019. "Aptamers: A Review of Their Chemical Properties." *Molecules* 24 (23): 4229. https://doi.org/10.3390/molecules24234229.

Afrasiabi, Shima, Maryam Pourhajibagher, Reza Raoofian, and Maryam Tabarzad. 2020. "Therapeutic Applications of Nucleic Acid Aptamers in Microbial Infections." *Journal of Biomedical Science* 27 (6). https://doi.org/10.1186/s12929-019-0611-0.

Bao, Gang, Won Jong Rhee, and Andrew Tsourkas. 2009. "Fluorescent Probes for Live-Cell RNA Detection." *Annual Review of Biomedical Engineering* 11: 25–47. https://doi.org/10.1146/annurev-bioeng-061008-124920.

Bast, Robert C., M. Feeney, H. Lazarus, L. M. Nadler, R. B. Colvin, and R. C. Knapp. 1981. "Reactivity of a Monoclonal Antibody with Human Ovarian Carcinoma." *Journal of Clinical Investigation*, 68 (5): 1331–1337. https://doi.org/10.1172/jci110380.

Bauer, Michelle, Joanna Macdonald, Justin Henri, Wei Duan, and Sarah Shigdar. 2016. "The Application of Aptamers for Immunohistochemistry." *Nucleic Acid Therapeutics* 26 (3): 120–126. https://doi.org/10.1089/nat.2015.0569.

Bhalla, Nikhil, Pawan Jolly, Nello Formisano, and Pedro Estrela. 2016. "Introduction to Biosensors." Edited by Pedro Estrela. *Essays in Biochemistry* 60 (1): 1–8. https://doi.org/10.1042/ebc20150001.

Briones, Carlos. 2011. "Aptamer." In Gargaud Muriel, et al. (eds.), *Encyclopedia of Astrobiology*, 56–56. Springer, Berlin Heidelberg. https://doi.org/10.1007/978-3-642-11274-4_403.

Byun, Jonghoe. 2021. "Recent Progress and Opportunities for Nucleic Acid Aptamers." *Life* 11 (3): 193. https://doi.org/10.3390/life11030193.

Chang, Yun Min, Michael J. Donovan, and Weihong Tan. 2013. "Using Aptamers for Cancer Biomarker Discovery." *Journal of Nucleic Acids* 1–7. https://doi.org/10.1155/2013/817350.

Chen, Hao, Sung-Gyu Park, Namhyun Choi, Hyung-Jun Kwon, Taejoon Kang, Mi-Kyung Lee, and Jaebum Choo. (2021). Sensitive detection of SARS-CoV-2 using a SERS-based aptasensor. *ACS Sensors* 6 (6), 2378–2385. https://doi.org/10.1021/acssensors.1c00596

Chen, Kai, and Xiaoyuan Chen. 2010. "Design and Development of Molecular Imaging Probes." *Current Topics in Medicinal Chemistry* 10 (12): 1227–1236. https://doi.org/10.2174/156802610791384225.

Cheng, Alan K. H., Huaipeng Su, Y. Andrew Wang, and Hua-Zhong Yu. 2009. "Aptamer-Based Detection of Epithelial Tumour Marker Mucin 1 with Quantum Dot-Based Fluorescence Readout." *Analytical Chemistry* 81 (15): 6130–6139. https://doi.org/10.1021/ac901223q.

Coppedè, Fabio. 2014. "Genetic and Epigenetic Biomarkers for Diagnosis, Prognosis and Treatment of Colorectal Cancer." *World Journal of Gastroenterology* 20 (4): 943. https://doi.org/10.3748/wjg.v20.i4.943.

De Matos, Leandro Luongo, Damila Cristina Trufelli, Maria Graciela Luongo De Matos, and Maria Aparecida Da Silva Pinhal. 2010. "Immunohistochemistry as an Important Tool in Biomarkers Detection and Clinical Practice." *Biomarker Insights* 5: 9–20. https://doi.org/10.4137/bmi.s2185.

Dhar, Shanta, Frank X. Gu, Robert Langer, Omid C. Farokhzad, and Stephen J. Lippard. 2008. "Targeted Delivery of Cisplatin to Prostate Cancer Cells by Aptamer Functionalized Pt(IV) Prodrug-PLGA–PEG Nanoparticles." *Proceedings of the National Academy of Sciences* 105 (45): 17356–17361. https://doi.org/10.1073/pnas.0809154105.

Duo, Jia, Camelia Chiriac, Richard Y.-C. Huang, John Timothy Mehl, Adrienne A. Tymiak, Peter Sabbatini, Renuka Pillutla, and Yan J Zhang. 2018. "Slow Off-Rate Modified Aptamer (SOMAmer) as a Novel Reagent in Immunoassay Development for Accurate Soluble Glypican-3 Quantification in Clinical Samples." *Analytical Chemistry* 90 (8): 5162–5170. https://doi.org/10.1021/acs.analchem.7b05277.

Farokhzad, Omid C., Jianjun Cheng, Benjamin A. Teply, Ines Sherifi, Sangyong Jon, Philip W. Kantoff, Jerome P. Richie, and Robert Langer. 2006. "Targeted Nanoparticle-Aptamer Bioconjugates for Cancer Chemotherapy In Vivo." *Proceedings of the National Academy of Sciences* 103 (16): 6315–6320. https://doi.org/10.1073/pnas.0601755103.

Fesseha, Haben, Tadelech Yilma, and Nato Hundessa. 2020. "Aptamers : Diagnostic and Therapeutic Applications." *Biomedical Journal of Scientific and Technical Research* 28 (4): 21735–21747. https://doi.org/10.26717/BJSTR.2020.28.004672.

Germer, Katherine, Marissa Leonard, and Xiaoting Zhang. 2013. "RNA Aptamers and Their Therapeutic and Diagnostic Applications." *International Journal of Biochemistry and Molecular Biology* 4 (1): 27–40.

Gold, Larry, Nebojsa Janjic, Thale Jarvis, Dan Schneider, Jeffrey J. Walker, Sheri K. Wilcox, and Dom Zichi. 2012. "Aptamers and the RNA World, Past and Present." *Cold Spring Harbor Perspectives in Biology* 4 (3): a003582. https://doi.org/10.1101/cshperspect.a003582.

Guan Baozhang, and Zhang Xingwang. 2020. "Aptamers as Versatile Ligands for Biomedical and Pharmaceutical Applications." *International Journal of Nanomedicine* 15: 1059-1071. doi: 10.2147/IJN.S237544. PMID: 32110008; PMCID: PMC7035142.

Han, Myoung-Eun, Sungmin Baek, Hyun-Jung Kim, Jung Hwan Lee, Sung-Ho Ryu, and Sae-Ock Oh. 2014. "Development of an Aptamer-Conjugated Fluorescent Nanoprobe for MMP2." *Nanoscale Research Letters* 9 (1): 104. https://doi.org/10.1186/1556-276x-9-104.

Han, Yong-Xu, Cheng, Jun-Hu, Sun, Da-Wen. 2019. "Changes in activity, structure and morphology of horseradish peroxidase induced by cold plasma". *Food chemistry* 301: 125240. doi: 10.1016/j.foodchem.2019.125240. Epub 2019 Jul 23. PMID: 31387040.

Hofman, Florence M., and Clive R. Taylor. 2013. "Immunohistochemistry." *Current Protocols in Immunology.* https://doi.org/10.1002/0471142735.im2104s103.

Huang, Jie, Xinxin Chen, Xuekun Fu, Zheng Li, Yuhong Huang, and Chao Liang. 2021. "Advances in Aptamer-Based Biomarker Discovery." *Frontiers in Cell and Developmental Biology* 9: 1–11. https://doi.org/10.3389/fcell.2021.659760.

Itzkovitz, Shalev, van Oudenaarden, Alexander. 2011. "Validating transcripts with probes and imaging technology." *Nature methods.* 8 (4 Suppl): S12–9. doi: 10.1038/nmeth.1573. Epub 2011 Mar 30. PMID: 21451512; PMCID: PMC3158979.

Jaffer, Shabnam, and Ira J. Bleiweiss. 2004. "Beyond Hematoxylin and Eosin—The Role of Immunohistochemistry in Surgical Pathology." *Cancer Investigation* 22 (3): 445–465. https://doi.org/10.1081/cnv-200034896.

Jain, Kewal K. 2010. *The Handbook of Biomarkers*. Humana Press. https://doi.org/10.1007/978-1-60761-685-6.

Jankowski, Wojciech, H. A. Daniel Lagassé, William C. Chang, Joseph Mcgill, Katarzyna I. Jankowska, Amy D. Gelinas, Nebojsa Janjic, and Zuben E. Sauna. 2020. "Modified Aptamers as Reagents to Characterize Recombinant Human Erythropoietin Products." *Scientific Reports* 10: 18593. https://doi.org/10.1038/s41598-020-75713-2.

Jones, Henry. 1848. "III. On a New Substance Occurring in the Urine of a Patient with Mollities Ossium." *Philosophical Transactions of the Royal Society of London* 138: 55–62. https://doi.org/10.1098/rstl.1848.0003.

Kaur, Harleen, John G. Bruno, Amit Kumar, and Tarun Kumar Sharma. 2018. "Aptamers in the Therapeutics and Diagnostics Pipelines." *Theranostics* 8 (15): 4016–4032. https://doi.org/10.7150/thno.25958.

Keefe, Anthony D., Supriya Pai, and Andrew Ellington. 2010. "Aptamers as Therapeutics." *Nature Reviews Drug Discovery* 9: 537–550. https://doi.org/10.1038/nrd3141.

Kim, Brianna. 2017. "Western Blot Techniques." In Espina, Virginia *Methods in Molecular Biology*, 133–139. Springer, New York. https://doi.org/10.1007/978-1-4939-6990-6_9.

Lakhin, A. V., Vyacheslav Zalmanovich Tarantul, and Lleonid Vladimirovich Gening. 2013. "Aptamers : Problems, Solutions and Prospects." *Acta Naturae* 5 (4): 34–43.

Lee, Seram, Young Sook Kim, Minjung Jo, Moonsoo Jin, Dong-Ki Lee, and Soyoun Kim. 2007. "Chip-Based Detection of Hepatitis C Virus Using RNA Aptamers That Specifically Bind to HCV Core Antigen." *Biochemical and Biophysical Research Communications* 358 (1): 47–52. https://doi.org/10.1016/j.bbrc.2007.04.057.

Leong, Anthony S.-Y. 2004. "Pitfalls in Diagnostic Immunohistology." *Advances in Anatomic Pathology* 11 (2): 86–93. https://doi.org/10.1097/00125480-200403000-00002.

Li, Feng, Jingjing Li, Chuan Wang, Jing Zhang, Xing-Fang Li, and X. Chris Le. 2011. "Competitive Protection of Aptamer-Functionalized Gold Nanoparticles by Controlling the DNA Assembly." *Analytical Chemistry* 83 (17): 6464–6467. https://doi.org/10.1021/ac201801k.

Li, Long, Shujuan Xu, He Yan, Xiaowei Li, Hoda Safari Yazd, Xiang Li, Tong Huang, Cheng Cui, Jianhui Jiang, and Weihong Tan. 2021. "Nucleic Acid Aptamers for Molecular Diagnostics and Therapeutics: Advances and Perspectives." *Angewandte Chemie International Edition* 60 (5): 2221–31. https://doi.org/10.1002/ange.202003563.

Lin, Jun Sheng, and Kenneth P McNatty. 2009. "Aptamer-Based Regionally Protected PCR for Protein Detection." *Clinical Chemistry* 55 (9): 1686–1693. https://doi.org/10.1373/clinchem.2009.127266.

Malik, Nazia, Tanvir Arfin, and Azhar U. Khan. 2019. "Graphene Nanomaterials: Chemistry and Pharmaceutical Perspectives." In Grumezescu, Alexandru Mihai (Ed.). *Nanomaterials for Drug Delivery and Therapy*, 373–402. Elsevier. https://doi.org/10.1016/B978-0-12-816505-8.00002-3.

Mayeux, Richard. 2004. "Biomarkers: Potential Uses and Limitations." *NeuroRX* 1 (2): 182–188. https://doi.org/10.1602/neurorx.1.2.182.

McDermott, Jason E., Jing Wang, Hugh Mitchell, Bobbie-Jo Webb-Robertson, Ryan Hafen, John Ramey, and Karin D. Rodland. 2012. "Challenges in Biomarker Discovery: Combining Expert Insights with Statistical Analysis of Complex Omics Data." *Expert Opinion on Medical Diagnostics* 7 (1): 37–51. https://doi.org/10.1517/17530059.2012.718329.

Meyer, Cindy, Ulrich Hahn, and Andrea Rentmeister. 2011. "Cell-Specific Aptamers as Emerging Therapeutics." *Journal of Nucleic Acids* 2011. https://doi.org/10.4061/2011/904750.

Meyer, Michael, Thomas Scheper, and Johanna-Gabriela Walter. 2013. "Aptamers: Versatile Probes for Flow Cytometry." *Applied Microbiology and Biotechnology* 97 (16): 7097–7109. https://doi.org/10.1007/s00253-013-5070-z.

Mishra, Manish, Shuchita Tiwari, Anita Gunaseelan, Dongyang Li, Bruce D. Hammock, and Aldrin V. Gomes. 2019. "Improving the Sensitivity of Traditional Western Blotting via Streptavidin Containing Poly-horseradish Peroxidase (PolyHRP)." *Electrophoresis* 40 (12–13): 1731–1739. https://doi.org/10.1002/elps.201900059.

Nagarkatti, Rana, Vaibhav Bist, Sirena Sun, Fernanda Fortes de Araujo, Hira L. Nakhasi, and Alain Debrabant. 2012. "Development of an Aptamer-Based Concentration Method for the Detection of Trypanosoma Cruzi in Blood." *PLoS One* 7 (8): e43533. doi:10.1371/journal.pone.0043533.

New, Roger R. C., and Tam T. T. Bui. 2020. "Binding Interactions of Peptide Aptamers." *Molecules* 25 (24): 6055. https://doi.org/10.3390/molecules25246055.

Ni, Shuaijian, Zhenjian Zhuo, Yufei Pan, Yuanyuan Yu, Fangfei Li, Jin Liu, Luyao Wang, et al. 2021. "Recent Progress in Aptamer Discoveries and Modi Fi Cations for Therapeutic Applications." *ACS Applied Materials and Interfaces* 13 (8): 9500–9519. https://doi.org/10.1021/acsami.0c05750.

Ni, Xiaohua, Mark Castanares, Amarnath Mukherjee, and Shawn Lupold. 2011. "Nucleic Acid Aptamers: Clinical Applications and Promising New Horizons." *Current Medicinal Chemistry* 18 (27): 4206–4214. https://doi.org/10.2174/092986711797189600.

Nimjee, Shahid M, Rebekah R. White, Richard C. Becker, Bruce A. Sullenger, and North Carolina. 2017. "Aptamers as Therapeutics." *Annual Review of Pharmacology and Toxicology* 57: 61–79. https://doi.org/10.1146/annurev-pharmtox-010716-104558.

Nybo, Kristie. 2012. "Western Blot: Protein Migration." *BioTechniques* 53 (1): 23–24. https://doi.org/10.2144/000113887.

Pan, Yuliang, Manli Guo, Zhou Nie, Yan Huang, Chunfeng Pan, Kai Zeng, Yu Zhang, and Shouzhuo Yao. 2010. "Selective Collection and Detection of Leukaemia Cells on a Magnet-Quartz Crystal Microbalance System Using Aptamer-Conjugated Magnetic Beads." *Biosensors & Bioelectronics* 25 (7): 1609–1614. https://doi.org/10.1016/j.bios.2009.11.022.

Pearce, Alison, Marion Haas, Rosalie Viney, Sallie-Anne Pearson, Philip Haywood, Chris Brown, and Robyn Ward. 2017. "Incidence and Severity of Self-Reported Chemotherapy Side Effects in Routine Care: A Prospective Cohort Study." Edited by Apar Kishor Ganti. *PLoS One* 12 (10): e0184360. https://doi.org/10.1371/journal.pone.0184360.

Penner, Gregory 2012. "Commercialization of an Aptamer-Based Diagnostic Test". *IVD Technology* 18: 31–37.

Pu, Ying, Zhenxu Liu, Yi Lu, Peng Yuan, Jun Liu, Bo Yu, Guodong Wang, Chaoyong James Yang, Huixia Liu, and Weihong Tan. 2015. "Using DNA Aptamer Probe for Immunostaining of Cancer Frozen Tissues." *Analytical Chemistry* 87 (3): 1919–1924. https://doi.org/10.1021/ac504175h.

Ramos-Vara, J. A., and M. A. Miller. 2013. "When Tissue Antigens and Antibodies Get Along: Revisiting the Technical Aspects of Immunohistochemistry—the Red, Brown, and Blue Technique." *Veterinary Pathology* 51 (1): 42–87. https://doi. org/10.1177/0300985813505879.

Ren, Lifen, Melissa A. Marquardt, and John J. Lech. 1997. "Estrogenic Effects of Nonylphenol on PS2, ER and MUC1 Gene Expression in Human Breast Cancer Cells-MCF-7." *Chemico-Biological Interactions* 104 (1) (April): 55–64. https://doi.org/10.1016/ s0009-2797(97)03767-8.

Reverdatto, Sergey, David Burz, and Alexander Shekhtman. 2015. "Peptide Aptamers : Development and Applications." *Current Topics in Medicinal Chemistry* 15 (12): 1082–1101. https://doi.org/10.2174/1568026615666150413153143.

Sandoval, Juan, Lorena Peiró-Chova, Federico V. Pallardó, and José Luis García-Giménez. 2013. "Epigenetic Biomarkers in Laboratory Diagnostics: Emerging Approaches and Opportunities." *Expert Review of Molecular Diagnostics* 13 (5) (June): 457–471. https:// doi.org/10.1586/erm.13.37.

Scaros, Olivia, and Richard Fisler. 2005. "Biomarker Technology Roundup: From Discovery to Clinical Applications, a Broad Set of Tools Is Required to Translate from the Lab to the Clinic." *BioTechniques*, no. 4S: S30–S32. https://doi.org/10.2144/05384su01.

Shin, Seonmi, Il-Hyun Kim, Wonchull Kang, Jin Kuk Yang, and Sang Soo Hah. 2010. "An Alternative to Western Blot Analysis Using RNA Aptamer-Functionalized Quantum Dots." *Bioorganic & Medicinal Chemistry Letters* 20 (11): 3322–3325. https://doi. org/10.1016/j.bmcl.2010.04.040.

Song, Kyung-mi, Seonghwan Lee, and Changill Ban. 2012. "Aptamers and Their Biological Applications." *Sensors* 12: 612–631. https://doi.org/10.3390/s120100612.

Song, Shiping, Lihua Wang, Jiang Li, Chunhai Fan, and Jianlong Zhao. 2008. "Aptamer-Based Biosensors." *TrAC Trends in Analytical Chemistry* 27 (2): 108–117. https://doi. org/10.1016/j.trac.2007.12.004.

Song, Yanling., Jia Song, Xinyu Wei, Mengjiao Huang, Miao Sun, Lin Zhu, Bingqian Lin, Haicong Shen, Zhi Zhu, and Chaoyong Yang. 2020. "Discovery of Aptamers Targeting the Receptor-Binding Domain of the SARS-CoV-2 Spike Glycoprotein." *Analytical Chemistry* 92 (14): 9895–9900. doi:10.1021/acs.analchem.0c01394.

Spitz, Margaret R., and Melissa L. Bondy. 2009. "The Evolving Discipline of Molecular Epidemiology of Cancer." *Carcinogenesis* 31 (1): 127–134. https://doi.org/10.1093/ carcin/bgp246.

Srikantan, Vasantha, Zhiqiang Zou, Gyorgy Petrovics, Linda Xu, Meena Augustus, Leland Davis, Jeffrey R. Livezey, et al. 2000. "PCGEM1, a Prostate-Specific Gene, Is Overexpressed in Prostate Cancer." *Proceedings of the National Academy of Sciences* 97 (22): 12216–12221. https://doi.org/10.1073/pnas.97.22.12216.

Srivastava, Shruti, Philip Raj Abraham, and Sangita Mukhopadhyay. 2021. "Aptamers: An Emerging Tool for Diagnosis and Therapeutics in Tuberculosis." *Frontiers in Cellular and Infection Microbiology* 11. https://doi.org/10.3389/fcimb.2021.656421.

Strimbu, Kyle, and Jorge A. Tavel. 2010. "What Are Biomarkers?" *Current Opinion in HIV and AIDS* 5 (6): 463–466. https://doi.org/10.1097/coh.0b013e32833ed177.

Taylor-Papadimitriou J, Burchell J, Miles DW, Dalziel M. 1999. "MUC1 and cancer." *Biochimica et Biophysica Acta* 1455 (2–3): 301–13. https://doi.org/ 10.1016/s0925-4439(99)00055-1. PMID: 10571020.

Tombelli, Sara, Maria Minunni, Ettore Luzi, and Marco Mascini. 2005. "Aptamer-Based Biosensors for the Detection of HIV-1 Tat Protein." *Bioelectrochemistry (Amsterdam, Netherlands)* 67 (2): 135–141. https://doi.org/10.1016/j.bioelechem.2004.04.011.

Tong, Pan, and Hua Li (2016). "Mining Massive Genomic Data for Therapeutic Biomarker Discovery in Cancer: Resources, Tools, and Algorithms." In Wong, Ka-Chun. (eds) *Big Data Analytics in Genomics*, 337–355. Springer International Publishing, Cham. http:// doi.org/10.1007/978-3-319-41279-5_10.

Wang, Jinli, Renji Lv, Jingjuan Xu, Danke Xu, and Hongyuan Chen. 2008. "Characterizing the Interaction between Aptamers and Human IgE by Use of Surface Plasmon Resonance." *Analytical and Bioanalytical Chemistry* 390 (4): 1059–1065. https://doi.org/10.1007/s00216-007-1697-x.

Wang, Tao, Changying Chen, Leon M. Larcher, Roberto A. Barrero, and Rakesh N. Veedu. 2019. "Three Decades of Nucleic Acid Aptamer Technologies : Lessons Learned, Progress and Opportunities on Aptamer Development." *Biotechnology Advances* 37 (1): 28–50. https://doi.org/10.1016/j.biotechadv.2018.11.001.

Wang, Tianjiao, and Judhajeet Ray. 2012. "Aptamer-Based Molecular Imaging." *Protein & Cell* 3 (10): 739–754. https://doi.org/10.1007/s13238-012-2072-z.

Wang, Yao, Zhe Li, and Hanyang Yu. 2020. "Aptamer-Based Western Blot for Selective Protein Recognition." *Frontiers in Chemistry*. https://doi.org/10.3389/fchem.2020.570528.

Weigand, Julia E., and Beatrix Suess. 2009. "Aptamers and Riboswitches: Perspectives in Biotechnology." *Applied Microbiology and Biotechnology* 85: 229–236. https://doi.org/10.1007/s00253-009-2194-2.

White, Rebekah R., Bruce A. Sullenger, Christopher P. Rusconi, Rebekah R. White, Bruce A. Sullenger, and Christopher P. Rusconi. 2000. "Developing Aptamers into Therapeutics." *The Journal of Clinical Investigation* 106 (8): 929–934. https://doi.org/10.1172/JCI11325.

Wu, Jia-Yo, Chen Yi, Ho-Ren Chung, Duen-Jeng Wang, Wen-Chien Chang, Sheng-Yang Lee, Che-Tung Lin, Yueh-Chao Yang, and Wei-Chung Vivian Yang. 2010. "Potential Biomarkers in Saliva for Oral Squamous Cell Carcinoma." *Oral Oncology* 46 (4): 226–231. https://doi.org/10.1016/j.oraloncology.2010.01.007.

Yu, Chenchen, Yan Hu, Jinhong Duan, Wei Yuan, Chen Wang, Haiyan Xu, and Xian-Da Yang. 2011. "Novel Aptamer-Nanoparticle Bioconjugates Enhances Delivery of Anticancer Drug to MUC1-Positive Cancer Cells In Vitro." Edited by Tarl Wayne Prow. *PLoS One* 6 (9): e24077. https://doi.org/10.1371/journal.pone.0024077.

Zhou, Jiehua, Maggie L. Bobbin, John C. Burnett, and John J. Rossi. 2012. "Current Progress of RNA Aptamer-Based Therapeutics." *Frontiers in Genetiocs* 3: 1–14. https://doi.org/10.3389/fgene.2012.00234.

Zhu, Qinchang, Ge Liu, and Masaaki Kai. 2015. "DNA Aptamers in the Diagnosis and Treatment of Human Diseases." *Molecules* 20 (12): 20979–20997. https://doi.org/10.3390/molecules201219739.

3 Designing and synthesis of aptamer via various approaches (SELEX and ExSELEX)

Arpana Parihar, Kritika Gaur, Ayushi Singhal and Raju Khan

3.1 INTRODUCTION

An aptamer is a novel form of single-stranded RNA or DNA, generated in vitro using the SELEX approach which is a comprehensive evolutionary method of synthesis of ligands by exponential enhancement mode (Petersen and Wengel, 2003). The random sequences have been derived from a nucleic acid database with 10^{15} varying species and subjected to the SELEX method. Aptamers are recognized as just a substitute for antibodies in numerous biotechnological and biological sciences activities, having targets ranging from small compounds to proteins and peptides to entire cells (Figure 3.1). Unlike antibodies, would both be immunogenic and heat stable (Pendergrast et al., 2005). Mechanisms of antibody binding with target molecules happen via electrostatic, hydrophobic, van der Waals forces, hydrogen bonding, base stacking, and complementarily interactions. Because of their mobility, compact size, and low steric hindrance, certain functional RNA and DNA molecules (aptamers) may easily detect biomolecules presenting enormous promise in diagnostic, therapies, or drug-delivery methods (Catuogno et al., 2016). An aptamer's physical arrangement is composed of two sections, the first possessing nucleotides at both ends hybridizing together to form a strand for secondary structure stabilization (Churcher et al., 2020) and the other nucleotides forming an anomalous loop to recognize the destination particularly, with the structural components of the loop determining its chemical attraction and sensor performance (Kwon et al., 2014). Aptamer-based biological recognition devices have indeed been extensively used to identify proteins, chemicals, and metabolites in biological samples, environmental pollutants, and eatables (Parihar et al., 2023). Previous research has shown that the duration of the sequences has a significant impact on the sensitivity of the aptamer detection approach (Han et al., 2014). Some key challenges with DNA aptamers for practical diagnostic and therapeutic applications include insufficient selectivity for objectives and resistance towards nucleases.

DOI: 10.1201/9781003304227-3

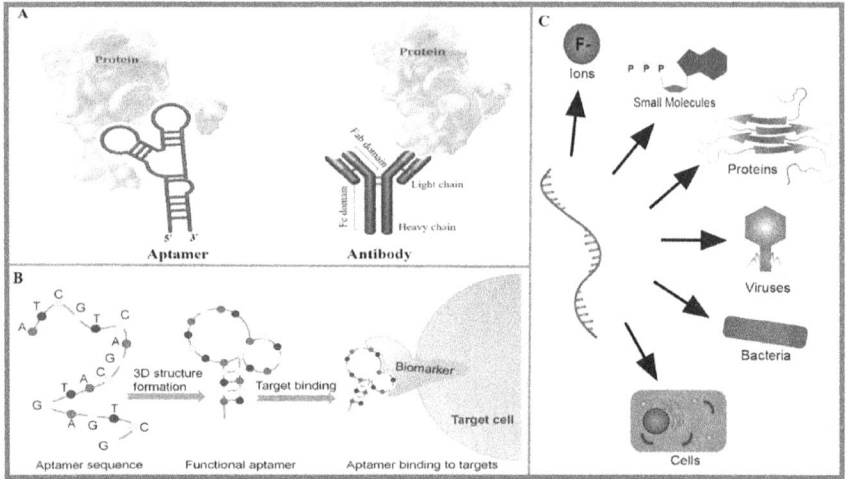

FIGURE 3.1 (a) Interaction of aptamer and antibody to target analyte (Kim et al., 2021). (b) 3D structures of Aptamers which are carefully designed with oligonucleotide sequences that attach to their targets with high affinity and specificity. (c) Versatility of aptamer (Wu and Kwon, 2016).

To address these difficulties, multiple strategies for modifying including aptamer synthesis were documented. The structure and chemical diversity of DNA aptamers in SELEX can be increased by expanding the biological analogue by producing unnatural base pairs (UBPs) (Matsunaga et al., 2017). Regardless of the downstream application, avidity, specificity, strong affinity, and/or selectivity are required for aptamers since they ultimately define the development of sensitive and targeted tests. It should be remembered that affinity and specificity are critical characteristics in any diagnostic or therapeutic application. Even though various academics have tried hard to explore the connection between attraction and distinctiveness no substantial association has been found. In this chapter, we have attempted to discuss methods of aptamer synthesis along with their effective approaches. Provide a better understanding of the advancement in the field of aptamer synthesis along with their application in therapeutics and diagnosis. This chapter ends up with the future goals and current challenges in this field.

3.2 APTAMER: POTENTIAL AND ADVANTAGES

Aptamers are high-affinity DNA or RNA molecules the Latin name means "to fit". Even though the biological significance of folded RNA had also long been known, in vitro development of molecules of nucleic acids with Inorganic functions had only been feasible when it was produced massively. The number of the degenerate short nucleic acid chain by the solid-phase formation and amplified individual moieties using molecular photocopying (PCR) allowed us to explore their usage. Such an approach enables the isolation of functioning nucleic acid molecules that can attach to a specific objective or catalyze a chemical change (Wilson and Szostak,

1999). To circumvent the low chemical diversity of nucleotides, nucleobases use testing approaches, particularly polymerase chain reaction (PCR). These modifications increase the structural diversity of nucleic acid libraries and, the association capacities of the aptamer.

So even though aptamers recognize and attach objectives of concern in the same way that antibodies do, they do have a few advantages over antibodies, including a shortened growth cycle, cheaper production costs, no processing variability, greater changeability, improved heat stability, and a broader target possibility (through ion to living organisms). The Fc tails of an antibody cause target cell death by increased phagocytosis or opsonization obstructing the translations. If generated via the PCR, many aptamer conjugates hold the potential of becoming extremely affordable and "wonder drug" for immunological disorders. For passive immunity using aptamers in vitro and in vivo experiments, various groups have successfully proven the avoidance or delay of bacterial and viral illnesses or biotoxin-mediated adverse consequences Even NASA has proposed that using aptamers as a potential option for the future space station to fight the consequences of dangerous and deadly extra-terrestrial "Andromeda strain" microbiota or latent viruses in astronauts, which could now enforce disease consequences even though cosmonauts were exposed in the space environment of Interstellar space for an extended length of time (Bruno, 2013).

3.3 APTAMER SYNTHESIS METHODS

3.3.1 SELEX

Tuerk and Gold (Tuerk and Gold, 1990) and Ellington and Szostak (Ellington and Szostak, 1990) independently discovered the mechanism of aptamer selection, entitled Systematic Evolution of Ligands by Exponential Enrichment (SELEX), in 1990. SELEX is a technique for determining nucleic acid aptamers which bind to a target with binding specificity and precision. Aptamer synthesis with the SELEX method entails numerous rounds of selection and enrichment procedures that are chance and labour-intensive, with cost-effective rates and production (Komarova and Kuznetsov, 2019). The process of SELEX is illustrated in Figure 3.2. SELEX may be used alongside advanced sequencing techniques, a procedure known as HT-SELEX or HTS (Zhuo et al., 2017).

3.3.2 CONVENTIONAL SELEX

SELEX was investigated separately by two laboratories in 1990. Ever since many changes and enhancements have now been made. The traditional SELEX approach comprises primarily the three phases listed below: Amplification, segmentation, and collection. In the selection process, the initial step is to set up an oligonucleotide library, which is then followed by the selection process. The initial stage in many standardsSELEX approach is a counter-selection against a grid with the objective immobile, following the elimination of non-specifically bound aptamers, the target is incubated in the pool of short nucleic acid. Unbound sequences are eliminated, collected from the bounded one, and converted into DNA by using a reverse transcription

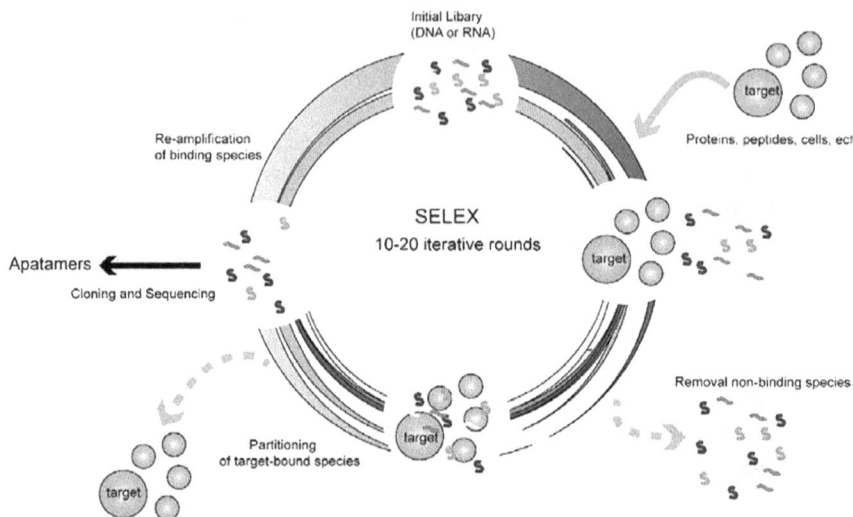

FIGURE 3.2 Schematic illustration of the SELEX process for the synthesis of DNA aptamers (Zhuo et al., 2017).

process (only for RNA aptamers), and then amplified by PCR (Figure 3.3). Following this, multiple rounds of selection, gene cloning, and gene sequencing processes are carried out, along with an assessment of the target affinity of the enriched aptamers.

The affinity and specificity of the chosen oligonucleotides, as shown by the number of screening cycles necessary for aptamer extraction should be effective (Komarova and Kuznetsov, 2019). For aptamer selection, a chemically generated oligonucleotide library is often employed. This collection comprises up to 60 random oligonucleotides bordered by brief constant sections, which are often a technique for annealing primer before PCR. Depending on the type of aptamer sought, standard SELEX introduces many selection processes (Darmostuk et al., 2015). It can take several weeks to months to get particular aptamer candidates, by PCR method and the hit rates are low. As a result, obtaining high-quality aptamers against important targets continues a problem. Numerous modified SELEX algorithms were created to reduce short listing time and increase hit rates. Although traditional SELEX is a proven and effective technology, the explosive growth of other approaches for aptamer choices seems to have become inescapable due to their significant time and effort demands.

3.3.3 Capillary electrophoresis SELEX

CE SELEX (capillary electrophoresis SELEX), which was initially demonstrated in 2004, serves as one of the most often used SELEX techniques (Mendonsa and Bowser, 2004a). In this technology after incubating a preliminary pool of oligonucleotides well with targets, the combination is segregated based on the mobility shift. These attached sequences are gathered, duplicated using PCR, and employed for cloning, proofreading, and calculating the affinity of the generated aptamers as shown in Figure 3.3 (Mendonsa and Bowser, 2004b).

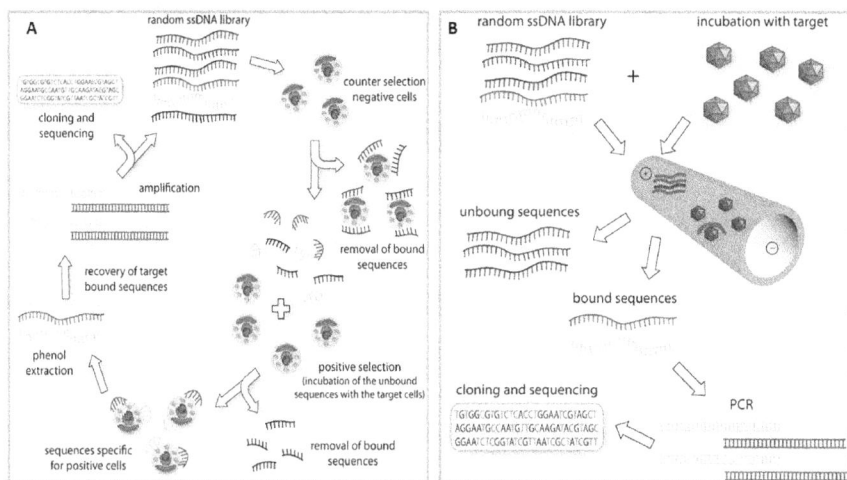

FIGURE 3.3 (a) The basic principle of aptamer generation by conventional SELEX. Selection starts from the construction of an initial oligonucleotide library, which is directly proceeded to the selection process. In many conventional SELEX protocols, the first step is a counter-selection against a matrix on which the target is immobilized. After the removal of non-specifically bound aptamers, a pool of oligonucleotides is incubated with the target. Unbound sequences are removed; the target-bound oligonucleotides are collected, reverse transcribed into DNA (only for RNA aptamers), and forwarded to PCR amplification. After several selection rounds, cloning and sequencing steps are performed followed by an evaluation of the target affinity of the enriched aptamers. (b) Schematic illustration of capillary electrophoresis-SELEX technology. An initial pool of oligonucleotides is first incubated with the target, and then the mixture is separated based on the mobility shift. The bound sequences are collected, amplified by PCR, and used for cloning, sequencing, and evaluation of the affinity of obtained aptamers (Darmostuk et al., 2015).

3.3.4 Magnetic-bead-based SELEX

In 1997, a SELEX approach for focus immobilization using magnetic beads was disclosed (Bruno, 1997). The first libraries of magnetic beads that have been loaded well with the targeted chemical are incubated. Next, using magnetization, oligonucleotides attached to the target are separated from loose sequences. Extracted DNA-bound oligonucleotides are subsequently amplified through PCR, and the cycle is repeated. Aptamers are being multiplied, cloned, and tested for affinity after thousands of rounds of selection.

3.3.5 Cell SELEX

Many of the SELEX approaches discussed previously are predicated on working in the sector of the destination for aptamer shortlisting. The only exception to this is the Cell-SELEX method which is illustrated in Figure 3.4 This well-developed strategy does not need prior information about the target. The first Cell-SELEX experiment used a live pathogenic organism, Trypanosoma brucei (Homann and Goringer,

1999). The results of this research revealed the development of three distinct kinds of elevated RNA aptamers for the parasite's infective circulatory stage of the life cycle. The aptamers were chosen to attach to the parasite's flagellar pocket, and none of the detected aptamers were connected to VSG protein, which was one of the most abundant polypeptides on the Trypanosoma interface. Daniels et al. pioneered it in 2003, and by utilizing a glioblastoma-derived cell line, researchers developed a DNA aptamer against tenascin-C U251 (Daniels et al., 2003). Several modified Cell-SELEX approaches are now being developed to increase the success rate of aptamer screenings.

By using technology, whole cells, both eukaryotic and prokaryotic, may be employed to manufacture highly selective aptamers. In a counter-selection process, a chemically produced oligonucleotide library is cultured with cells dissimilar to the target cells. Unbound oligonucleotides are collected and treated with target cells. Bound sequences and their destinations are distinguished by phenol extraction, amplified by PCR, and submitted to the following round of choosing. Following selection, enhanced aptamers are employed in further phases of cloning, sequencing, and target affinity assessment. Cell-SELEX may need 35 rounds for selection and 8–10 rounds for high affinity. This approach produced several aptamers against various cancer cell types (Ninomiya et al., 2013).

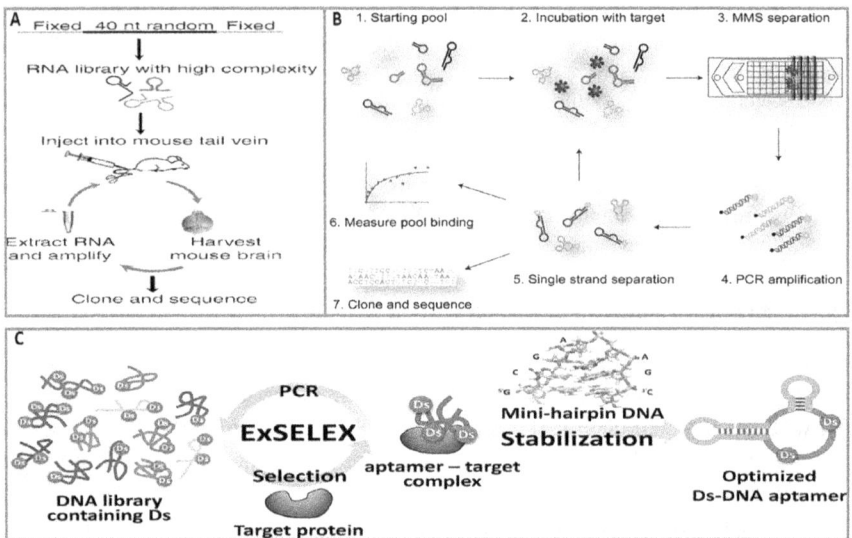

FIGURE 3.4   (a) In vivo SELEX for aptamers (Cheng et al., 2013). (b) Schematic showing the major steps of M-SELEX. The starting pool (1) is incubated with magnetic beads coated with the target protein (2) After incubation, the sample is loaded onto the micro-magnetic separation (MMS) device, which traps the beads for high-stringency washing (3) The eluted beads are then PCR-amplified to generate double-stranded DNA (4) The fluorescently labelled forward strand is recovered during a single-strand separation step (5), and can then be used for the next selection round, binding measurements (6), or cloning and sequencing (7) (Ahmad et al., 2011). (c) DNA aptamer generation by ExSELEX using genetic alphabet expansion with a mini-hairpin DNA stabilization method (Hirao et al., 2018).

3.3.6 MICROFLUIDIC **SELEX**

Many advantages are maintained by microfluidic SELEX approach. For starters, since most isolation technologies primarily work at the contacting surfaces, shrinking the system to achieve a better surface-to-volume ratio dramatically improves detachment effectiveness while also lowering substance utilization. This length decrease reduces the risk of non-specific binding then-off adhesion in chromatographic techniques based on affinity, permitting adverse choices to still be removed in several cases. Second, limiting the number of targets (therefore boosting the overall consistency of the selection) leads to quicker converging of the aptamer pool to a small sequence pool. Microfluidic techniques specialize in controlling small amounts of liquid chemicals, increasing consistency while decreasing manufacturing costs. Furthermore, a major drawback of SELEX in principle is that every phase of the process may be labour-intensive, time-consuming, and require professional skills (Figure 3.4). Microfluidic techniques provide a more effective and efficient automation technology and are multiplexed, reducing the time and energy spent within every novel aptamer and streamlining the SELEX process. This is what has developed in so many microfluidic SELEX separation technologies, and also as capillary electrophoresis, microfluidic bead-based separations, and sol–gel encapsulating method (Dembowski and Bowser, 2018).

3.3.7 IN VIVO **SELEX**

Recognizing that aptamers selected in culture might not even necessarily be successful in vivo, the researcher developed an in vivo-based SELEX technique for quick synthesis of tissue-penetrating aptamers using lab animals of target illnesses. Mi et al. attempted to pick aptamers inside a living organism's tumour for the first time in 2010 (Mi et al., 2010). In the first infectious pool of HIV-1 DNA genotypes used as in vivo SELEX experiment, an infectious pool of HIV-1 DNA genotypes with genetic changes was transplanted into CD4+ T cells. This process included numerous stages of viral replication, cloning, and sequencing. The main selection process in this in vivo SELEX is fairly similar to traditional SELEX, with the difference of employing live organisms for selection rather than isolated targets as in conventional SELEX. In in vivo SELEX, mice with intrahepatic colorectal metastases were used for aptamer synthesis. This can be employed as a modelling approach for RNA aptamers.

3.3.8 EX SELEX

The improved aptamer advancement strategies (XNA-aptamers) display lower nM to pM range dissolution values and hence ultra-high affinities as parts of the Artificially Expanded Genetic Information System (AEGIS) and genetic alphabet extension SELEX (ExSELEX) employing "unusual" or synthesized nucleotide process as depicted in paste Figure 3.4 here (Kimoto et al., 2016). This technique, nevertheless, is significantly reliant on polymerases' capacity to take modified or artificial nucleotide triphosphates as precursors, as well as their capacity to "deep sequence" those XNA aptamers. DNA libraries in ExSELEX contain the very hydrophobic Ds bases as a fifth letter.

Also, when UBPs are present in the libraries, PCR can successfully duplicate or amplify them as a duplex in the existence of Ds or Px triphosphate precursors in addition to the natural base substrate. Using ExSELEX, one can produce a large number of elevated Ds-containing DNA (Ds-DNA) aptamers that contact protein (Sefah et al., 2014). The extremely hydrophobic Ds bases in the aptamers significantly increase their affinities towards target proteins' hydrophobic regions. Kimoto and colleagues were among the first to develop aptamers containing a fifth base (dDs). SELEX is an abbreviation for Genetic Alphabet Expansion (ExSELEX). They built many libraries, each with 1–3 dDs scattered over a random region. Every library featured a different two or three-nucleotide index at the end of the forward primer, allowing the decoded clones to be allocated towards the collection from which they had derived and consequently the positions of the dDs to be identified.

ExSELEX aptamers for the proteins interferon-g (IFN-g) come with different modifications The affinities of these modified aptamers are at least 100-fold higher than those of previously reported aptamers for both targets containing only the four natural bases (Kimoto et al., 2016).

3.4   ADVANCED METHODS

It stands that increasing the quantity and kind of aptamer-target contacts would allow for the development of aptamers with a shorter off-rate or even a higher affinity (Hasegawa et al., 2016). The most evident weakness in traditional SELEX is to create. The minimum environmental influenced variety of typical DNA/RNA collections which leads to high-affinity aptamers. Proteinaceous antibodies, on the other hand, to diversify their binding locations, may mix and combine 20 different hydrophobic and hydrophilic amino acids. Typical aptamers lack or have weak hydrophobic interactions with the target due to their hydrophilic polyanionic cornerstone, trying to limit their fully functioning contact details and conditional abilities. To resolve the above issues, Gorenstein's laboratory invented different SELEX speculative methodologies including X-aptamers and Xeno Nucleic Acids or XNAs (Pinheiro and Holliger, 2014). Further, SOMAmers, LNAs (Hernandez et al., 2009), etc. are being investigated for their ability to improve aptamer affinity by utilizing nucleotides which do not present in surroundings.

XNA-based aptamers offer better results and have indeed been successfully created by a variety of changes to the nucleotide bases, sugar rings in the random phosphate backbone, and primer-binding regions of oligonucleotides (Lipi et al., 2016).

Hydrophobicity, which seems to be common in the interaction of two proteins (Chanphai et al., 2015), however uncommon between aptamers and their target molecules. This constraint has been solved using a novel selection approach that employs SOMAmers (Slow Off-rate Modified Aptamers) as a new generation of aptamers. SOMAmers contain deoxyuridine residues that have been thermally changed to have amino acid-like side chains. The 13 "difficult" human proteins that rejected conventional DNA SELEX showed a strong affinity to slow-off-rate aptamers.

Locked Nucleic Acids (LNAs) LNAs increased avidin-binding aptamer binding affinity by 8.5 folds when purine nucleotides were replaced with LNAs These nucleotides have many sugar modifications. The 20-O-40 C-methylene-b-d-ribofuranose moiety is perhaps the most often utilized derivative. Nucleotides having this altera-tion have been recognized to significantly raise the melting temperature of substi-tuted RNAs. The substituting of RNAs with LNAs improves thermo stability.

An alternate option to SELEX that has already been presented in the last nearly a decade is to create aptamers for varied applications using bioinformatics computa-tional tools such as molecular dynamics (MD) and molecular docking. Of course, the technique may be utilized in conjunction with SELEX and HTS to improve research efficacy. Some computational biology technique is used to design and analyze the HTS experimental data

Next-generation sequencing (NGS) is rapidly expanding and integrating it allows for the performance of current high research and the development of novel screen-ing strategies. The methods for aptamer ripening in silico are as follows SELEX-derived aptamers are tested for target selectivity using an aptamer blot assay. The duplication of aptamer sequences is done in silico and spontaneously added with other sequences, followed by crossing over and two-point mutations. The specific characteristics of the unique nucleotide sequences are then evaluated once more, and selected aptamers go through a second phase of in silico maturation.

Dausse et al. have offered an intriguing and unusual way to test aptamer affinity following picking (2011). This HAPIscreen approach (high-throughput aptamer iden-tification) is based on PerkinElmer's AlphaScreen® technology, which was originally characterized as luminescence oxygen channelling immunoassay HAPI screen tech-nology works by associating the target molecule and potential aptamer with donor and acceptor microbeads. Whenever an aptamer binds with its target analysis, a fluo-rescent sensor recognizes a fluorescent signal created by microbeads. Because this approach has been automated, hundreds of responses can run at the same time. The aptamer scanning enables a rapid selection of aptamers. Other important advanced methods and modification approaches are shown in Table 3.1.

3.5 APPLICATION OF APTAMER

Aptamers have been researched as a biocompatible material in several studies includ-ing its usage as a diagnostic and therapeutic tool and biosensing probe, as well as in the creation of novel medications, pharmaceutical delivery systems, etc.

3.5.1 DIAGNOSTIC APPROACH

Cancer is the world's second-largest cause of mortality. Accurate tumour diagnos-tic technology has practical implications since it allows clinicians to propose treat-ment methods, evaluate therapy results at an early stage, track tumour recurrence and metastasis, and estimate prognosis (Parihar et al., 2022c). Currently, antibodies are widely utilized in clinical tumour diagnostics, such as flow cytometry, tumour marker detection, immunohistochemistry, in vivo imaging, and so on (Zhang et al., 2014). However, because of disadvantages such as high immunogenicity, poor stability, com-plex chemical modification, restricted production techniques, and high production costs, antibodies' clinical applicability has been limited to some extent. Aptamers, like antibodies, offer great affinity and specificity for binding to the target Figure 3.5.

TABLE 3.1

Advanced modification in SELEX Methodology for aptamer

Method	Description
Fluorescence activated cell sorting-SELEX (FACS-SELEX)	In a modified FACS-SELEX technique, fluorescently tagged oligonucleotide libraries are incubated with a variety of different types of cells (e.g. vital and dead cells).
	Aptamers that have exclusively bonded to the cells of interest. Aptamers linked to a specific cell phenotypic basis are selected in both live and decaying cells.
3D Cell-SELEX	It is equivalent to the natural atmosphere wherein cells develop and adapt, taking the aptamer procedure closer to the clinical.
	To make 3D cell cultures, the method takes some time and necessitates laboratory competence.
Negative SELEX	In general, the target molecules are bound to the immobilization matrix, allowing partitioning. Some of the sequences may unintentionally attach to the immobilization matrix during the selection process, resulting in false positive findings.
	Ellington and Szostak proposed a novel approach termed negative SELEX in 1992 to remove such a possibility.
Counter SELEX	Counter SELEX is identical to the negative SELEX technique. The counter SELEX uses similar target molecules as incubation subjects.
	Jenison et al. created the counter SELEX technique to increase aptamer specificity in 1994.
On-chip selection	This approach combines microarray technology with point mutations of specified sequences using a genetic algorithm. First, using the CombiMatrix device, silico-generated random sequences are synthesized and incubated with the target.
	The sequence with the highest specificity is chosen as a "mother". In silico single and double mutations are applied to the sequence and round repeats. The first-generation aptamer is immobilized on an SPR chip and used in binding assays to determine the aptamer/target complex Kd.
	This method enables the rapid and automated selection of aptamers .against a diverse set of targets.
Cell-internalization SELEX	This aptamer (s) not only binds towards the cell membrane but is also absorbed.
	It takes time to research and obtain intracellularly delivered aptamer sequences.
TECS-SELEX	Cell-SELEX is used by TECS-SELEX (target generated on the surface of the cell) is used to discover proteins that are overexpressed on the surface of the cell.
	Positive selection rounds against cells of interest alternate with counter-selection rounds employing cells that do not produce the protein of interest employed in this approach. Aptamers with nanomolar Kd are chosen after eleven rounds of screening.
Cross-over SELEX	The rigorous selection method aids in increasing selection efficiency.
	The procedure is time-consuming due to the additional selection step.

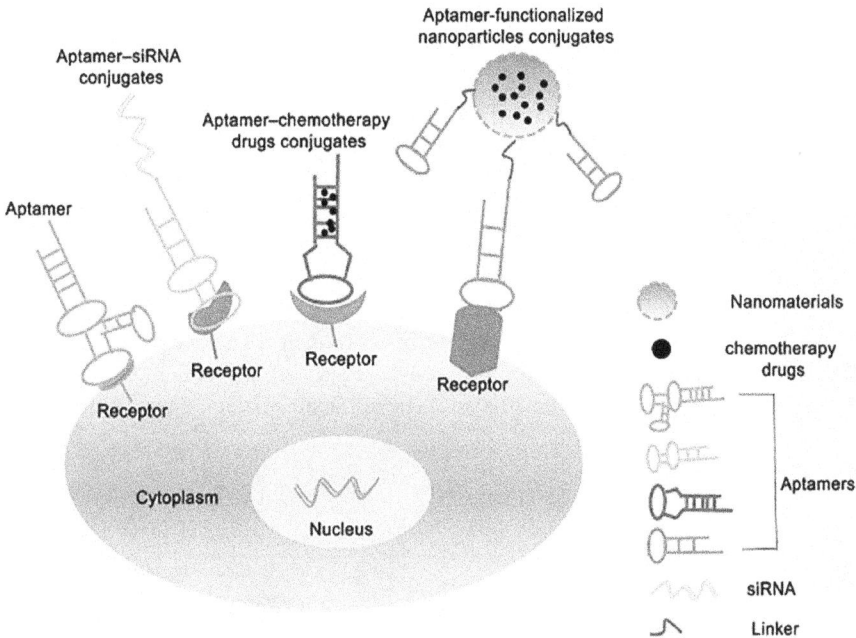

FIGURE 3.5 Aptamer-based cancer therapy options. The aptamers can be utilized in conjunction with siRNA, chemotherapeutic medicines, and nanoparticles to eradicate malignant cells rather than being employed as a treatment (Han et al., 2014).

It has been widely employed in numerous domains of tumour diagnostics, including the identification of circulating tumour cells (CTCs), immunohistochemical analysis, and in vivo imaging.

Aptamers can also be employed in lateral flow assays (LFAs), a rapid processing technology for locating and quantifying particles in different molecules LFAs also currently used in residence or perhaps in diagnostic, such as widespread pregnancy tests; many experiments are inexpensive, easy to use, that utilize antibodies as either an image detection ingredient (Koczula and Gallotta, 2016).

Traditional imaging techniques, such as X-rays in CAT scans and radiolabeled substances (e.g. fluorodeoxyglucose) PET, Magnetic resonance, and ultrasounds all rely heavily on diversity and abundance. These approaches are commonly employed in clinical settings, such as cancer screening measures. Aptamers also were used as different fluorescent dye containers during imaging diagnosis that may be identified by spectroscopic methods, such as fluorescein or rhodamine (Xu et al., 2006). Several examples of molecular probes for typical clinical imaging applications are shown, accompanied by a quick review of fundamental conjugation procedures applicable to Aptamers of RNA and DNA designed for detection.

The epidemic of a new coronavirus (SARS-CoV-2) reached pandemic proportions in 2019. However, the process of coronavirus infection is not well known. Furthermore, no common treatment medicines or vaccines exist to combat this condition. Strong intensity aptamers addressing the receptor-binding region (RBD) of the severe acute respiratory spikes glycoprotein were created utilizing SELEX in vitro assays supplemented with and in computational studies. The in vitro SELEX DNA pools were examined using SMART-Aptamer-2. Furthermore, molecular docking and MD were employed to investigate aptamer/RBD binding. The remarkable affinity of the two optimized RBD aptamers for SARS-CoV-2 was proven by their Kd values. As a result, the developed aptamers are effective for SARS-CoV-2 diagnoses and antiviral therapy (Figure 3.6).

Traditional diagnostic approaches, such as immunological tests ELISA and PCR, requires pathogen extraction, culturing for development, and microscopic identification. Several aptamers are now commonly utilized in the diagnosis of infectious illness. Suh et al. (2018), for example, created a Sandwich test using DNA aptamers to collect and identify *L. monocytogenes*. The application of aptamers is enlisted in Table 3.2.

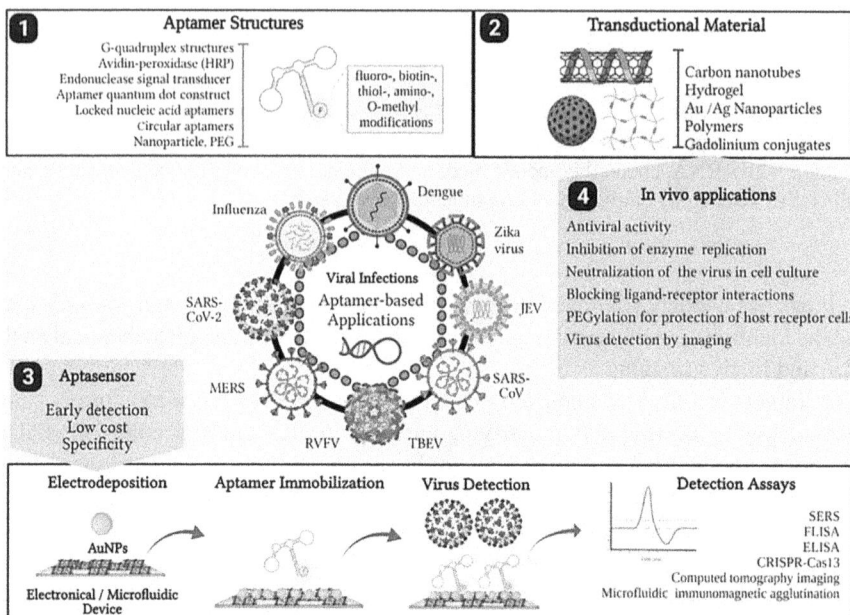

FIGURE 3.6 Aptamer against viral diseases. Aptamers chosen using in vitro SELEX technology were utilized to diagnose numerous human pathogenic viruses, including influenza, MERS, SARS-CoV, SARS-CoV-2, dengue, Zika virus, Rift Valley fever virus (RVFV), Japanese Encephalitis virus (JEV), and tick-borne encephalitis virus (TBEV). (1) Aptamers with changed structures can be immobilized using (2) designed transduction material, such as Au-nanoparticles (AuNPs) based on detection tests, as (3) aptasensors, or (4) in vivo research to limit cell infection or viral multiplication. PEG stands for polyethylene glycol (Krüger et al., 2021).

TABLE 3.2

Aptamer usage in diagnostic application

Application	Aptamer	Target	Result	References
Cancer cells detection	AS1411	MCF-7 breast cancer cells	Colour identification of breast cancer cells with a detectable limit of ten cells.	Borghei et al. (2016)
	Sgc8	leukemia cells	Amine-labelled aptamers were conjugated to carboxyl-modified fluorescent silica nanoparticles to detect malignant cells in a highly precise and discriminatory way.	
	R13	Ovarian cancer Cells	The R13 aptamer had a strong affinity for various ovarian cancer cell lines.	Li et al. (2018)
Infectious diseases diagnosis	AU1 and AD1	*Candida albicans*	The aptamers AU1 and AD1 were utilized to detect the—d-glucans discovered with significant specificity and affinity inside the cellular membrane of the fungus *Candida albicans.*	Borghei et al. (2016)
	A8 and A20	Influenza viruses (H3N2 and H1N1)	A8 and A20 DNA aptamers, as well as their shortened counterparts, were employed to detect type A influenza virus with significant specificity and affinity (H3N2 and H1N1).	Bai et al. (2018)
	S15	Dengue virus 2 (DENV)	aptamer S15 exhibits dengue virus 2 envelope protein domain III (ED3) (DENV)	
Imaging/ diagnosis	A10	PSMA	CT imaging contrast Agents	Kim et al. (2010)
	sgc8c	CCRF-CEM cells	Stimulus-responsive contrast agent in ultrasound imaging	Wang et al. (2011)
	99mTc	MUC1 protein	a tumour biomarker for ultrasound imaging	Pieve et al. (2009)
	TA29	Human α-thrombin	Fluorescence polarization research has been used to identify aptamer-protein contacts.	Zhang et al. (2011)

3.5.2 THERAPEUTIC APPROACH

Aptamers derived from XNAs were successfully synthesized (Pinheiro et al., 2012) opening up new possibilities for aptamers resulting in a significant. Changes to the phosphate-sugar backbone, for example, may boost aptamer absorption and pharmacokinetics, which in itself is interesting for medicinal applications.

Aptamers' suitability for in vivo applications has been increased. Aptamers may be used in treatment to prevent viral particles from fighting without host receptor molecules or viral entryway proteins for entrance into host cells. Intracellular viral targeting with aptamers, on the other hand, is a promising method. Aptamers have been created to disrupt nucleocapsid assembly or to target proteins involved in viral replication, such as SARS-CoV NTPase/helicase, HIV reverse transcriptase, and hepatitis C virus (HCV) RNA polymerase.

Patients' lives are being ruined by neurodegenerative illnesses. Although the cause of these disorders is unknown, they are defined by an unfolded protein synthesis in the central nervous system. As a result, developing viable methods to reduce or prevent the onset of these illnesses is critical. As technology progresses, aptamers have created new prospects therefore in the scientific sector has advanced. Aptamers might attach to certain specific molecules that are linked and disrupt their accumulation, thereby inhibiting or delaying neurodegenerative disease progression.

The delicate nature of eye illnesses necessitates extremely specialized, targeted, long-lasting, adaptable, and nontoxic therapy techniques. As a result, aptamers are the most ideal family of molecules for treating eye problems, owing to their great specificity to their target molecules and nonimmunogenic character. Furthermore, because aptamers are substantially bigger than tiny molecular therapies, their stay in the eye is extended. This improved accessibility and controllability overcome several problems encountered by conventional single molecule or protein-based treatments. Pegaptanib is a VEGF-specific anti-angiogenesis aptamer, a 40 kDa dimeric glycoprotein, that is responsible for angiogenesis in the majority of eye diseases, making it an important therapeutic target. Several aptamers have currently been investigated for the treatment of eye-related disorders, including one approach found beneficial in therapy. There are various other FDA-approved under clinical trial aptamers for therapeutic applications enlisted in Table 3.3.

TABLE 3.3
Therapeutic uses of aptamer for several diseases

Aptamer	Target	Application	References
Pegaptanib sodium (Macugen) RNA (27 nt)	VEGF	AMD Diabetic macular oedema Diabetic retinopathy	
NU172 DNA (26 nt)	Thrombin	Heart disease	Zavyalova et al. (2019)
ARC1905 (Zimura) RNA (38 nt)	C5	Dry AMD IPCV	Biesecker et al. (1999)
ApolloDx's	Specific targets of pathogens found in water and foods	Food safety testing for commercialization	CibusDx, Inc.
Thrombin-specific aptamers	Thrombin	estimate prothrombin fragment	
SOMAScan	Human proteins within body fluids at sub-pg amounts	Proteomics	

3.6 CHALLENGES IN APTAMER SYNTHESIS

Since its launch in 1990, aptamer and SELEX technologies have revolutionized biological sectors (Sun and Zu, 2015), and their wide application is illustrated in Figure 3.7. Because aptamers are quickly washed out of the body, modifications (or greater concentrations) are required to extend their time in the body. Susceptibility to nuclease breakdown, particularly in vivo clinical effects of these drugs has been limited by their ability to adequate excretion. Aptamer alterations and conjugations have therefore been developed to address constraints in the deployment of aptamer-based therapeutics.

Because phosphate backbone alterations are sensitive to nuclease degradation, they must be used. According to nuclease-mediated disintegration, the in vivo half-lives of unmodified aptamers are typically shorter about 10 minutes (Soldevilla et al., 2015). Some targets will not connect with aptamers owing to a lack of functional groups or other features. Target molecule bonds are often weaker than antibody bonds. Enzymes may readily digest aptamers. SELEX objectives are generally obtained through prokaryotic and eukaryotic cells identifying the correct by chromatographic purification. Aptamers synthesized targeting prokaryotic targets would

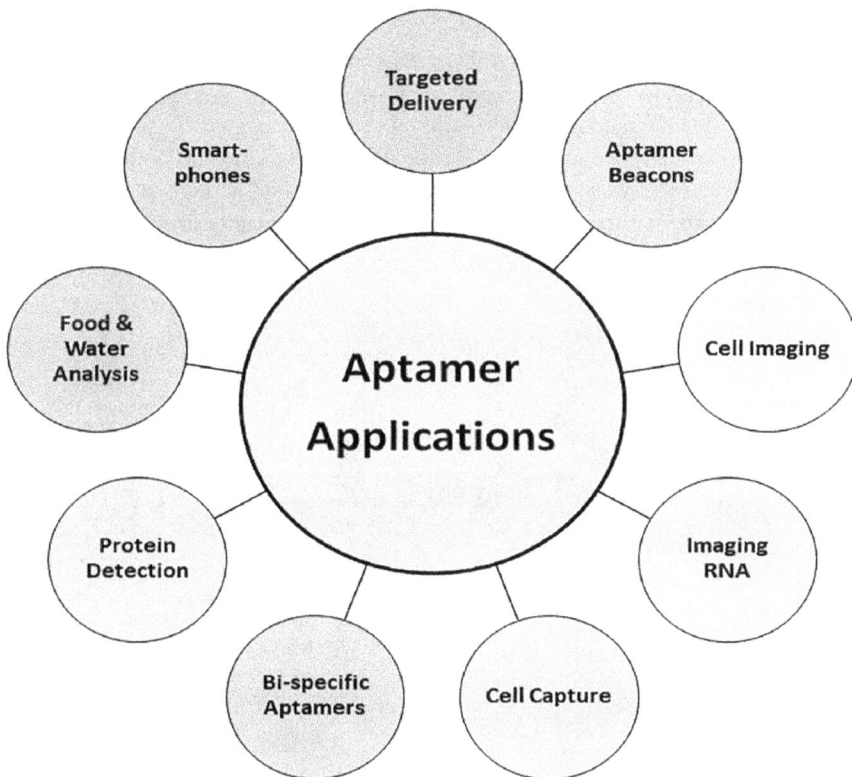

FIGURE 3.7 Applications of aptamers in various fields.

not necessarily attach to the identical receptor synthesized in eukaryotic cells. It could be because subsequent cells lacked post-translational changes.

A variety of limitations prevent aptamers from being used more widely as treatments. The first is the fast breakdown of aptamers in blood by nucleases. Aptamer toxicity and control over their function are still unknown. To conduct a clinical study another problem in aptamer therapeutic uses is controlling their effect.

Costs might be high in comparison to traditional approaches because it is still a continually expanding discipline of research. Even though monoclonal-specific antibody treatments are still dominating the marketplaces for targeted diagnosis and therapies, antibody immunology and cost of production remain the fundamental hurdles to widespread clinical application (Sun and Zu, 2015). Aptamers, which are small, flexible oligonucleotide ligands, hold a lot of potential as replacements or additions to monoclonal antibodies. Aptamer research and applications overlap substantially, and in certain circumstances, Aptamers outperformed antibodies specifically in biomarkers identification, in vitro and in vivo diagnostics, and precisely regulated therapeutic targets, among other applications shown in Figure 3.8.

Several clinically studied aptamers are typically prepared by capping the 3¢ end using reversed thymidine. It's challenging to choose aptamers against the protein of interest which is less abundant mostly on the cell membranes. Furthermore, to prevent non-specific aptamer absorption and attachment during the aptamer selection technique, the living cells would have to be approachable. So yet, no optimal SELEX procedure exists, and researchers must pick from a range of SELEX modifications, each with its own set of restrictions and problems. First and foremost, the expense of an aptamer methodology should indeed be considered. To begin the selection procedure, researchers must first create a huge DNA oligonucleotide library of around 10^{15} sequences (Darmostuk et al., 2015). Because of their capacity to fold into more complex 3D structures, RNA aptamers are frequently favoured over DNA

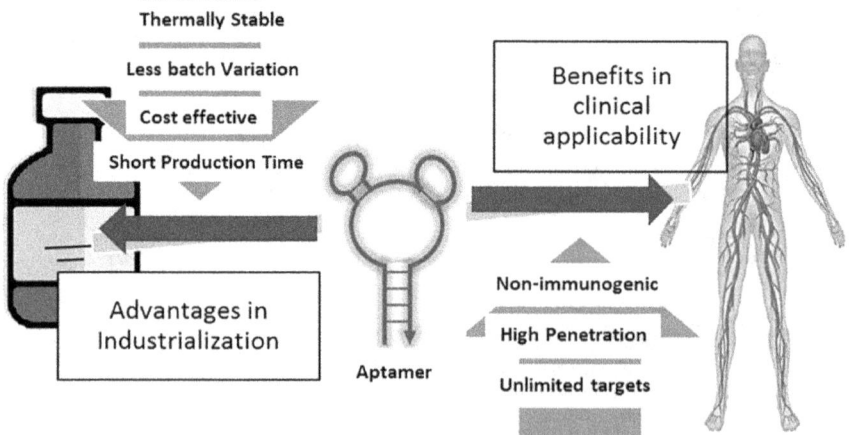

FIGURE 3.8　Advantages of aptamer and its benefits for clinical applications (Razali et al., 2020).

aptamers. SELEX sequence identification still seems to be stagnant. After immobilization of the target molecule, approximately one-third of the target surface may be lost or inaccessible. Immobilization procedures are not always appropriate for tiny molecular targets, especially when the compounds lack functional groups (Kudłak and Wieczerzak, 2020). Amongst the most serious problems with existing cancer treatments is that most of them destroy both healthy and malignant cells. Delivery of drugs experts today face the problem and potential of increasing the therapeutic index and, ultimately, delivering tailored medicines to cancerous cells while minimizing off-target adverse effects (Buglak et al., 2020). Recently, 2D nanomaterial-enabled improved biosensors have shown promise in cancer detection. MXene-enabled electrochemical aptasensors with a femtomolar limit of detection have shown considerable potential in the detection of cancer biomarkers. Furthermore, the stability, simplicity of synthesis, repeatability, and high specificity provided by MXene-enabled aptasensors indicate that they have the potential to become the standard diagnostic technique (Parihar et al., 2022c).

3.7   CONCLUSION AND FUTURE OUTLOOK

We review in this chapter technical advances in the synthesis approaches and development of aptamer-based technologies in the field of health care such as aptamer-enabled biosensors with enhanced sensitivity and selectivity, as well as the actualization of newly emerging real-time and in-field detection applications, along with therapeutic applications of aptamer (Bird et al., 1995; Kaur, 2018; Liu et al., 2017; Onoa and Tinoco, 2004; Ranjan et al., 2020; Siegel et al., 2016; Tan et al., 2017; Yoo et al., 2020).

Aptamers have demonstrated remarkable success in the disease diagnostic field, and the industry recently celebrated 25 years of aptamer technological advancement. However, when compared to antibodies, this approach appears to be in its infancy (Kalra et al., 2018).

Whereas the efficient implementation of aptamer-based medications remains a few decades away, academics including biopharmaceutical firms are optimistic about the promising potential. Even though antibodies have a broader clinical application in terms of therapeutic and diagnostic intervention, aptamers have features such as simple chemical functionalization, thermal conductivity, and accelerated synthesis, as well as particular target recognition, that make them appropriate tools for clinical diagnosis of various illness (Khan et al., 2021; Parihar et al., 2020, 2022a, 2022b, 2023).

The framework of a SELEX experiment has a huge influence on the effectiveness of aptamer creation. Aptamer separation capability is enhanced by a wide and physiologically significant starting library as well as suitable adsorption and dissociation methods, magnification, and pool regeneration processes. The likelihood of isolating aptamers with increased affinity rises with the original nucleic acid library's structural complexity and target concentration.

Aptamers appear to also be artificially edited oligonucleotide libraries. Negative and counter selections may be used to fine-tune the specificity of the chosen aptamers. Despite advances in tumour therapeutic research, aptamers concentration needs to be optimized, among other things; the drug concentration, targeted effectiveness, sustained release, and compatibility are all other factors to be considered.

More study is needed on aptamer-pharmaceutical combos as well as aptamer-mediated nanocarrier alteration. SELEX technology and chemical modification techniques for aptamers synthesis are predicted to play a larger role in future cancer applications. SELEX's basic operations have been considerably optimized, involving the creation of a starting patterns collection (e.g., nucleic acid chain modifications), and aptamer categorizations with computerized functioning (e.g., microfluidic devices) (e.g., HTS). Researchers now have an ever-expanding arsenal of aptamer discovery tools at their disposal, and Alternative techniques are also being explored to enhance selecting hit rates simultaneously reducing the time and cost required to generate novel aptamers.

However, technological developments will profit from the quick production of extremely specific aptamers along with a decrease in manufacturing costs, which will be lower than that of antibodies but still significant. The rapid advancement of artificial intelligence (AI), particularly in quantitative reasoning and big data extraction, could have been addressed, as they can be helpful for the prediction of aptamer structure and its interaction with target molecules. Sophisticated records can aid in the creation of libraries and selections. With an ever-expanding sequence library of known aptamers, in vitro selection utilizing computational methods might be a viable future option for aptamer research. This aptamer dataset will contain compositional information from previous aptamer-ligand combinations and will be used in the next phase of SELEX innovation.

Determining the affinity amongst compounds including using perpetual motion estimations might result in a method of running SELEX computationally without the expensive and time-consuming processes of experimental in vitro selection. Computational aptamer selection, also known as in silico selection, has lately been researched using several programmes.

This chapter discusses present technologies as well as approaches for the production and deployment of aptamers, with a focus on the diagnostic and medicinal areas. The emergence of several methods and strategies for aptamer synthesis and deployment should be fully explored, which can be of interest to readers.

ACKNOWLEDGEMENTS

The authors would like to thank the Director of CSIR-Advanced Materials and Process Research AMPRI Bhopal, India, for his attention and encouragement in this effort. Arpana Parihar's fellowship under the DST-WoS-B (DST/WOS-B/HN-4/2021) initiative is gratefully acknowledged. Raju Khan would like to thank the Science and Engineering Research Board SERB for funding the IPA/2020/000130 study.

REFERENCES

Ahmad, K. M., Oh, S. S., Kim, S., McClellen, F. M., Xiao, Y., & Soh, H. T. (2011). Probing the limits of aptamer affinity with a microfluidic SELEX platform. *PLoS ONE*, *6*(11), e27051. https://doi.org/10.1371/journal.pone.0027051

Bai, C., Lu, Z., Jiang, H., Yang, Z., Liu, X., Ding, H., Li, H., Dong, J., Huang, A., Fang, T., Jiang, Y., Zhu, L., Lou, X., Li, S., & Shao, N. (2018). Aptamer selection and application in multivalent binding-based electrical impedance detection of inactivated H1N1 virus. *Biosensors and Bioelectronics, 110*, 162–167. https://doi.org/10.1016/j.bios.2018.03.047

Biesecker, G., Dihel, L., Enney, K., & Bendele, R. A. (1999). Derivation of RNA aptamer inhibitors of human complement C5. *Immunopharmacology, 42*(1–3), 219–230. https://doi.org/10.1016/S0162-3109(99)00020-X

Bird, A. C., Bressler, N. M., Bressler, S. B., Chisholm, I. H., Coscas, G., Davis, M. D., de Jong, P. T. V. M., Klaver, C. C. W., Klein, B. E. K., Klein, R., Mitchell, P., Sarks, J. P., Sarks, S. H., Soubrane, G., Taylor, H. R., & Vingerling, J. R. (1995). An international classification and grading system for age-related maculopathy and age-related macular degeneration. *Survey of Ophthalmology, 39*(5), 367–374. https://doi.org/10.1016/S0039-6257(05)80092-X

Borghei, Y.-S., Hosseini, M., Dadmehr, M., Hosseinkhani, S., Ganjali, M. R., & Sheikhnejad, R. (2016). Visual detection of cancer cells by colorimetric aptasensor based on aggregation of gold nanoparticles induced by DNA hybridization. *Analytica Chimica Acta, 904*, 92–97. https://doi.org/10.1016/j.aca.2015.11.026

Bruno, J. G. (2013). A review of therapeutic aptamer conjugates with emphasis on new approaches. *Pharmaceuticals (Basel, Switzerland), 6*(3), 340–357. https://doi.org/10.3390/ph6030340

Bruno, J. G., Carrillo, M. P., & Crowell, R. (2009). Preliminary development of DNA aptamer-Fc conjugate opsonins. *Journal of Biomedical Materials Research Part A, 90A*(4), 1152–1161. https://doi.org/10.1002/jbm.a.32182

Buglak, A. A., Samokhvalov, A. V., Zherdev, A. V., & Dzantiev, B. B. (2020). Methods and applications of in silico aptamer design and modeling. *International Journal of Molecular Sciences, 21*(22), E8420. https://doi.org/10.3390/ijms21228420

Catuogno, S., Esposito, C., & de Franciscis, V. (2016). Aptamer-mediated targeted delivery of therapeutics: An update. *Pharmaceuticals, 9*(4), 69. https://doi.org/10.3390/ph9040069

Chanphai, P., Bekale, L., & Tajmir-Riahi, H. A. (2015). Effect of hydrophobicity on protein–protein interactions. *European Polymer Journal, 67*, 224–231. https://doi.org/10.1016/j.eurpolymj.2015.03.069

Cheng, C., Chen, Y. H., Lennox, K. A., Behlke, M. A., & Davidson, B. L. (2013). In vivo SELEX for identification of brain-penetrating aptamers. *Molecular Therapy – Nucleic Acids, 2*, e67. https://doi.org/10.1038/mtna.2012.59

Chu, T. C., Marks, J. W., Lavery, L. A., Faulkner, S., Rosenblum, M. G., Ellington, A. D., & Levy, M. (2006). Aptamer: Toxin conjugates that specifically target prostate tumor cells. *Cancer Research, 66*(12), 5989–5992. https://doi.org/10.1158/0008-5472.CAN-05-4583

Churcher, Z. R., Garaev, D., Hunter, H. N., & Johnson, P. E. (2020). Reduction in dynamics of base pair opening upon ligand binding by the cocaine-binding aptamer. *Biophysical Journal, 119*(6), 1147–1156. https://doi.org/10.1016/j.bpj.2020.08.012

Daniels, D. A., Chen, H., Hicke, B. J., Swiderek, K. M., & Gold, L. (2003). A tenascin-C aptamer identified by tumor cell SELEX: Systematic evolution of ligands by exponential enrichment. *Proceedings of the National Academy of Sciences, 100*(26), 15416–15421. https://doi.org/10.1073/pnas.2136683100

Darmostuk, M., Rimpelova, S., Gbelcova, H., & Ruml, T. (2015). Current approaches in SELEX: An update to aptamer selection technology. *Biotechnology Advances, 33*(6), 1141–1161. https://doi.org/10.1016/j.biotechadv.2015.02.008

Dausse, E., Taouji, S., Evadé, L., Di Primo, C., Chevet, E., & Toulmé, J.-J. (2011). HAPIscreen, a method for high-throughput aptamer identification. *Journal of Nanobiotechnology, 9*(1), 25. https://doi.org/10.1186/1477-3155-9-25

Dembowski, S. K., & Bowser, M. T. (2018). Microfluidic methods for aptamer selection and characterization. *The Analyst, 143*(1), 21–32. https://doi.org/10.1039/C7AN01046J

Dimitrov, D. S. (2004). Virus entry: Molecular mechanisms and biomedical applications. *Nature Reviews Microbiology*, *2*(2), 109–122. https://doi.org/10.1038/nrmicro817

Ellington, A. D., & Szostak, J. W. (1990). In vitro selection of RNA molecules that bind specific ligands. *Nature*, *346*(6287), 818–822. https://doi.org/10.1038/346818a0

Förster, C., Zydek, M., Rothkegel, M., Wu, Z., Gallin, C., Geßner, R., Lisdat, F., & Fürste, J. P. (2012). Properties of an 'LNA'-modified ricin RNA aptamer. *Biochemical and Biophysical Research Communications*, *419*(1), 60–65. https://doi.org/10.1016/j.bbrc.2012.01.127

Gold, L., Ayers, D., Bertino, J., Bock, C., Bock, A., Brody, E. N., Carter, J., Dalby, A. B., Eaton, B. E., Fitzwater, T., Flather, D., Forbes, A., Foreman, T., Fowler, C., Gawande, B., Goss, M., Gunn, M., Gupta, S., Halladay, D., … Zichi, D. (2010). Aptamer-based multiplexed proteomic technology for biomarker discovery. *PLoS ONE*, *5*(12), e15004. https://doi.org/10.1371/journal.pone.0015004

Han, S. R., Yu, J., & Lee, S.-W. (2014). In vitro selection of RNA aptamers that selectively bind danofloxacin. *Biochemical and Biophysical Research Communications*, *448*(4), 397–402. https://doi.org/10.1016/j.bbrc.2014.04.103

Hasegawa, H., Savory, N., Abe, K., & Ikebukuro, K. (2016). Methods for improving aptamer binding affinity. *Molecules*, *21*(4), 421. https://doi.org/10.3390/molecules21040421

Hernandez, F. J., Kalra, N., Wengel, J., & Vester, B. (2009). Aptamers as a model for functional evaluation of LNA and 2′-amino LNA. *Bioorganic & Medicinal Chemistry Letters*, *19*(23), 6585–6587. https://doi.org/10.1016/j.bmcl.2009.10.039

Hirao, I., Kimoto, M., & Lee, K. H. (2018). DNA aptamer generation by ExSELEX using genetic alphabet expansion with a mini-hairpin DNA stabilization method. *Aptamer Technology and Applications*, *145*, 15–21. https://doi.org/10.1016/j.biochi.2017.09.007

Homann, M., & Goringer, H. U. (1999). Combinatorial selection of high affinity RNA ligands to live African trypanosomes. *Nucleic Acids Research*, *27*(9), 2006–2014. https://doi.org/10.1093/nar/27.9.2006

Kalra, P., Dhiman, A., Cho, W. C., Bruno, J. G., & Sharma, T. K. (2018). Simple methods and rational design for enhancing aptamer sensitivity and specificity. *Frontiers in Molecular Biosciences*, *5*, 41. https://doi.org/10.3389/fmolb.2018.00041

Kaur, H. (2018). Recent developments in cell-SELEX technology for aptamer selection. *Biochimica Et Biophysica Acta. General Subjects*, *1862*(10), 2323–2329. https://doi.org/10.1016/j.bbagen.2018.07.029

Khan, R., Parihar, A., & Sanghi, S. K. (Eds.). (2021). *Biosensor based advanced cancer diagnostics: From lab to clinics*. Academic Press.

Kim, D., Jeong, Y. Y., & Jon, S. (2010). A drug-loaded aptamer-gold nanoparticle bioconjugate for combined CT imaging and therapy of prostate cancer. *ACS Nano*, *4*(7), 3689–3696. https://doi.org/10.1021/nn901877h

Kim, D.-H., Seo, J.-M., Shin, K.-J., & Yang, S.-G. (2021). Design and clinical developments of aptamer-drug conjugates for targeted cancer therapy. *Biomaterials Research*, *25*(1), 42. https://doi.org/10.1186/s40824-021-00244-4

Kimoto, M., Matsunaga, K., & Hirao, I. (2016). DNA aptamer generation by genetic alphabet expansion SELEX (ExSELEX) using an unnatural base pair system. In G. Mayer (Ed.), *Nucleic acid aptamers* (Vol. 1380, pp. 47–60). Springer, New York. https://doi.org/10.1007/978-1-4939-3197-2_4

Koczula, K. M., & Gallotta, A. (2016). Lateral flow assays. *Essays in Biochemistry*, *60*(1), 111–120. https://doi.org/10.1042/EBC20150012

Komarova, N., & Kuznetsov, A. (2019). Inside the Black box: What makes SELEX better? *Molecules*, *24*(19), 3598. https://doi.org/10.3390/molecules24193598

Krüger, A., de Jesus Santos, A. P., de Sá, V., Ulrich, H., & Wrenger, C. (2021). Aptamer applications in emerging viral diseases. *Pharmaceuticals*, *14*(7), 622. https://doi.org/10.3390/ph14070622

Kudłak, B., & Wieczerzak, M. (2020). Aptamer based tools for environmental and therapeutic monitoring: A review of developments, applications, future perspectives. *Critical Reviews in Environmental Science and Technology, 50*(8), 816–867. https://doi.org/10.1080/10643389.2019.1634457

Kwon, Y. S., Ahmad Raston, N. H., & Gu, M. B. (2014). An ultra-sensitive colorimetric detection of tetracyclines using the shortest aptamer with highly enhanced affinity. *Chemical Communications, 50*(1), 40–42. https://doi.org/10.1039/C3CC47108J

Lee, K. H., Hamashima, K., Kimoto, M., & Hirao, I. (2018). Genetic alphabet expansion biotechnology by creating unnatural base pairs. *Current Opinion in Biotechnology, 51,* 8–15. https://doi.org/10.1016/j.copbio.2017.09.006

Li, F., Wang, Q., Zhang, H., Deng, T., Feng, P., Hu, B., Jiang, Y., & Cao, L. (2018). Characterization of a DNA aptamer for ovarian cancer clinical tissue recognition and in vivo imaging. *Cellular Physiology and Biochemistry, 51*(6), 2564–2574. https://doi.org/10.1159/000495925

Lipi, F., Chen, S., Chakravarthy, M., Rakesh, S., & Veedu, R. N. (2016). *In vitro* evolution of chemically-modified nucleic acid aptamers: Pros and cons, and comprehensive selection strategies. *RNA Biology, 13*(12), 1232–1245. https://doi.org/10.1080/15476286.2016.1236173

Liu, D., Jia, S., Zhang, H., Ma, Y., Guan, Z., Li, J., Zhu, Z., Ji, T., & Yang, C. J. (2017). Integrating target-responsive hydrogel with pressuremeter readout enables simple, sensitive, user-friendly, quantitative point-of-care testing. *ACS Applied Materials & Interfaces, 9*(27), 22252–22258. https://doi.org/10.1021/acsami.7b05531

Matsunaga, K., Kimoto, M., & Hirao, I. (2017). High-affinity DNA aptamer generation targeting von Willebrand factor A1-domain by genetic alphabet expansion for systematic evolution of ligands by exponential enrichment using two types of libraries composed of five different bases. *Journal of the American Chemical Society, 139*(1), 324–334. https://doi.org/10.1021/jacs.6b10767

Meek, K. N., Rangel, A. E., & Heemstra, J. M. (2016). Enhancing aptamer function and stability via in vitro selection using modified nucleic acids. *Methods, 106,* 29–36. https://doi.org/10.1016/j.ymeth.2016.03.008

Mendonsa, S. D., & Bowser, M. T. (2004a). In vitro evolution of functional DNA using capillary electrophoresis. *Journal of the American Chemical Society, 126*(1), 20–21. https://doi.org/10.1021/ja037832s

Mendonsa, S. D., & Bowser, M. T. (2004b). In vitro selection of high-affinity DNA ligands for human IgE using capillary electrophoresis. *Analytical Chemistry, 76*(18), 5387–5392. https://doi.org/10.1021/ac049857v

Mi, J., Liu, Y., Rabbani, Z. N., Yang, Z., Urban, J. H., Sullenger, B. A., & Clary, B. M. (2010). In vivo selection of tumor-targeting RNA motifs. *Nature Chemical Biology, 6*(1), 22–24. https://doi.org/10.1038/nchembio.277

Ninomiya, K., Kaneda, K., Kawashima, S., Miyachi, Y., Ogino, C., & Shimizu, N. (2013). Cell-SELEX based selection and characterization of DNA aptamer recognizing human hepatocarcinoma. *Bioorganic & Medicinal Chemistry Letters, 23*(6), 1797–1802. https://doi.org/10.1016/j.bmcl.2013.01.040

Onoa, B., & Tinoco, I. (2004). RNA folding and unfolding. *Current Opinion in Structural Biology, 14*(3), 374–379. https://doi.org/10.1016/j.sbi.2004.04.001

Parihar, A., Choudhary, N. K., Sharma, P., & Khan, R. (2022a). MXene-based aptasensor for the detection of aflatoxin in food and agricultural products. *Environmental Pollution, 316,* 120695.

Parihar, A., Pandita, V., & Khan, R. (2022b). 3D printed human organoids: High throughput system for drug screening and testing in current COVID-19 pandemic. *Biotechnology and Bioengineering, 119*(10), 2669–2688.

Parihar, A., Ranjan, P., Sanghi, S. K., Srivastava, A. K., & Khan, R. (2020). Point-of-care biosensor-based diagnosis of COVID-19 holds promise to combat current and future pandemics. *ACS Applied Bio Materials*, *3*(11), 7326–7343. https://doi.org/10.1021/acsabm.0c01083

Parihar, A., Singhal, A., Kumar, N., Khan, R., Khan, Mohd. A., & Srivastava, A. K. (2022c). Next-generation intelligent MXene-based electrochemical aptasensors for point-of-care cancer diagnostics. *Nano-Micro Letters*, *14*(1), 100. https://doi.org/10.1007/s40820-022-00845-1

Parihar, A., Yadav, S., Sadique, M. A., Ranjan, P., Kumar, N., Singhal, A., ... & Srivastava, A. K. (2023). Internet-of-medical-things integrated point-of-care biosensing devices for infectious diseases: Toward better preparedness for futuristic pandemics. *Bioengineering & Translational Medicine, 8*, e10481.

Pendergrast, P. S., Marsh, H. N., Grate, D., Healy, J. M., & Stanton, M. (2005). Nucleic acid aptamers for target validation and therapeutic applications. *Journal of Biomolecular Techniques: JBT*, *16*(3), 224–234.

Petersen, M., & Wengel, J. (2003). LNA: A versatile tool for therapeutics and genomics. *Trends in Biotechnology*, *21*(2), 74–81. https://doi.org/10.1016/S0167-7799(02)00038-0

Pfeiffer, F., Rosenthal, M., Siegl, J., Ewers, J., & Mayer, G. (2017). Customised nucleic acid libraries for enhanced aptamer selection and performance. *Current Opinion in Biotechnology*, *48*, 111–118. https://doi.org/10.1016/j.copbio.2017.03.026

Pieve, C. D., Perkins, A. C., & Missailidis, S. (2009). Anti-MUC1 aptamers: Radiolabelling with 99mTc and biodistribution in MCF-7 tumour-bearing mice. *Nuclear Medicine and Biology*, *36*(6), 703–710. https://doi.org/10.1016/j.nucmedbio.2009.04.004

Pinheiro, V. B., & Holliger, P. (2014). Towards XNA nanotechnology: New materials from synthetic genetic polymers. *Trends in Biotechnology*, *32*(6), 321–328. https://doi.org/10.1016/j.tibtech.2014.03.010

Pinheiro, V. B., Taylor, A. I., Cozens, C., Abramov, M., Renders, M., Zhang, S., Chaput, J. C., Wengel, J., Peak-Chew, S.-Y., McLaughlin, S. H., Herdewijn, P., & Holliger, P. (2012). Synthetic genetic polymers capable of heredity and evolution. *Science*, *336*(6079), 341–344. https://doi.org/10.1126/science.1217622

Ranjan, P., Parihar, A., Jain, S., Kumar, N., Dhand, C., Murali, S., Mishra, D., Sanghi, S. K., Chaurasia, J. P., & Srivastava, A. K. (2020). Biosensor-based diagnostic approaches for various cellular biomarkers of breast cancer: A comprehensive review. *Analytical Biochemistry*, *610*, 113996.

Sefah, K., Yang, Z., Bradley, K. M., Hoshika, S., Jiménez, E., Zhang, L., Zhu, G., Shanker, S., Yu, F., Turek, D., Tan, W., & Benner, S. A. (2014). In vitro selection with artificial expanded genetic information systems. *Proceedings of the National Academy of Sciences*, *111*(4), 1449–1454. https://doi.org/10.1073/pnas.1311778111

Shraga, R., Amir, O., & Gal, A. (2020). Learning to characterize matching experts. *arXiv*. http://arxiv.org/abs/2012.01229

Siegel, R. L., Miller, K. D., & Jemal, A. (2016). Cancer statistics, 2016. *CA: A Cancer Journal for Clinicians*, *66*(1), 7–30. https://doi.org/10.3322/caac.21332

Soldevilla, M. M., Villanueva, H., Bendandi, M., Inoges, S., López-Díaz de Cerio, A., & Pastor, F. (2015). 2-Fluoro-RNA oligonucleotide CD40 targeted aptamers for the control of B lymphoma and bone-marrow aplasia. *Biomaterials*, *67*, 274–285. https://doi.org/10.1016/j.biomaterials.2015.07.020

Song, J., Zheng, Y., Huang, M., Wu, L., Wang, W., Zhu, Z., Song, Y., & Yang, C. (2020). A Sequential multidimensional analysis algorithm for aptamer identification based on structure analysis and machine learning. *Analytical Chemistry*, *92*(4), 3307–3314. https://doi.org/10.1021/acs.analchem.9b05203

Song, Y., Song, J., Wei, X., Huang, M., Sun, M., Zhu, L., Lin, B., Shen, H., Zhu, Z., & Yang, C. (2020). Discovery of aptamers targeting the receptor-binding domain of the SARS-CoV-2 spike glycoprotein. *Analytical Chemistry*, *92*(14), 9895–9900. https://doi.org/10.1021/acs.analchem.0c01394

Sun, H., & Zu, Y. (2015). A highlight of recent advances in aptamer technology and its application. *Molecules*, *20*(7), 11959–11980. https://doi.org/10.3390/molecules200711959

Tan, C., Cao, X., Wu, X.-J., He, Q., Yang, J., Zhang, X., Chen, J., Zhao, W., Han, S., Nam, G.-H., Sindoro, M., & Zhang, H. (2017). Recent advances in ultrathin two-dimensional nanomaterials. *Chemical Reviews*, *117*(9), 6225–6331. https://doi.org/10.1021/acs.chemrev.6b00558

Tuerk, C., & Gold, L. (1990). Systematic evolution of ligands by exponential enrichment: RNA ligands to bacteriophage T4 DNA polymerase. *Science*, *249*(4968), 505–510. https://doi.org/10.1126/science.2200121

Ullman, E. F., Kirakossian, H., Switchenko, A. C., Ishkanian, J., Ericson, M., Wartchow, C. A., Pirio, M., Pease, J., Irvin, B. R., Singh, S., Singh, R., Patel, R., Dafforn, A., Davalian, D., Skold, C., Kurn, N., & Wagner, D. B. (1996). Luminescent oxygen channeling assay (LOCI): Sensitive, broadly applicable homogeneous immunoassay method. *Clinical Chemistry*, *42*(9), 1518–1526.

Wang, C.-H., Huang, Y.-F., & Yeh, C.-K. (2011). Aptamer-conjugated nanobubbles for targeted ultrasound molecular imaging. *Langmuir*, *27*(11), 6971–6976. https://doi.org/10.1021/la2011259

Webber, J., Stone, T. C., Katilius, E., Smith, B. C., Gordon, B., Mason, M. D., Tabi, Z., Brewis, I. A., & Clayton, A. (2014). Proteomics analysis of cancer exosomes using a novel modified aptamer-based array (SOMAscanTM) platform. *Molecular & Cellular Proteomics*, *13*(4), 1050–1064. https://doi.org/10.1074/mcp.M113.032136

Wilson, D. S., & Szostak, J. W. (1999). In vitro selection of functional nucleic acids. *Annual Review of Biochemistry*, *68*(1), 611–647. https://doi.org/10.1146/annurev.biochem.68.1.611

Wu, Y. X., & Kwon, Y. J. (2016). Aptamers: The "evolution" of SELEX. *Methods (San Diego, Calif.)*, *106*, 21–28. https://doi.org/10.1016/j.ymeth.2016.04.020

Xu, Y., Yang, L., Ye, X., He, P., & Fang, Y. (2006). An aptamer-based protein biosensor by detecting the amplified impedance signal. *Electroanalysis*, *18*(15), 1449–1456. https://doi.org/10.1002/elan.200603566

Yoo, H., Jo, H., & Oh, S. S. (2020). Detection and beyond: Challenges and advances in aptamer-based biosensors. *Materials Advances*, *1*(8), 2663–2687. https://doi.org/10.1039/D0MA00639D

Zavyalova, E., Legatova, V., Alieva, R., Zalevsky, A., Tashlitsky, V., Arutyunyan, A., & Kopylov, A. (2019). Putative mechanisms underlying high inhibitory activities of bimodular DNA aptamers to thrombin. *Biomolecules*, *9*(2), 41. https://doi.org/10.3390/biom9020041

Zhang, D., Lu, M., & Wang, H. (2011). Fluorescence anisotropy analysis for mapping aptamer–protein interaction at the single nucleotide level. *Journal of the American Chemical Society*, *133*(24), 9188–9191. https://doi.org/10.1021/ja202141y

Zhang, X., Soori, G., Dobleman, T. J., & Xiao, G. G. (2014). The application of monoclonal antibodies in cancer diagnosis. *Expert Review of Molecular Diagnostics*, *14*(1), 97–106. https://doi.org/10.1586/14737159.2014.866039

Zhou, J., & Rossi, J. (2017). Aptamers as targeted therapeutics: Current potential and challenges. *Nature Reviews Drug Discovery*, *16*(3), 181–202. https://doi.org/10.1038/nrd.2016.199

Zhuo, Z., Yu, Y., Wang, M., Li, J., Zhang, Z., Liu, J., Wu, X., Lu, A., Zhang, G., & Zhang, B. (2017). Recent advances in SELEX technology and aptamer applications in biomedicine. *International Journal of Molecular Sciences*, *18*(10), 2142. https://doi.org/10.3390/ijms18102142

4 A comparative study of aptasensor versus immunosensor for biomarker detection

Priya Chauhan, Annu Pandey,
Ayushi Singhal and Raju Khan

4.1 INTRODUCTION

In recent times, marked changes in lifestyle have posed a transformation in dietary patterns, involving enhanced consumption of saturated fat as well as reduced fruits, vegetables, air pollutants, stress, different waves, etc. However, such types of major elements have shown augmented occurrence of non-communicable diseases such as cardiovascular disease, cancer, diabetes, etc (Kelley 2017; Kelley et al. 2014; Wu et al. 2019). The abrupt as well as the unrestrained progress of cells in a part of the body instigated through genetics and inheritance, few viruses, environmental threats like smoking, ionizing radiation, and chemicals or pattern and lifestyle in the form of diet, the declined time of exercise and enhanced stress have been known as the interrelated risk factors of several types of cancers (Borrebaeck 2017; Edgell et al. 2010; Henry and Hayes 2012).

Thus, the chief aim of the research is to find out the biomarkers in order to detect various diseases at early stages (Peters et al. 2005; Verma 2012). Typically, biomarkers have been known as a group of measurable indicators of some biological circumstances (Ravelli et al. 2015). Biomarkers have been often assessed for the purpose of studying natural biological phenomena, to diagnose different pathogenic processes or the reaction to a specific treatment. Currently, the distinctive biomarkers have been utilized widely so as to recognize several diseases. Conversely, non-invasive, sensitive, and cost-effective measurement, stability in the samples, specified diagnosis, and early detection prior to the commencing of symptoms, have been known as the chief characteristics which may be anticipated for a biomarker (Brody and Gold 2000). Since last three periods, the usage of synthetic DNA or RNA single-stranded oligonucleotides (aptamers) have been extended in different fields of biology as well as in medicine by numerous ways (Nilsen-Hamilton 2009; Mascini 2009).

Nowadays, protein biomarkers have gradually become a significant tool from a clinical point of view not only in the field of oncology but as well as in order to direct

DOI: 10.1201/9781003304227-4

the clinical treatment of various infections (Huang et al. 2014). Recently, the boards of protein biomarkers have been certainly suggested as prognostic factors both from merely accessible biological fluids such as serum and from tissues. Because of their importance as well as consolidated application in clinics, protein biomarkers are well known as an attractive object of miniaturized biosensor-based assays. In the case of clinical diagnostics, the prompt recognition of disease biomarkers is prominently effective. Moreover, biosensors that use nanomaterials, such as conducting polymer nanowires, semiconductor nanowires, carbon nanotubes, as well as graphene, holds attractive expedient properties for the detection of biomarker (Gooding and Gaus 2016).

Therefore, this proposes that there is a huge requisite to propose sensitive, reliable, time-efficient, inexpensive, specific diagnostic, as well as cost-effective methods for the analysis of cancer-related proteins, small molecules, and cells. Accordingly, the growth of biosensors has attracted huge attention nowadays as auspicious substitute to traditional diagnostic approaches. Biosensors hold distinct advantages over other conventional methods such as rapidity, ease of use, cost, simplicity, portability, and ease-of-mass manufacture as well as diagnosis. A biosensor is recognized as a compact analytical device which comprises a biorecognition element as well as a transducer (Chung et al. 2014). Here, a biorecognition element recognizes the existence of a target through intermingling with the sample, and thus the transducer helps in converting the biological signal into an electrical signal. In a specific way, the biosensor is said to be the type of molecular diagnostic technique that helps in sensing the presence or concentration of cells or biomarkers by the interpretation of a biochemical interaction at the surface of the probe into a calculable physical signal. The biorecognition molecules have been known as the highest precarious fraction of a biosensor as the precision of the sensor highly relies on the solid affinity as well as specificity of the recognition molecules with its target. It signifies the specificity as well as the sensitivity of the fabricated sensor (Giljohann and Mirkin 2009). Different ranges of molecules have been employed as recognition probes like enzymes, antibodies, or nanoparticles. Several types of sensors have been developed for the purpose of detecting cancer. Therefore, the biosensors based on antibodies possess few limitations related to stability. As the antibodies are proteinoids in nature, they are highly sensitive to changes in pH, ionic strength, as well as temperature, which might affect their activity. Therefore, the maximum number of antibody-based sensors have been known for single-use sensors and are costly as well. Consequently, in order to overcome such types of limitations, the substitute recognition molecule, i.e. the aptamers, has been extensively applied to develop cancer diagnostic tools (Severi et al. 2014).

The objective of biosensors in the case of medical diagnostic applications is to analyze biomarker molecules in body fluids that are convoyed through a high selectivity and a quick response time. Thus, such three benchmarks have been known as the major challenges for developing an effective biosensor and may be cautiously considered. A rapid response time may be gained with the help of acceleration of the mass transport of the analyte molecule onto the biosensor surface, wherever the diffusion distance must be reduced. Lastly, selectivity, which reports the ability to recognize the existence of the biomarker as it is outnumbered by nontarget species with the help of various orders of magnitude, must be enhanced by the minimization of the cross-reactivity (Downs et al. 2021; Tian et al. 2017).

Aptamers comprised a novel category of bioreceptors which delivers auspicious platforms for several biosensing-related applications. Aptamers have shown a varied range of benefits over several prevailing biological recognition elements related to stability, design flexibility, robustness, as well as cost-effectiveness. The aptamers are greatly stable and are impervious to denaturation as well as degradation. Therefore, they possess several advantages and are known to be highly emerging perfect aspirants in terms of application as the recognition elements in biosensors (Luu et al. 2020). Besides, the biosensors with aptamers as a biorecognition element are often called "Aptasensor". However, in the last few eras, several aptasensors have been designed through the exploitation of the target binding affinity of aptamers as well as ligand-induced structural reorganization in aptamers. Usually, aptamers experience the modification in their conformation on binding sites with their target (Mascini and Tombelli 2008). Such type of property possesses the benefits of scheming the novel switchable aptasensors that cannot be attained with the antibodies. Aptamers may be reformed with various reporter molecules like fluorophores, quantum dots, methylene blue, etc. deprived of affecting their affinity. Such an aspect gives a suppleness in order to design different detection schemes for aptasensor. Aptasensors are known to be highly stable as compared to immunosensors as well as may be certainly regenerated for reusable purposes. Nevertheless, aptasensors have released a novel route for the development of rapid, sensitive, as well as point-of-care diagnostics (Sawyers 2008; Verma 2012). Aptasensors are generally such types of biosensors where aptamers might function as the biorecognition element in their structure. However, aptasensors might identify analytes in very small amounts where such minimal amounts cannot be detected with various other existing approaches. Additionally, the low cost in order to design the aptasensors in comparison to different diagnostics techniques must be regarded as one of the less expensive methods, including low detection time as well as a fast detecting process (Ronkainen et al. 2010).

Numerous types of aptamer-based biosensors like the quartz crystal microbalance, electrochemiluminescence, fluorescent, as well as electrochemical sensor have been efficaciously smeared to analyze proteins. Amongst such methods, the electrochemical biosensors have attracted huge attention due to short assay time, simple handling, low cost, small sample requisite, probability of multiplexing and miniaturization, and showing superior performance in complex samples along with nominal pre-treatments, which helps in validating their applicability for point of care (POC) use (Hermann and Patel 2000; Mascini 2009).

However, the proficient alternatives in order to attain sensitive, fast, cheap, and POC measurements biosensors have been recognized as better tools.The electrochemical immunosensors, which are among the distinct types of biosensors, depending on the transduction of an electrochemical signal developed in the interface between antibodies and antigens in body fluids, have attracted great attention, due to their high sensitivity, specificity, and accuracy as well as the probability of miniaturization of the sensing platform that is the crucial need for a portable device (Ellington and Szostak 1990; Mills 2011). The application of nanotechnology in immunogens permits to increase biodevices properties; particularly miniaturization and sensitivity, thereby dropping detection limits. Various conventional immunoassay methods like enzyme-linked immunosorbent assay (ELISA), radioimmunoassay, fluorescent immunoassay, chemiluminescence immunoassay, electrophoretic immunoassay, and mass spectrometry-based proteomics have been proposed since the last few periods for quantitative detection of the biomarker. On the contrary, the electrochemical immunoassay greatly counts on the electrochemical detection of the labelled immunogens or markers such as enzymes, metal nanoparticles, or different electroactive compounds that displayed improved detection sensitivity. Amongst the electrochemical immunoassays, paper-based electrochemical detection is extremely simple, cost-effective, as well as easy to attain along with less complex fabrication procedures (Tuerk and Gold 1990; Zhuo et al. 2017).

Therefore the detection of biomarkers may be beneficial in various ways including risk assessment, diagnosis, prognosis, foreseeing the treatment efficiency, toxicity, recurrence of any type of tumour, and many more. Currently, biosensors-based advanced diagnostic approaches have exposed a huge potential for the early detection of cancer and various lethal diseases. Various methods employed for the detections are optical, electrochemical, and piezoelectric. The electrochemical-based detection of different biomarkers like EpCAM, CD44, VEGF, Mucin 1, and CEA has drawn huge attention (Iliuk et al. 2011; Nilsen-Hamilton 2009; Tombelli et al. 2005).

4.2   APTASENSORS AND IMMUNOSENSORS

In early 1990, since the discovery aptamers have known to be appeared as a novel category of target ligands which helps in binding with their target site along with great affinity as well as specificity. However, the name aptamer has been derived from the Latin word i.e. "aptus" which means "fit", and the Greek word "meros" which denotes a "part". Usually, aptamers have been known to composed of a short single-stranded oligonucleotide, either of RNA or DNA, which have the capability to develop into well-defined 3D structures as well as binds explicitly with their corresponding ligands through complementary interaction of shape (Stoltenburg et al. 2007; Zhuo et al. 2017).

In last few decades, alongside a great variety of targets the aptamers have been selected, ranging from insignificant inorganic molecules to entire organisms (Nimjee et al. 2005). Thus the aptamers possess huge binding affinity towards their particular targets along with dissociation constants ranging from μM to pM. Generally, aptamers are equivalent to antibodies because of their explicit biorecognition properties, and they possess several qualities which makes them highly superior to antibodies. In comparison to antibodies, aptamers are extremely steady over a huge temperature range as well as pH (Ma et al. 2015). Such exclusive physical as well as chemical properties make aptamers an excellent candidate for biorecognition elements for the purpose of designing novel biosensors.

Biosensors are such type of analytical devices that help in transforming a biological response into an electrical signal. Usually, it comprises a biorecognition element which helps in the recognition of the analyte or the target molecule, a transducer which helps in transforming the biorecognition event into a measurable signal, An amplifier which is used to amplify the signal and lastly a processor which assists in displaying the result (Bhalla et al. 2016). An aptamer-based sensor i.e. an aptasensor is composed of aptamers as biorecognition elements. The biochemical interaction that is known to occur between an analyte and the aptamers has been transformed by a transducer into an electric or digital signal which may be measured, displayed, as well as analyzed (Proske et al. 2005). The produced intensity of the signals is known to be directly or inversely proportional to the concentration of the analyte. Consequently, to the transducing elements, biosensors may be grouped as electrochemical, optical, piezoelectric, as well as thermal sensors. Amongst several aptamer-based transduction methods, electrochemicals have been widely examined because of their huge sensitivity, modest instrumentation, low cost of production, quick response, and compactness as well (Xu et al. 2009). However, the schemes involved for the purpose of detection in the aptasensors might be either label-free methods, like surface plasmon resonance (SPR) and quartz crystal microbalance (QCM) measurements, Raman spectroscopy, electrochemical impedance spectroscopy, or may be labelled detection schemes like fluorescence, chemiluminescence, electrochemiluminescence (ECL), and field-effect transistors, nanoparticles (Chen et al. 2020).

In order to fabricate any type of sensor, the vital term includes the process of the immobilization of biorecognition element onto the surface of the transducer platform (Balamurugan et al. 2008). Occasionally aptamers are fastened onto the surface of the electrode through some of the linkers like linkers that are derived from oligonucleotide (Chandra et al. 2013; Goda et al. 2015; Vorobyeva et al. 2016) i.e., oligo(A), oligo(U) or oligo(T) repeats, linkers from Polyethylene glycol (PEG) (Riese et al. 2016), alkanethiol (Tian and Heyduk 2009), phosphorothioate etc. Thereby, the essential role of linkers is to assist in the affluence of convenience of analyte onto the site of binding of aptamers as well as prevent steric hindrance. Usually, the function of electrochemical biosensors depends on the immobilization of a recognition element onto the electrode surface. However, the phase of immobilization is generally arduous as well as time-consuming (Jia et al. 2014; Odeh et al. 2019; Shaver et al. 2020). Remarkably, based on vicinity hybridization assay various electrochemical immunoassays have been developed that don't include immobilization of biorecognition element onto the surface of the electrode (Hou et al. 2015; Sun et al. 2014; Xu et al. 2015).

However, aptamers possess the capability to bind with their targets along with great affinity as well as specificity which assists in developing the ultrasensitive aptasensor. Thus, the sensor based on aptamer may analyze nearly a very small concentration of marker proteins and range up to picomolar as well in the existence of several infecting proteins (Boltz et al. 2011; Xia et al. 2020). On the other hand, aptamers bid the prospect to design "label-free" sensors, and such type of sensors that don't require any covalent labelling to either the analyte or to the recognition element. Though, "Label-free" methods have been known to be highly nominal as well as auspicious approaches for quicker, simpler, and more convenient detection, it may also evade costly and cumbersome process of labelling as well. Similarly, it also stimulates labelling reactions as on holding the uppermost active degree and affinity for the recognition element as well. Thus, "Label-free" sensors have been considered highly auspicious biosensors for future directions (Gao et al. 2017; Zhou et al. 2017).

Generally, aptamers have been known as artificial antibodies that may function equally to antibodies and offer great benefits. The reason behind equating aptamers and antibodies is that both the molecules' functions are like affinity agents. Furthermore, antibodies possess the ability to bind with larger molecules, although aptamers may interact with smaller molecules (Pugh et al. 2018). However, the comparison between aptamers and antibodies has been conferred below (Table 4.1).

Immunosensors have been designed for the purpose to recognize the binding of antigens or antibodies (Abs) due to their wonderful target specificity along with affinity (Sharma et al. 2016). However, the antibody-based biosensor is known as an extensive approach for the purpose of development of new tools to diagnose cancer by a resourceful application, as antibodies may be united with various biomaterials and thus may possess an application in a varied range of approaches such as for optical as well as electrochemical biosensors (Du et al. 2013; Wang et al. 2017a).

The utmost salient property of immunosensors, involves the specificity of reaction between antigen and antibody making them very good candidates for the purpose of developing as a diagnostic tool. Several additional advantages of immunosensors are as follows: reduced cost of medicines by decreasing the period of hospitalization because of quick analysis response; ease of use as well as diminishment, and making it suitable for "in-home" or "POC" application, thus enhancing the amenability of patients in follow-up therapy; as well as rapid 176 Biosensors – Micro and Nanoscale Applications response, that might possess a decisive role in life-threatening diseases such as myocardial infarction or infectious diseases (Müller et al. 2007). A general description representing the MC-LR aptasensor and β-LG immunosensor has been discussed below (Figure 4.1; Eissa et al. 2020):

In last two decades, various aptamer-based biosensors has been reported including several studies that highlight their advancement over immunosensors. However, only a few studies have experimentally compared immunosensors and aptasensors under similar conditions which shows inconsistent performance of the sensor. Thus the biosensing performance related to selectivity and sensitivity is similar for both

TABLE 4.1
Comparative chart of aptamers and antibodies

Features	Aptamers	Antibodies
Material	Nucleic acid	Polypeptides
Time of synthesis	Few days or weeks	Few months
Stability	Ambient temperature	Low temperature
Size	Smaller	Larger
Chemical modification	Easy	Difficult or limited
Production	In vitro	In vivo
Cost	Low	Expensive
Toxicity	No humoral response	High
Affinity	High	High
Potential target	Wide range	Limited to immunogenic molecules
Specificity	High	High

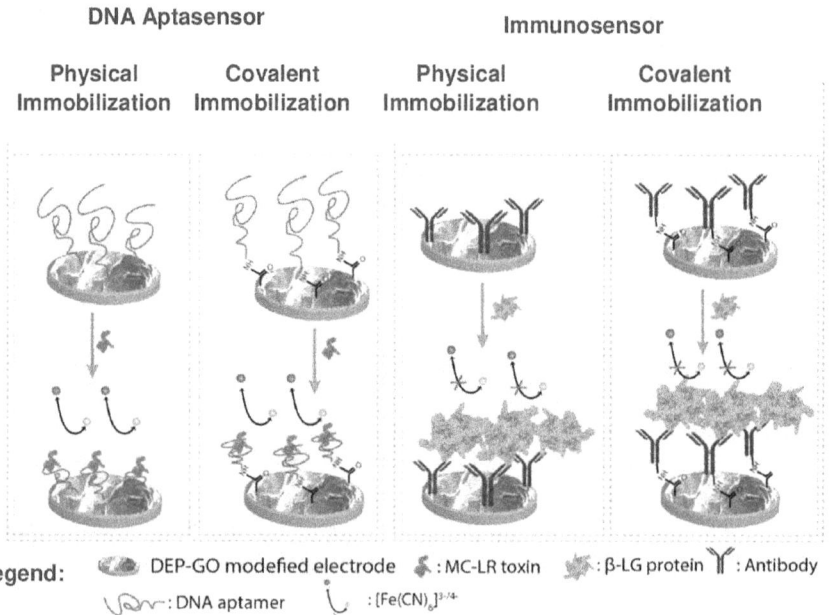

FIGURE 4.1 Representation of the MC-LR aptasensors and β-LG immunosensors (Eissa et al. 2020).

the sensors in the case of various types of transducers likewise based on quartz crystal, nanogap impedance, nano-modified screen printed electrodes, and for porous silicon thin films also (Sharma et al. 2016). Although the factor affecting the performance of the sensor is the immobilization route of the several capturing probes, The comparison between aptasensor and immunosensor has been discussed below:

a. Aptasensor possess enhanced stability and versatile design, and are reusable as compared to immunosensor.
b. The shelf life of aptasensor is significantly longer in comparison to immunosensor.
c. Aptasensors can be stored for several weeks without any sensitivity loss as well as in dry conditions while immunosensors are usually limited to several days though under refrigeration and in wet conditions (Wang et al. 2017).
d. Regeneration of aptasensors can be easily acheived without hampering their activity, thus permitting them to be reusable biosensors. However, in the case of immunosensors regeneration is quite more challenging and the condition must be probed tediously. If the bound target is released from the immunosensor a significant loss in performance has been generally seen because of irreversible damage to the antibodies. Therefore, its regeneration greatly depends upon the specific antibody as well as on its durability (Gao et al. 2017).

e. As compared to immunosensors, in the case of aptasensors the small size of aptamers permits their immobilization in a dense receptor layer on the surface of the biosensor. This helps in extending the biosensor's detection range, enhancing the response of the biosensor as well as the target binding capacity.

4.3 FUNDAMENTALS OF ELECTROCHEMICAL DETECTION OF BIOMARKER

However, the significant principle involved behind the various detection methods of biomarkers is the specific binding that permits to internment of specific targets through natural selection. However, extensively utilized biomarker detection approaches is usually the biomarker sensor based on electrochemistry which has been utilized in various detection areas, such as safety of food (Manikandan et al. 2018) and environment fortification, as well as in space assessment. Depending on the different detection approaches, the biomarker sensors relying on electrochemistry comprise voltammetry-linear sweep, differential pulse, square wave, stripping, and amperometry (Ma et al. 2020). In current scenario years, few biomarker sensors based on electrochemistry have been developed as well as fabricated, which may be categorized into two groups based on enhancing strategy: First, to enhance the apprehension efficacy onto the device surface. Preferably, the biomarker sensor may merely capture biomarkers through precise binding while not capturing several additional contaminations. However, always some predictable factors, and many more factors such as contaminations in the buffer solution, vibrations, as well as changes in temperature may be involved within the detection environment. Second, in the presence of the same concentration of biomarkers the intensity of the signal is enhanced (Sone et al. 2010).

4.4 ELECTROCHEMICAL BEHAVIOUR OF APTASENSOR AND IMMUNOSENSOR

Several studies have generally engrossed on the development of electrochemical aptasensors involving the purpose of identifying cancer biomarkers. However, in the case of a conventional voltametric aptasensor, the aptamers of the biorecognition element have been generally immobilized onto the surface of the electrode in order to identify the target molecules which have been required to be overtly detected (Kunst et al. 2011). As the aptamers bind to the target biomarker and thus the result is a change in electrochemical current, which is then measured. In electrochemical methods, several methods have been engaged for the sensing of aptamer, involving the use of labelling of catalysts like enzymes or redox enzymes, inorganic or organic catalysts, and nanoparticles as well. Labelling of electroactive agents like ferricyanide $[Fe(CN)_6]^{4-/3-}$, ferrocene, methylene blue (MB) bis-anthraquinone modified propanediol have been smeared as the redox-active reporting units within the aptasensor. However, the redox molecule ensues at a definite distance away from the aptamers in the absence of a target, as on generating the electrochemical current

(McQueen 2016). However, in another case, if the analyte or target molecule is present, the analyte molecules are then apprehended as well as absorbed by the aptamer molecules, which leads to the assignment of redox molecules by distinct distances. Such methodology generates as well as records the variances in the electrochemical current which is usually relational to the number of analytes (Shankar and Srivastava 2015).

Usually, the electrochemical aptasensors rely on the process of ligand-induced conformation variation of aptamers or sandwich architecture similar to the antibody-target-antibody sandwich assays. Furthermore, the electrochemical sensors may be either potentiometric or amperometric. Generally, in the potentiometric biosensors the ion-selective electrodes have been utilized for the purpose of signal transduction of a biological reaction into a potential signal through the amperometric biosensors functions through smearing the constant potential as well as monitors the current followed by a reduction or oxidation of an electroactive species intricated in the process of recognition (Stanner et al. 2008). Usually, depending on the change in the mechanistic response of aptasensors, they may be categorised into "signal off" as well as "signal on" approach. Once the target, i.e., a tumour marker protein or cancerous cell meets the aptamers established on the transducer surface, the reaction of the sensor whichever may be reduced or enhanced comprise the "signal off" and "signal on" mechanism, correspondingly (Wu et al. 2016).

The electrochemical aptasensors was first proposed in 2004 and in recent era, it has been known as extremely used biosensors for tumour imaging purposes. They have been known to offer low-power as well as ultra-low detection limits of target analytes. As it offers huge accuracy along with good reproducibility, such a type of sensor may be often applicable as a slightly offensive device. Usually, in this sensor the aptamer has been attached to the surface of the electrode that acts like a biological recognition element With the assistance of the explicit binding of the aptamer with the target, the change in the capacitance instigated by the binding of the analyte and thus the current as well as the potential response produced through the oxidation and reduction reactions onto the surface of the electrode have been evaluated (Qu et al. 2010).

Electrochemical biosensors possess several advantages, like simplicity, low cost, high selectivity as well as high sensitivity. Thus, such types of sensors became prevailing implements in different biomedical areas, particularly in disease diagnosis. It is composed of three main components, i.e., a biological recognition element (aptamer), a transducer as well as a detector. The purpose to select biorecognition element mainly depends on possessing a greater affinity against the analyte. However, the redox behaviour plays an important ant role in the diagnosis of electrochemical aptasensors. In order to record the electrochemical current, the redox molecules have been located at a definite distance just near the aptamer, because of the absence of analyte within the environment. As if, the analyte molecules have been present in the environment, the analyte molecules are then captured as well as absorbed by the aptamer molecules because of the specific affinity among aptamer and analyte, leading to the assignment of redox molecules at various distinct places; such a method makes as well as records various electrochemical currents. Through assessing as well as comparing recorded electrochemical currents, it is highly probable to identify analytes quantitatively though in very lesser amounts with the help of such types of electrochemical aptasensors (Xu et al. 2017; Stanner 2008).

Currently, the electrochemical immunosensors relying on EIS (Electrochemical Impedance Spectroscopy) have attracted huge attention in the field of biosensor developments. However, EIS is a known successful technique as it is generally applied for the study of biosensing systems response at various frequencies. Such type of responses has been instigated by various reactions occurring on the electrode surface. Moreover, EIS is an influential technique due to its non-destructive properties. Likewise, it offers substantial information through directly transforming biological reactions into electrical signals. Furthermore, the EIS system is lesser as well as highly portable as compared to the optic system, additionally, such property gives on-site analysis (Wang et al. 2017).

Electrochemical immunosensor is considered as an tremendous podium for the purpose of analysing cancer biomarkers at the early stage, providing quick results through the tumour profiles, possessing high sensitivity, offering small consumption of sample, as well as its a non-invasive method as compared to classical diagnostic methods. Such properties make it exceptional aspirants for annexation in point-of-care applications which merges the benefits of biosensor devices, electroanalytical methods, as well as the specific reaction of immunorecognition (Sun et al. 2015). Thus, potentially it is likely to accomplish analytical tests outside the amenities of the clinical reference laboratory, as well as decrease the execution time and response of analytical tests as well. Since the last ten years, the aim of electrochemistry has consequently been the apprehension of analyzing and quantifying systems for the greatest pervasive as well as vital tumour markers comprising carcinoma antigen CA (CA125, CA15-3, CA19-9, CA242), prostate-specific antigen (PSA), carcinoembryonic antigen (CEA), α-fetoprotein (AFP) and cytokeratin 19 fragment 211 (CYFRA211) (Fan et al. 2015).

4.5 ROLE OF BIOSENSOR AS DIAGNOSTIC TOOL

The biosensor is referred to as a compact analytical device to detect and quantify a target analyte; first, it is composed of three elements i.e., of a biological receptor like DNA, antibodies, enzymes, cells which precisely analyze the target molecule; second it consists of a transducer, which helps in interpreting the biological recognition event as well as interprets it into a measurable signal; and third it consists of a display unit for the purpose of processing a signal. The upsurge of biosensors is just because of the limitations that the techniques used recently possess high costs, require qualified personnel, and long response time. Such type of complications is incompatible with the initial stage prompt diagnosis (Wang et al. 2017).

In the case of medical applications, biosensors have been fabricated in order to detect as well as quantify biomedical analytes. At the present time, biosensors that are implantable have already been established as well as generally are in use for a few patients, i.e., for continuous observation of glucose. Biosensors may be categorized either through their bioreceptor element or maybe through the transducing mechanism. Hereon, if the antibodies have been employed as bioreceptors they are generally known as immunosensors (Stanner et al. 2008). Usually, antibodies have been known as the highly essential bioreceptors for targeting specific analytes, which grosses benefits of the greatly specific non-covalent interaction among antibodies and antigens. Based on the transducer type, they are generally classified as optical, mechanical, and electrochemical. In addition, the electrochemical technique may be sectioned as amperometric, potentiometric, conductometric, and impedimetric (Sone et al. 2010).

4.5.1 OPTICAL BIOSENSORS

As a response to the biorecognition process, optical transducers are known to have mostly relied on the variations in the phase, amplitude, polarization, or frequency of the input light. Usually, the general classes of optical biosensors comprised colorimetric, fluorescence luminescence, surface plasma resonance, and fibre-optics based biosensors. Hereon, the biorecognition element might be either labelled with the help of chromogenic or fluorescent dyes, or it may be label free. In addition to this, optical biosensors may be known as one of the highly sensitive methods which permit a limit of detection down to pg/ml. Moreover, the optical biosensor possesses bulky instrumentation, which is highly expensive and time-consuming, and needs sophisticated personnel in order to conduct the tests (Justino et al. 2010).

4.5.2 MECHANICAL BIOSENSORS

Transducers depending on the mechanical approaches can detect modifications in mechanical properties, such as mass, surface stress, effective Young's modulus, and visco elasticity in biorecognition interactions as well (Tamayo et al. 2013). Thus, such type of biosensors has not been well known as compared to optical as well as electrochemical sensors due to their intricacy. Amongst mechanical biosensors, the QCM sensors are known to be vastly established ones, which mostly rely on quartz crystal resonators (Lange et al. 2008). Here the electrical signal has been produced as the crystal being distorted through the piezoelectric technique. The change in mass befalls as the analyte binds to the biorecognition element which is then immobilized onto the surface of the crystal. Mechanical biosensors involve several advantages such as QCM which includes high sensitivity as well as vast dynamic range of recognition spanning that ranges between the nanomolar to femtomolar as well as the flexibility that is to be pertinent virtually at any coating surface for the purpose of assays. However, the chief detriment is somewhat an unwieldy method for handling samples i.e. the conversion of liquid phase to solid phase that may be vulnerable in order to produce measurement artefacts (Arlett et al. 2011).

4.5.3 ELECTROCHEMICAL BIOSENSORS

The electrochemical biosensor is extensively used sensor approach because of the less expensive, ease of use, portability, as well as possess simple fabrication. Using an electrochemical biosensor, as the target analyte, has been detected to frequently produce the current (amperometry), a charge accumulation or potential (potentiometry), or variation in conductivity (conductometry/impedimetry) (Justino et al. 2010). In voltammetric biosensors, the concentration of detecting agents, like the secondary

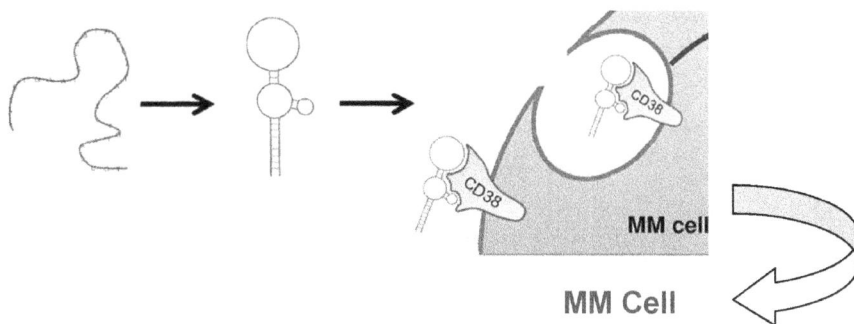

FIGURE 4.2   The binding mechanism of aptamers with the target (Yuspian et al. 2021).

antibody labelled with an enzyme or other reporter which might support the generation of electroactive species, doesn't affect the electrochemical signal which is generated. Consequently, the elimination of detecting agent which is not bound is not compulsory, which may expressively diminish the operation time. A typical voltammetric biosensor consists of whichever of a three-electrode system i.e., a working electrode, a reference electrode, and a counter electrode, or a two-electrode system composed only of a working electrode and a reference electrode (Lange et al. 2008). However, the two-electrode system is quite easy and is less expensive as a disposable sensor. The electrodes of biosensors might be merely miniaturized, as well as various nanomaterials such as nanowires, nanoparticles, and carbon nanotubes may be assimilated onto the sensor so that it enhances their sensitivity (Yuspian et al. 2021). However, the development of aptamers relying on voltammetric biosensors with different immobilization procedures as well as electrodes for the purpose of signal enhancement and amplification so as to identify various biomarkers have been shown below (Figure 4.2; Yuspian et al. 2021).

Moreover, a bioreceptor applied for the detection of samples and analytes, like enzymes, proteins, antibodies, cells, or several biochemistry compounds, thus in contrast, on aptasensor, aptamers have been utilized as bioreceptors. The bioreceptor selectively interrelated with a sample as well as an analyte thus producing the measuring specific signal (Maryam et al. 2021). The schematic depiction of the electrochemical biosensor is described below (Figure 4.3; Maryam et al. 2021)

4.6   DETECTION OF BIOLOGICAL ANALYTES USING APTASENSORS

Currently, various voltammetric aptasensors have been proposed so as to identify specific cells, biological molecules, biomarkers, proteins, genes, and enzymes along with hormones using different methods like EIS, SWV, DPV, CV, and chronocoulometric (Kavosi et al. 2015; Wang et al. 2015). Particularly, biomarkers have been found to be known as a substantial focus of aptasensors. The, biomarkers along with the cells, proteins, and nucleic acids, are known as such types of molecules that possess atypical expression, activity, as well as inactivity that might be perceived in pathologic situations. However, they may be used as indicators in order to evaluate

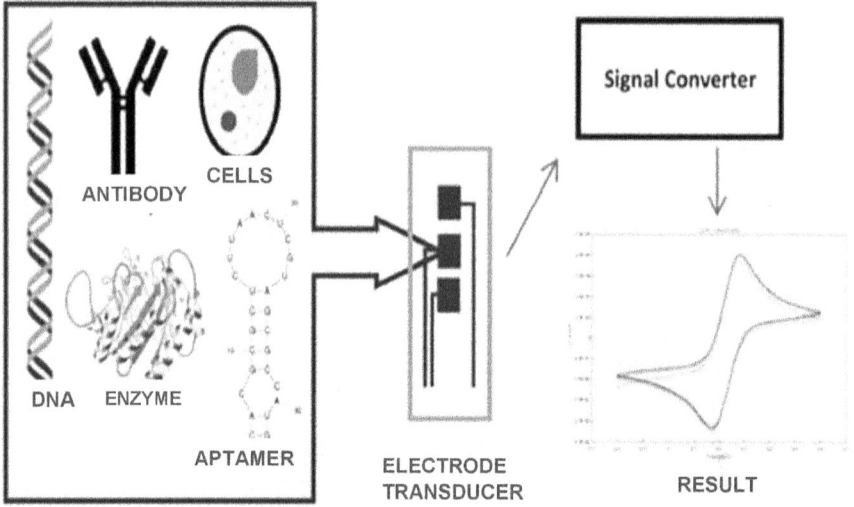

FIGURE 4.3   Electrochemical biosensor with several bioreceptors (Maryam et al. 2021).

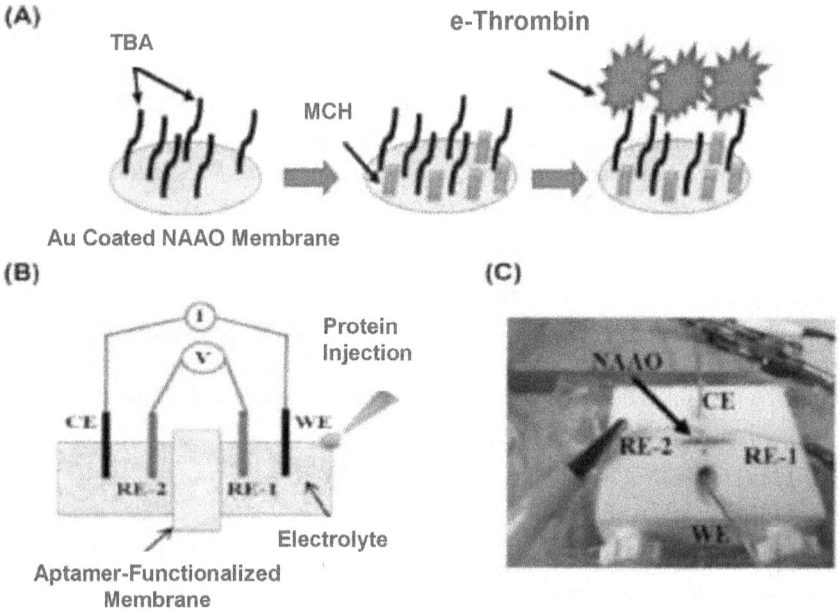

FIGURE 4.4 (a) Schematic showing membrane immobilization steps. (b) The four-electrode scheme is shown. (c) The Teflon cell as used in the electrochemical experiments with the Nanoporous anodized alumina or aluminum oxide (NAAO) membrane and the four-electrode set-up (Gosai et al. 2019).

either normal or pathologic conditions. However, the application of aptamers in the diagnosis of biomarker particularly relying in the case of cancer disease have risen because of their selective target affinity as well as allowing chemical modification (Ilkhani et al. 2015; Lu et al. 2015). Thus, aptamers might also identify insignificant differences among proteins having analogous structures, and such sole property permits aptamers to differentiate cancer cells from healthy ones. However, discernment till now has been known as an apprehension for cancer aptasensors due to the complexity of cancer cells. Moreover, the concentrations of disease-related biomarkers typically may not be identified in the initial stage of the disease (Chen at al. 2014; Heydari-Bafrooei and Shamszadeh 2017). Therefore, the detection of the disease-related biomarkers in a timely manner as possible along with the smaller concentrations has been found to be highly anticipated. To detect several classes of biological analytes along with their sensitivities, a few examples of aptasensosrs have been discussed below (Table 4.2) along with the schematic representation showing membrane immobilization and four-electrode systems (Figure 4.4; Gosai et al. 2019).

TABLE 4.2
Biological analyte detection using aptasensors

Technique	Biological analyte	Target analyte	Detection limit	References
DPV	HeLa	Cell	10 cell/mL	Wang et al. (2015)
DPV	K562	Cell	14 cell/mL	Lu et al. (2015)
DPV	CCRF-CEM (human leukaemic lymphoblast)	Cell	10 cell/Ml	Chen et al. (2015)
EIS, CV	MCF-7	Cell	8 cell/mL	Wang et al. (2017)
EIS	MCF-7	Cell	36 cell/mL	Zhou et al. (2019)
DPV, EIS	PSA	Biomarker	1 pg/mL	Heydari-Bafrooei and Shamszadeh (2017)
DPV	EGFR (epidermal growth factor receptor)	Biomarker	50 pg/mL	Ilkhani et al. (2015)
EIS	PSA	Biomarker	5 pg/mL	Kavosi et al. (2015)
CV, EIS	Serpin A12	Biomarker	0.031 ng/mL	Salek et al. (2020)
EIS, CV, DPV	MUC1 (Mucin 1)	Biomarker	0.62 ppb	Taleat et al. (2014)
EIS	Cardiac Troponin I	Biomarker	1.23 pM	Qiao et al. (2018)
DPV	Cardiac Troponin I	Biomarker	16 pg/mL	Sun et al. (2019)
Amperometry	Interleukin 6	Biomarker	0.33 pg/mL	Tertis et al. (2017)
Amperometry	Human factor IX	Biomarker	6 pM	Letchumanan et al. (2019)
DPV, EIS	Alpha-fetoprotein	Protein	61.8 fg/mL	Huang et al. (2019)
EIS	Thrombin	Protein	10 pM	Gosai et al. (2019)
DPV	Insulin	Hormone	0.18 fM	Tabrizi et al. (2017)
CV, EIS	Thyroxine(T4)	Hormone	10.33 pM	Park et al. (2020)
CV, EIS	Progesterone (P4)	Hormone	1.86 pM	Samie and Arvand (2020)

4.7   APPLICATION OF APTASENSORS TO DETECT SEVERAL BIOMARKERS

Though the study of biomarkers in blood, urine as well as in other body fluids is considered one of the approaches that may be incorporated in the early diagnose of diseases. However, aptasensors have been exploited for the diagnosis of biomarkers, like thrombin and immunoglobulin (Ig) E. However, the fabrication of the object-electrode along with the Transmission Electron Microscopy (TEM) micrograph for cocaine-encapsulated liposome helps in releasing the encapsulated cocaine into the numbering incubation beaker thus followed by adding SH-CBA2 in the incubation beaker to get the incubation sample, and after that the fabrication of measure-electrode and ECL response before and after binding with the cocaine, respectively has been explained schematically (Figure 4.5; Mao et al. 2011). The application of aptasensors to detect biomarkers has been described in Table 4.3.

4.8   APPLICATION OF APTASENSORS TO DETECT CANCER BIOMARKERS

Nowadays, cancers have posed a substantial menace for the human health around the world. The number of cases related to cancer is rising per year, however, the general

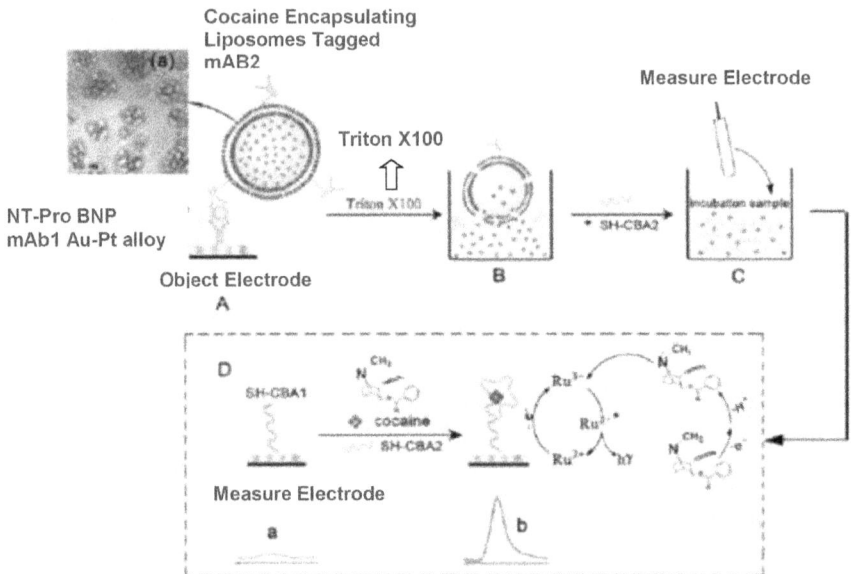

FIGURE 4.5   The schematic illustration for (a) The fabrication of the object-electrode and the TEM micrograph for cocaine-encapsulated liposome (A). (B) Releasing the encapsulated cocaine into the numbering incubation beaker. (C) Followed by adding SH-CBA2 in the incubation beaker to get the incubation sample. (D) The fabrication of measure-electrode and ECL response before (a) and after (b) binding with cocaine respectively (Mao et al. 2011).

TABLE 4.3
Aptasensors for biomarkers detection

Target biomarker	Aptamer	Type of detection	Limit of detection	References
Thrombin	DNA labelled with the hollow CoPt alloy nanoparticle onto a reduced graphene oxide sheet (HCoPt-RGs) conjugates	Sandwich-type	1.0×10^{-12} to 5.0×10^{-8} M/3.4×10^{-13} M	Wang et al. (2011)
Thrombin	DNA dual labelled with AuNPs and horseradish peroxidase (HRP)	Sandwich-type	0.1–60 Pm/30 Fm	Zhao et al. (2011)
Thrombin	DNA	Label-free detection	0–0.02 Mm/0.1 Nm	Pu et al. (2009)
Thrombin	DNA labelled with a hole injector, naphthalimide, and a fluorophore, Alexa532	DNA charge transport	5 Pm to 5 Nm/1.2 Pm	Zhao et al. (2011)
Thrombin	DNA SA-ALP and biotinylated labelled	Sandwich-type	1×10–15 to 1×10–8 M/0.33 Fm	Liao et al. (2011)
Immunoglobulin (IgE)	DNA streptavidin labelled	ELISA-like array	Not specified (n.s./n.s.)	Wang et al. (2008)
Immunoglobulin (IgE)	DNA labelled with avidin monolayer	Direct detection	2.5–200 µg/L/2.5 µg/L	Yao et al. (2009)
Immunoglobulin (IgE)	DNA labelled with single polypyrrole (PPy) nanowire-based microfluidic	One-step electrochemical deposition method	0.1–100 Nm/0.01 Nm	Huang et al. (2011)
Immunoglobulin (IgE)	DNA attached to carboxyl (COOH)-modified nanocrystalline diamond (NCD) surface	Direct and label-free detection	0.03–42.8 µg/ML/0.03 µg/ML	Tran et al. (2011)
Retinol binding protein (RBP4)	Single-stranded DNA	Label-free detection	0.2–0.5 µg/ML/75 Nm	Lee et al. (2008)
C-reactive protein (CRP)	RNA biotinylated	Direct detection	n.s./0.005 ppm	Bini et al. (2008)
C-reactive protein (CRP)	DNA	Sandwich-type	10 µg/L to 100 mg/L/n.s.	Pultar et al. (2009)
N-terminal pro-brain natriuretic peptide (NT-proBNP)	DNA with cocaine-binding	Sandwich-type	0.01–500 ng/ML/0.77 pg/ML	Mao et al. (2011)
Interferon (IFN) gamma	DNA thiolated/MB redox tag	Direct detection	10 Nm/0.06 Nm	Liu et al. (2010)

cause in several cases of mortality as well as morbidity across the world is the late detection of the disease. However, the recognition of tumour cells usually relies upon the identification of biomarkers of cancer (Yang et al. 2016). Cancer biomarkers are generally composed of various molecular origins, including free DNA, RNA, or protein/glycoproteins along with circulating tumour cells. In recent eras, cancer-derived exosomes have attained a huge consideration as a biomarker for the early detection as well as drug sensitivity analysis of cancer. Various current studies have efficaciously utilized aptamers to detect as well as to measure the expression and action of target molecules which effect the behaviour of tumour or may persuade an alteration in response to therapy (Borghei et al. 2016). Numerous aptasensors for the purpose of detecting different cancers have been discussed in the chapter. Although, the fabrication process of the electrochemical aptasensor for the determination of $VEGF_{165}$ is described (Figure 4.6; Amouzadeh et al. 2015). Table 4.4 describes the aptasensors for several cancer targets comprising the types of nucleic acid of the aptamer (DNA or RNA), the signal transduction mode.

Figure 4.6 depicts the fabrication process of the electrochemical aptasensor for the $VEGF_{165}$ determination using screen printed electrodes.

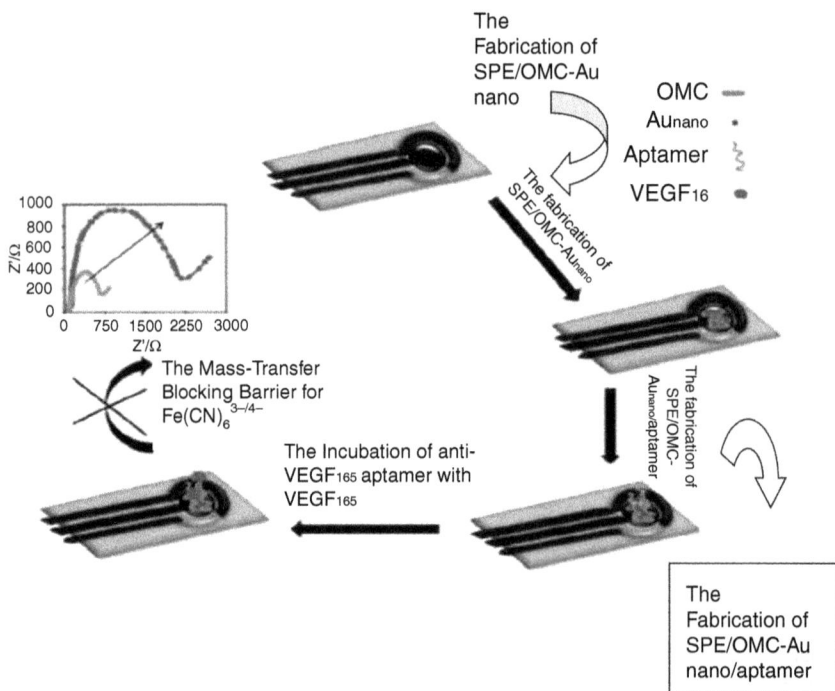

FIGURE 4.6   Fabrication process of electrochemical aptasensor for the $VEGF_{165}$ determination (Amouzadeh et al. 2015).

TABLE 4.4

Cancer biomarker detection using aptasensors

S. no.	Biomarker	Aptamer	Type of detection	Transduction mode	Limit of detection	References
1.	Human Burkitt's lymphoma Ramos cells	Amino-substituted DNA aptamer (TD05)	Sandwich assay	Electrochemical	55 cells/mL	Yang et al. (2016)
2.	Lung cancer protein	Thiolated DNA	Sandwich assay	Electrochemical	2.3 ng/mL	Zamay et al. (2016)
3.	MUC1	Thiolated DNA	Sandwich assay	Electrochemical	1pM	Chen et al. (2015)
4.	MCF7	DNA	Colorimetry Direct detection	Optical	10 cells	Borghei et al. (2016)
5.	VEGF$_{165}$	DNA labelled with the amino group	Label-free DPV	Electrochemical	0.32 pM, 0.48pM	Shamsipur et al. (2015)
6.	PSA	Thiolated DNA	Fluorescence	Optical	0.029 aM	Wu et al. (2015)
7.	CEA	CEA DNA aptamer linked to hemin aptamer using adenines linker	Chemiluminescence	Optical	0.58 ng/mL	Khang et al. (2017)
8.	ER α	RNA	Colorimetry	Optical	0.64 ng/mL	Ahirwar and Nahar (2016)
9.	VEGF	Thiolated DNA	Enzyme amplification	Electrochemical	30 nmol/L	Lim et al. (2010)
10.	VEGF$_{165}$	DNA labelled with a thiol group	Label-free, EIS, CV	Electrochemical	1.0 pg/mL	Amouzadeh et al. (2015)
11.	K562 cells	DNA labelled with amino and C6 linker	Indirectly by DNA-based assay	Electrochemical	14 cells/mL	Lu et al. (2015)
12.	MUC1 MCF7	DNA labelled with Cy3	Fluorescence	Optical	6.52 nmol/L (MUC1) 8500 cells/mL (MCF7)	Li et al. (2015)
13.	A549	DNA labelled with amino	Direct Chronoamperometric	Electrochemical	8 cells/mL	Mir et al. (2015)
14.	CCRF-CEM cells	DNA	Label-free visual detection, colorimetric	Optical	40 cells	Zhang et al. (2014)
15.	OPN	RNA labelled with Biotin	CV	Electrochemical	8 nM	Meirinho et al. (2015)

4.9 VOLTAMMETRIC IMMUNOSENSORS TO DETECT CANCER BIOMARKERS

Recently, various range of biomarkers have been applied as prognostic tools so as to diagnose cancer on an initial stages; for instance, breast cancer possess the human epidermal growth factor receptor 2 (HER2) as well as estrogen and progesterone receptors; colorectal cancer has the epidermal growth factor (EGFR), along with the KRAS gene as well as the UDP-glucuronosyltransferase1–1 (UGT-1A); leukaemia and lymphoma have and the CD20 and CD30 cytokines, the platelet-derived growth factor receptor (PDGFR) and the promyelocytic leukaemia protein; lung cancer involves the EGFR, KRAS gene and the echinoderm microtubule associated protein-like 4 (EML4); melanoma has the BRAF gene; pancreas cancer has elevated levels of leucine, isoleucine and valine; ovary cancer possess the cancer antigen 125 (CA125) whereas the prostate cancer includes PSA, vascular endothelial growth factor (VEGF) as well as transmembrane glycoprotein mucin type 1 (MUC1) (Marques et al. 2014). Moreover, the complete process of preparing immunosensor for alpha-fetoprotein has been described (Figure 4.7; Wang et al. 2017). Hereon, different types of biomarker detection especially the general protein biomarkers associated with cancer diagnosis have been discussed below (Table 4.5).

4.10 FUTURE DIRECTIONS

The progression in science and technology has exposed a drastic expansion in the analysis of cancer at an initial stage. The findings of novel biomarkers as well as the

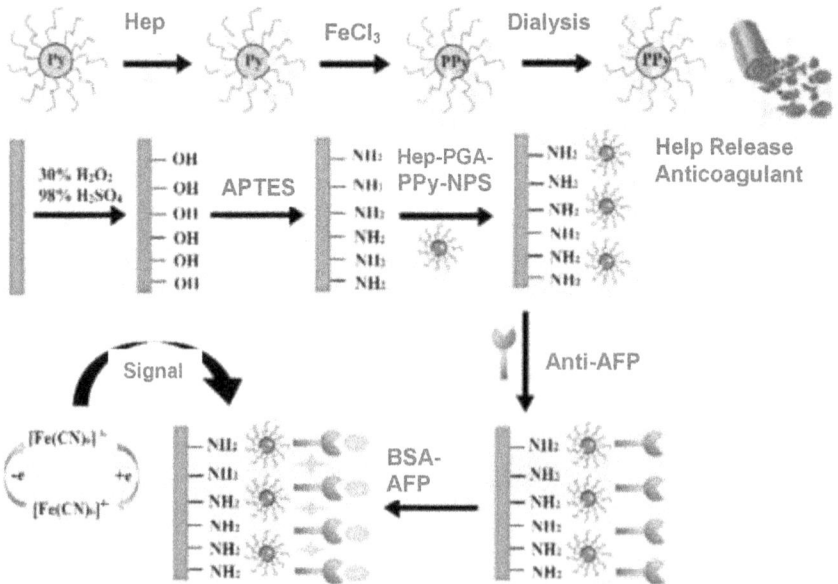

FIGURE 4.7 Preparation process of immunosensor for alpha-fetoprotein (Wang et al. 2017).

TABLE 4.5

Biomarkers detection using immunosensors

Cancer	Sample	Biomarker	Limit of detection	References
Prostate	Serum	PSA	7.0 pg/mL	Marques et al. (2014)
Liver	Blood	AFP	0.099 ng/mL	Qu et al. (2010)
Stomach	Spiked Serum Sample	CA 72–4	0.10 U/mL	Sun et al. (2015)
Breast	Spiked Human Serum	HER2	0.10 U/mL	Vashist and Luong (2018)
Colorectal	Serum	CA 19–9	0.0063 U/mL	Yang et al. (2015)
	PBS	EGFR	4 pg/mL	
	Human Plasma		0.34 pg/mL	
			0.88 pg/mL	
Lung	Serum	NSE	0.26 pg/mL	Wang et al. (2017)
Ovary	Serum	CA-125	0.0016 U/mL	Lennon et al. (2018)

expansion of profound diagnostic components have not merely enhanced the situation of cancer patients but it also exposed a significant upsurge in their endurance. Aptamers have been known as a novel class of bioreceptors due to their exceptional selectivity, sensitivity, as well as specificity to their target. Due to tremendous stability, easy reproducibility, design flexibility, robustness, as well as cost-effectiveness, aptasensors possess the perspectives to astound the deficient of most traditional biosensors. Since the last few periods, a large number of aptamer-based biosensors have been fabricated. Generally, the potential of aptasensor is highly enormous in the analysis of cancer.

Thus, novel techniques expending magnetic nanoparticles, quantum dots, carbon nanotubes, noble metal nanoparticles, or hybrid nanomaterials, either as labels or immobilization platforms, have enhanced the various electrochemical immunosensors as well as their applications in various fields. Because of their huge selectivity and sensitivity, as well as the prospect to reduce such systems, the application of electrochemical immunosensors aimed at the purpose of in vivo use is highly conceivable. Though several developments have been made in the areas of immunosensors, new approaches have been still required to progress the selectivity, sensitivity, as well as simplicity of such devices, which are all set to meet the crucial necessities of clinical analysis or for industrial purposes. Thus, the necessity to miniaturize as well as integrate into an electronic platform made them suitable to detect the biomarkers or pathogens at present are known as the additional challenges in such active regions of research.

REFERENCES

Ahirwar, R. and P. Nahar (2016) Development of a label-free gold nanoparticle-based colorimetric aptasensor for detection of human estrogen receptor alpha. *Anal. Bioanal. Chem* 408: 327–332.

Amouzadeh Tabrizi, M., M. Shamsipur and L. Farzin (2015) A high sensitive electrochemical aptasensor for the determination of VEGF(165) in serum of lung cancer patient. *Biosens. Bioelectron* 74: 764–769.

Arlett, J., E. Myers and M. Roukes (2011) Comparative advantages of mechanical biosensors. *Nat. Nanotechnol* 6: 203–215.

Borrebaeck, C. A. K. (2017) Precision diagnostics: moving towards protein biomarker signatures of clinical utility in cancer. *Nat. Rev. Cancer* 17: 199–204.

Brody, E. N. and L. Gold (2000) Aptamers as therapeutic and diagnostic agents. *J. Biotechnol* 74: 5–13.

Bhalla, N., P. Jolly, N. Formisano and P. Estrela (2016) Introduction to biosensors. *Essays Biochem* 60: 1–8.

Balamurugan, S., A. Obubuafo, S. A. Soper and D. A. Spivak (2008) Surface immobilization methods for aptamer diagnostic applications. *Anal. Bioanal. Chem* 390: 1009–1021.

Bini, A., S. Centi, S. Tombelli, M. Minunni and M. Mascini (2008) Development of an optical RNA-based aptasensor for C-reactive protein. *Anal. Bioanal. Chem* 390: 1077–1086.

Boltz, A., B. Piater, L. Toleikis, R. Guenther, H. Kolmar and B. Hock (2011) Bi-specific aptamers mediating tumor cell lysis. *J. Biol. Chem* 286: 21896–21905.

Borghei, Y. S., M. Hosseini, M. Dadmehr, S. Hosseinkhani, M. R. Ganjali and R. Sheikhnejad (2016) Visual detection of cancer cells by colorimetric aptasensor based on aggregation of gold nanoparticles induced by DNA hybridization. *Anal. Chim. Acta* 904: 92–97.

Chandra, P., J. Singh, A. Singh, A. Srivastava, R. N. Goyal and Y. B. Shim (2013) Gold nanoparticles and nanocomposites in clinical diagnostics using electrochemical methods. *J. Nanoparticles* 2013: 1–12.

Chen, M., Z. Tang, C. Ma and Y. Yan (2020) A fluorometric aptamer based assay for prostate specific antigen based on enzyme-assisted target recycling. *Sens. Actuators B Chem* 302: 127178.

Chen, X. J., Y. Z. Wang, Y. Y. Zhang, Z. H. Chen, Y. Liu, Z. L. Li and J. H. Li (2014) Sensitive electrochemical aptamer biosensor for dynamic cell surface n-glycan evaluation featuring multivalent recognition and signal amplification on a dendrimer-graphene electrode interface. *Anal. Chem* 86: 4278–4286.

Chen, X., Q. Zhang, C. Qian, N. Hao, L. Xu and C. Yao (2015) Electrochemical aptasensor for mucin 1 based on dual signal amplification of poly(o-phenylenediamine) carrier and functionalized carbon nanotubes tracing tag. *Biosens. Bioelectron* 64: 485–492.

Chung, L., K. Moore, L. Phillips, F. M. Boyle, D. J. Marsh and R. C. Baxter (2014) Novel serum protein biomarker panel revealed by mass spectrometry and its prognostic value in breast cancer. *Breast Cancer Res* 16: R63.

Downs, A. M., J. Gerson, M. N. Hossain, K. Ploense, M. Pham, H. B. Kraatz, T. Kippin and K. W. Plaxco (2021) Nanoporous gold for the miniaturization of in vivo electrochemical aptamer-based sensors. *ACS Sens* 6: 2299–2306.

Du, Y., B. Li and E. Wang (2013) Fitting makes "sensing" simple: label-free detection strategies based on nucleic acid aptamers. *Acc. Chem. Res* 46: 203–213.

Edgell, T. A., D. L. Barraclough, A. Rajic, J. Dhulia, K. J. Lewis, J. E. Armes, R. Barraclough, P. S. Rudland, G. E. Rice and D. J. Autelitano (2010) Increased plasma concentrations of anterior gradient 2 protein are positively associated with ovarian cancer. *Clin. Sci* 118: 717–725.

Ellington, A. D. and J. W. Szostak (1990) *In vitro* selection of RNA molecules that bind specific ligands. *Nature* 346: 818–822.

Eissa, S., J. N'diaye, P. Brisebois, R. Izquierdo, A. C. Tavares, and M. Siaj (2020) Probing the influence of graphene oxide sheets size on the performance of label-free electrochemical biosensors. *Sci. Rep* 10: 1–12.

Fan, H., Z. Guo, L. Gao, Y. Zhang, D. Fan, G. Ji, B. Du and Q. Wei (2015) Ultrasensitive electrochemical immunosensor for carbohydrate antigen 72–4 based on dual signal amplification strategy of nanoporous gold and polyaniline-Au asymmetric multicomponent nanoparticles. *Biosens. Bioelectron* 64: 51.

Gooding, J. J. and K. Gaus (2016) Single-molecule sensors: challenges and opportunities for quantitative analysis. *Angew. Chem. Int. Ed* 55: 11354–11366.

Giljohann, D. A. and C. A. Mirkin (2009) Drivers of biodiagnostic development. *Nature* 462: 461–464.

Goda, T., D. Higashi, A. Matsumoto, T. Hoshi, T. Sawaguchi and Y. Miyahara (2015) Dual aptamer-immobilized surfaces for improved affinity through multiple target binding in potentiometric thrombin biosensing. *Biosens. Bioelectron* 73: 174–180.

Gao, F., F. Zhou, S. Chen, Y. Yao, J. Wu, D. Yin, D. Geng and P. Wang (2017) Proximity hybridization triggered rolling-circle amplification for sensitive electrochemical homogeneous immunoassay. *Analyst* 142: 4308–4316.

Gosai, A., B. S. Hau Yeah, M. Nilsen-Hamilton and P. Shrotriya (2019) Label free thrombin detection in presence of high concentration of albumin using an aptamer-functionalized nanoporous membrane. *Biosens. Bioelectron* 126: 88–95.

Henry, N. L. and D. F. Hayes (2012) Cancer biomarkers. *Mol. Oncol* 6: 140–146.

Hermann, T. and D. J. Patel (2000) Adaptive recognition by nucleic acid aptamers. *Science* 287: 820–825.

Huang, H., R. C. Ideh, E. Gitau, M. L. Thézénas, M. Jallow, B. Ebruke, O. Chimah, C. Oluwalana, H. Karanja, G. Mackenzie, R. A. Adegbola, D. Kwiatkowski, B. M. Kessler, J. A. Berkley, S. R. C. Howie and C. Casals-Pascual (2014) Discovery and validation of biomarkers to guide clinical management of pneumonia in African children. *Clin. Infect. Dis* 58: 1707–1715.

Hou, L., X. Wu, G. Chen, H. Yang, M. Lu and D. Tang (2015) HCR-stimulated formation of DNAzyme concatamers on gold nanoparticle for ultrasensitive impedimetric immunoassay. *Biosens. Bioelectron* 68: 487–493.

Heydari-Bafrooei, E. and N. S. Shamszadeh (2017) Electrochemical bioassay development for ultrasensitive aptasensing of prostate specific antigen. *Biosens. Bioelectron* 91: 284–292.

Huang, X. Y., B. B. Cui, Y. S. Ma, X. Yan, L. Xia, N. Zhou, M. H. Wang, L. H. He and Z. H. Zhang (2019) Three-dimensional nitrogen-doped mesoporous carbon nanomaterials derived from plant biomass: cost-effective construction of label-free electrochemical aptasensor for sensitively detecting alpha-fetoprotein. *Anal. Chim. Acta* 1078: 125–134.

Huang, J., X. Luo, I. Lee, Y. Hu, X. T. Cui and M. Yun (2011) Rapid real-time electrical detection of proteins using single conducting polymer nanowire-based microfluidic aptasensor. *Biosens. Bioelectron* 30: 306–309.

Iliuk, A. B., L. Hu and W. A. Tao (2011) Aptamer in bioanalytical applications. *Anal. Chem* 83: 4440–4452.

Ilkhani, H., M. Sarparast, A. Noori, S. Z. Bathaie and M. F. Mousavi (2015) Electrochemical aptamer/antibody based sandwich immunosensor for the detection of EGFR, a cancer biomarker, using gold nanoparticles as a signaling probe. *Biosens. Bioelectron* 74: 491–497.

Jia, X., X. Chen, J. Han, J. Ma and Z. Ma (2014) A label-free immunosensor based on graphene nanocomposites for simultaneous multiplexed electrochemical determination of tumor markers. *Biosens. Bioelectron* 53: 65–70.

Justino, C. I., T. A. Rocha-Santos and A. C. Duarte (2010) Review of analytical figures of merit of sensors and biosensors in clinical applications. *Trends Anal. Chem* 29: 1172–1183.

Kavosi, B., A. Salimi, R. Hallaj and F. Moradi (2015) Ultrasensitive electrochemical immunosensor for PSA biomarker detection in prostate cancer cells using gold nanoparticles/PAMAM dendrimer loaded with enzyme linked aptamer as integrated triple signal amplification strategy. *Biosens. Bioelectron* 74: 915–923.

Kelley, S. O. (2017) What are clinically relevant levels of cellular and biomolecular analytes? *ACS Sens* 2: 193–197.

Kelley, S. O., C. A. Mirkin, D. R. Walt, R. F. Ismagilov, M. Toner and E. H. Sargent (2014) Advancing the speed, sensitivity and accuracy of biomolecular detection using multi-length-scale engineering. *Nat. Nanotechnol* 9: 969–980.

Khang, H., K. Cho, S. Chong and J. H. Lee (2017) All-in-one dual-aptasensor capable of rapidly quantifying carcinoembryonic antigen. *Biosens. Bioelectron* 90: 46–52.

Kunst, A., K. Stronks and C. Agyemang (2011) Non-communicable diseases. Migration and health in the European Union, 1(116).

Lange, K., B. E. Rapp and M. Rapp (2008) Surface acoustic wave biosensors: a review. *Anal. Bioanal. Chem* 391: 1509–1519.

Lee, S. J., B. S. Youn, J. W. Park, J. H. Niazi, Y. S. Kim and M. B. Gu (2008) ssDNA aptamer-based surface plasmon resonance biosensor for the detection of retinol binding protein 4 for the early diagnosis of type 2 diabetes. *Anal. Chem* 80: 2867–2873.

Letchumanan, I., S. C. B. Gopinath, M. K. Md Arshad, P. Anbu and T. Lakshmipriya (2019) Gold nano-urchin integrated label-free amperometric aptasensing human blood clotting factor IX: a prognosticative approach for "Royal disease". *Biosens. Bioelectron* 131: 128–135.

Lennon, R. P., K. A. Claussen and K. A. Kuersteiner (2018) State of the heart: an overview of the disease burden of cardiovascular disease from an epidemiologic perspective. *Prim. Care Clin. Pract* 45: 1–15.

Li, C., Y. Meng, S. Wang, M. Qian, J. Wang, W. Lu and R. Huang (2015) Mesoporous carbon nanospheres featured fluorescent aptasensor for multiple diagnosis of cancer *in vitro* and *in vivo*. *ACS Nano* 9: 12096–12103.

Liao, Y., R. Yuan, Y. Chai, Y. Zhuo, Y. Yuan, L. Bai, L. Mao and S. Yuan (2011) In-situ produced ascorbic acid as coreactant for an ultrasensitive solid-state tris(2,2'-bipyridyl) ruthenium(II) electrochemiluminescence aptasensor. *Biosens. Bioelectron* 26: 4815–4818.

Lim, D. K., K. S. Jeon, H. M. Kim, J. M. Nam and Y. D. Suh (2010) Nanogap-engineerable Raman-active nanodumbbells for single-molecule detection. *Nat. Mater* 9: 60–67.

Liu, Y., N. Tuleouva, E. Ramanculov and A. Revzin (2010) Aptamer-based electrochemical biosensor for interferon gamma detection. *Anal. Chem* 82: 8131–8136.

Lu, C. Y., J. J. Xu, Z. H. Wang and H. Y. Chen (2015) A novel signal-amplified electrochemical aptasensor based on supersandwich G-quadruplex DNAzyme for highly sensitive cancer cell detection. *Electrochem. Commun* 52: 49–52.

Luu, T. T. T., D. H. Bach, D. Kim, R. Hu, H. J. Park and S. K. Lee (2020) Overexpression of AGR2 is associated with drug resistance in mutant non-small cell lung cancers. *Anticancer Res* 40: 1855–1866.

Ma, H., J. Liu, M. M. Ali, M. A. I. Mahmood, L. Labanieh, M. Lu, S. M. Iqbal, Q. Zhang, W. Zhao and Y. Wan (2015) Nucleic acid aptamers in cancer research, diagnosis and therapy. *Chem. Soc. Rev* 44: 1240–1256.

Ma, H., B. Zhao, Z. Liu, C. Du and B. Shou (2020) Local chemistry–electrochemistry and stress corrosion susceptibility of X80 steel below disbonded coating in acidic soil environment under cathodic protection. *Constr. Build. Mater* 243: 118203.

Manikandan, V. S., B. R. Adhikari and A. Chen (2018) Nanomaterial based electrochemical sensors for the safety and quality control of food and beverages. *Analyst* 143: 4537–4554.

Mao, L., R. Yuan, Y. Chai, Y. Zhuo and Y. Xiang (2011) Signal-enhancer molecules encapsulated liposome as a valuable sensing and amplification platform combining the aptasensor for ultrasensitive ECL immunoassay. *Biosens. Bioelectron* 26: 4204–4208.

Marques, R. C. B., S. Viswanathan, H. P. A. Nouws, C. D. Matos and M. B. G. Garcia (2014) Electrochemical immunosensor for the analysis of the breast cancer biomarker HER2 ECD. *Talanta* 129: 599.

Maryam, N., H. Arnab, M. Mohsen, P. Marta, A. Jon and S. Yi (2021) A multivalent aptamer-based electrochemical biosensor for biomarker detection in urinary tract infection. *Electrochim. Acta* 389: 138644.

Mascini, M. (2009) *Aptamers in Bioanalysis.* (Vol. 314). New York: Wiley.

Mascini, M. and S. Tombelli (2008) Biosensors for biomarkers in medical diagnostics. *Biomarkers* 13: 637–657.

McQueen, D. V. (2016) Global Handbook on Noncommunicable Diseases and Health Promotion. New York: Springer.

Meirinho, S. G., L. G. Dias, A. M. Peres and L. R. Rodrigues (2015) Voltammetric aptasensors for protein disease biomarkers detection: a review. *Biosens. Bioelectron* 71: 332–341.

Mills, K. H. G. (2011) TLR-dependent T cell activation in autoimmunity. *Nat. Rev. Immunol* 11: 807–822.

Mir, T. A., J. H. Yoon, N. G. Gurudatt, M. S. Won and Y. B. Shim (2015) Ultrasensitive cytosensing based on an aptamer modified nanobiosensor with a bioconjugate: detection of human non-small-cell lung cancer cells. *Biosens. Bioelectron* 74: 594–600.

Müller, J., B. Wulffen, B. Potzsch and G. Mayer (2007) Multidomain targeting generates a high-affinity thrombin-inhibiting bivalent aptamer. *ChemBioChem* 8: 2223–2226.

Nilsen-Hamilton, M. (2009) Aptamers in bioanalysis. *J. Am. Chem. Soc* 131: 12018.

Nimjee, S. M., C. P. Rusconi and B. A. Sullenger (2005) Aptamers: an emerging class of therapeutics. *Annu. Rev. Med* 56: 555–583.

Odeh, F., H. Nsairat, W. Alshaer, M. A. Ismail, E. Esawi, B. Qaqish, A. Al Bawab, S. I. Ismail and A. A. B. Jo (2019) Aptamers chemistry: chemical modifications and conjugation strategies. *Molecules* 25: 3.

Park, S. Y., J. Kim, G. Yim, H. Jang, Y. Lee, S. M. Kim, C. Park, M. H. Lee and T. Lee (2020) Fabrication of electrochemical biosensor composed of multi-functional DNA/rhodium nanoplate heterolayer for thyroxine detection in clinical sample. *Colloids Surf. B: Biointerfaces* 195: 111240.

Peters, K. E., K. E. Peters, C. C. Walters and J. Moldowan (2005) *Biomarkers and Isotopes in the Environment and Human History. Volume 2: Biomarkers and Isotopes in Petroleum Exploration and Earth History.* 2nd ed. Cambridge: Cambridge University Press.

Proske, D., M. Blank, R. Buhmann and A. Resch (2005) Aptamers—basic research, drug development, and clinical applications. *App. Microbiol. Biotech* 69: 367–374.

Pugh, G. C., J. R. Burns and S. Howarka (2018) Comparing proteins and nucleic acids for next-generation biomolecular engineering. *Nat. Rev. Chem* 2: 113–130.

Pu, F., Z. Huang, D. Hu, J. Ren, S. Wang and X. Qu (2009) Sensitive, selective and label-free protein detection using a smart polymeric transducer and aptamer/ligand system. *Chem. Commun. (Camb)* 47: 7357–7359.

Pultar, J., U. Sauer, P. Domnanich and C. Preininger (2009) Aptamer-antibody on-chip sandwich immunoassay for detection of CRP in spiked serum. *Biosens. Bioelectron* 24: 1456–1461.

Qiao, X. J., K. X. Li, J. Q. Xu, N. Cheng, Q. L. Sheng, W. Cao, T. L. Yue and J. B. Zheng (2018) Novel electrochemical sensing platform for ultrasensitive detection of cardiac troponin I based on aptamer-mos2 nanoconjugates. *Biosens. Bioelectron* 113: 142–147.

Qu, B., L. Guo, X. Chu, D. H. Wu, G. L. Shen and R. Q. Yu (2010) An electrochemical immunosensor based on enzyme-encapsulated liposomes and biocatalytic metal deposition. *Anal. Chim. Acta* 663: 147.

Ravelli, A., J. M. Reuben, F. Lanza, S. Anfossi, M. R. Cappelletti and L. Zanotti (2015) Breast cancer circulating biomarkers: advantages, drawbacks, and new insights. *Tumour Biol* 36: 6653–6665.

Riese, S. B., K. Buscher, S. Enders, C. Kuehne, R. Tauber and J. Dernedde (2016) Structural requirements of mono- and multivalent L-selectin blocking aptamers for enhanced receptor inhibition in vitro and in vivo. *Nanomedicine* 12: 901–908.

Ronkainen, N. J., H. B. Halsall and W. R. Heineman (2010) Electrochemical biosensors. *Chem. Soc. Rev* 39: 1747–1763.

Sawyers, C. L. (2008) The cancer biomarker problem. *Nature* 452: 548–552.

Salek Maghsoudi, A., S. Hassani, M. Rezaei Akmal, M. R. Ganjali, K. Mirnia, P. Norouzi and M. Abdollahi (2020) An electrochemical aptasensor platform based on flower-like gold microstructure-modified screen-printed carbon electrode for detection of serpin A12 as a type 2 diabetes biomarker. *Int. J. Nanomed* 15: 2219–2230.

Samie, H. A. and M. Arvand (2020) Label-free electrochemical aptasensor for progesterone detection in biological fluids. *Bioelectrochemistry* 133: 107489.

Severi, G., L. M. FitzGerald, D. C. Muller, J. Pedersen, A. Longano, M. C. Southey, J. L. Hopper, D. R. English, G. G. Giles and J. Mills (2014) A three-protein biomarker panel assessed in diagnostic tissue predicts death from prostate cancer for men with localized disease. *Cancer Med* 3: 1266–1274.

Shamsipur, M., L. Farzin, M. Amouzadeh Tabrizi and F. Molaabasi (2015) Highly sensitive label free electrochemical detection of $VGEF_{165}$ tumor marker based on "signal off" and "signal on" strategies using an anti-$VEGF_{165}$ aptamer immobilized BSA-gold nanoclusters/ionic liquid/glassy carbon electrode. *Biosens. Bioelectron* 74: 369–375.

Shaver, A., S. D. Curtis and N. Arroyo-Curras (2020) Alkanethiol monolayer end groups affect the long-term operational stability and signaling of electrochemical, aptamer-based sensors in biological fluids. *ACS Appl. Mater. Interfaces* 12: 11214–11223.

Sharma, S., H. Byrne and R. J. O. Kennedy (2016) Antibodies and antibody-derived analytical biosensors. *Essays Biochem* 60: 9.

Shankar, S. and R. K. Srivastava (2015) Nutrition, Diet and Cancer. Netherlands: Springer.

Sone, Y., O. Kawasaki, N. Immamura, T. Inoue and H. Yoshida (2010) Performance of the lithium-ion secondary cells targeting space exploration missions. *Electrochemistry* 78: 489–492.

Stoltenburg, R., C. Reinemann and B. Strehlitz (2007) SELEX—a (r)evolutionary method to generate high-affinity nucleic acid ligands. *Biomol. Eng* 24: 381–403.

Stanner S, Foundation BN (2008) *Cardiovascular Disease: Diet, Nutrition and Emerging Risk Factors (The Report of the British Nutrition Foundation Task Force)*. Wiley.

Sun, B., F. Qiao, L. Chen, Z. Zhao, H. Yin and S. Ai (2014) Effective signal-on photoelectrochemical immunoassay of subgroup J avian leukosis virus based on Bi2S3 nanorods as photosensitizer and in situ generated ascorbic acid for electron donating. *Biosens. Bioelectron* 54: 237–243.

Sun, G., H. Liu, Y. Zhang, J. Yu, M. Yan, X. Song and W. He (2015) Gold nanorods-paper electrode based enzyme-free electrochemical immunoassay for prostate specific antigen using porous zinc oxide spheres–silver nanoparticles nanocomposites as labels. *New J. Chem* 39: 6062.

Sun, D., Z. Luo, J. Lu, S. Zhang, T. Che, Z. Chen and L. Zhang (2019) Electrochemical dual-aptamer-based biosensor for nonenzymatic detection of cardiac troponin I by nanohybrid electrocatalysts labeling combined with DNA nanotetrahedron structure. *Biosens. Bioelectron* 134: 49–56.

Tabrizi, M. A., M. Shamsipur, R.,Saber, S. Sarkar and M. Besharati (2017) An electrochemical aptamer-based assay for femtomolar determination of insulin using a screen printed electrode modified with mesoporous carbon and 1,3,6,8-pyrenetetrasulfonate. *Mikrochim. Acta* 185: 59.

Taleat, Z., C. Cristea, G. Marrazza, M. Mazloum-Ardakani and R. Sandulescu (2014) Electrochemical immunoassay based on aptamer–protein interaction and functionalized polymer for cancer biomarker detection. *J. Electroanal. Chem* 717: 119–124.

Tamayo, J., P. M. Kosaka and J. J. Ruz (2013) Biosensors based on nanomechanical systems. *Chem. Soc. Rev* 42: 1287–1311.

Tertis, M., B. Ciui, M. Suciu, R. Sandulescu and C. Cristea (2017) Label-free electrochemical aptasensor based on gold and polypyrrole nanoparticles for interleukin 6 detection. *Electrochim. Acta* 258: 1208–1218.

Tian, L. and T. Heyduk (2009) Bivalent ligands with long nanometer-scale flexible linkers. *Biochemistry* 48: 264–275.

Tian, S. B., K. X. Tao, J. Hu, Z. B. Liu, X. L. Ding, Y. N. Chu, J. Y. Cui, X. M. Shuai, J. B. Gao, K. L. Cai, J. L. Wang, G. B. Wang, L. Wang and Z. Wang (2017) The prognostic value of AGR2 expression in solid tumours: a systematic review and meta-analysis. *Sci. Rep* 7: 15500.

Tombelli, S., M. Minunni and M. Mascini (2005) Analytical applications of aptamers. *Biosens. Bioelectron* 20: 2424–2434.

Tuerk, C. and L. Gold (1990) Systematic evolution of ligands by exponential enrichment: RNA ligands to bacteriophage T4 DNA polymerase. *Science* 249: 505–510.

Tran, D. T., V. Vermeeren, L. Grieten, S. Wenmackers, P. Wagner, J. Pollet, K. P. Janssen, L. Michiels, and J. Lammertyn (2011) Nanocrystalline diamond impedimetric aptasensor for the label-free detection of human IgE. *Biosens. Bioelectron.* 26, 2987–2993.

Vashist, S. K. and J. H. T. Luong (2018) *Quartz Crystal Microbalance Based Sensors, in Handbook of Immunoassay Technologies.* Amsterdam: Elsevier.

Verma, M. (2012) Epigenetic biomarkers in cancer epidemiology. *Methods Mol. Biol.* 863: 467–480.

Vorobyeva, M., P. Vorobjev and A. Venyaminova (2016) Multivalent aptamers: versatile tools for diagnostic and therapeutic applications. *Molecules* 21: 1613.

Wang, C., Y. Qian, Y. Zhang, S. Meng, S. Wang, Y. Li and F. Gao (2017a) A novel label-free and signal-on electrochemical aptasensor based on the autonomous assembly of hemin/G-quadruplex and direct electron transfer of hemin. *Sens. Actuators B Chem* 238: 434–440.

Wang, H., H. Han and Z. Ma (2017b) Conductive hydrogel composed of 1,3,5-benzenetricarboxylic acid and Fe^{3+} used as enhanced electrochemical immunosensing substrate for tumor biomarker. *Bioelectrochemistry* 144: 48.

Wang, T. S., J. Y. Liu, X. X. Gu, D. Li, J. Wang and E. Wang (2015) Label-free electrochemical aptasensor constructed by layer-by-layer technology for sensitive and selective detection of cancer cells. *Anal. Chim. Acta* 882: 32–37.

Wang, K., M. Q. He, F. H. Zhai, R. H. He and Y. L. Yu (2017c) A novel electrochemical biosensor based on polyadenine modified aptamer for label-free and ultrasensitive detection of human breast cancer cells. *Talanta* 166: 87–92.

Wang, Y., R. Yuan, Y. Chai, Y. Yuan, L. Bai and Y. Liao (2011) A multi-amplification aptasensor for highly sensitive detection of thrombin based on high-quality hollow CoPt nanoparticles decorated graphene. *Biosens. Bioelectron* 30: 61–66.

Wang, J., R. Lv, J. Xu, D. Xu and H. Chen (2008) Characterizing the interaction between aptamers and human IgE by use of surface plasmon resonance. *Anal. Bioanal. Chem* 390: 1059–1065.

Wu, Y., R. D. Tilley and J. J. J. Gooding (2019) Challenges and solutions in developing ultrasensitive biosensors. *Am. Chem. Soc* 141: 1162–1170.

Wu, S., S. Powers, W. Zhu and Y. A. Hannun (2016) Substantial contribution of extrinsic risk factors to cancer development. *Nature* 529: 43–47.

Wu, X., F. Gao, L. Xu, H. Kuang, L. Wang and C. Xu (2015) A fluorescence active gold nanorod–quantum dot core–satellite nanostructure for sub-attomolar tumor marker biosensing. *RSC Adv* 5: 97898–97902.

Xia, X., Q. He, Y. Dong, R. Deng and J. Li (2020) Aptamer-based homogenous analysis for food control. *Curr. Anal. Chem* 16: 4–13.

Xu, Y., G. Cheng, P. He and Y. A. Fang (2009) A review: electrochemical aptasensors with various detection strategies. *Electroanalysis* 21: 1251–1259.

Xu, T., H. Zhang, X. Li, Z. Xie and X. Li (2015) Enzyme-triggered tyramine-enzyme repeats on prussian blue-gold hybrid nanostructures for highly sensitive electrochemical immunoassay of tissue polypeptide antigen. *Biosens. Bioelectron* 73: 167–173.

Xu, T., B. Chi, J. Gao, M. Chu, W. Fan, M. Yi, H. Xu and C. Mao (2017) Novel electrochemical immune sensor based on Hep-PGA-PPy nanoparticles for detection of α-Fetoprotein in whole blood. *Anal. Chim. Acta* 977: 36–43.

Yao, C., Y. Qi, Y. Zhao, Y. Xiang, Q. Chen and W. Fu (2009) Aptamer-based piezoelectric quartz crystal microbalance biosensor array for the quantification of IgE. *Biosens. Bioelectron* 24: 2499–2503.

Yang, F., Z. Yang, Y. Zhuo, Y. Chai and R. Yuan (2015) Ultrasensitive electrochemical immunosensor for carbohydrate antigen 19-9 using Au/porous graphene nanocomposites as platform and Au@Pd core/shell bimetallic functionalized graphene nanocomposites as signal enhancers. *Biosens. Bioelectron* 66: 356.

Yang, H., Q.Yang, Z. Li, Y. Du and C. Zhang (2016) Sensitive Electrogenerated Chemiluminescence Aptasensor for the Detection of Ramos Cells Incorporating Polyamidoamine Dendrimers and Oligonucleotide. *Sens. Actuators B Chem* 236: 712–717.

Yuspian, N., G. Shabarni, H. Yeni Wahyuni and S. Toto (2021) Applications of electrochemical biosensor of aptamers-based (APTASENSOR) for the detection of leukemia biomarker. *Sens. Biosens. Res* 32: 100416.

Zamay, G. S., T. N. Zamay, V. A. Kolovskii, A. V. Shabanov, Y. E. Glazyrin, D. V. Veprintsev, A. V. Krat, S. S. Zamay, O. S. Kolovskaya, A. Gargaun, A. E. Sokolov, A. A. Modestov, I. P. Artyukhov, N. V. Chesnokov, M. M. Petrova, M. V. Berezovski and A. S. Zamay (2016) Electrochemical aptasensor for lung cancer-related protein detection in crude blood plasma samples. *Sci. Rep* 6: 34350.

Zhang, X., K. Xiao, L. Cheng, H. Chen, B. Liu, S. Zhang and J. Kong (2014) Visual and highly sensitive detection of cancer cells by a colorimetric aptasensor based on cell-triggered cyclic enzymatic signal amplification. *Anal. Chem* 86: 5567–5572.

Zhao, J., Y. Zhang, H. Li, Y. Wen, X. Fan, F. Lin, L. Tan and S. Yao (2011) Ultrasensitive electrochemical aptasensor for thrombin based on the amplification of aptamer-AuNPs-HRP conjugates. *Biosens. Bioelectron* 26: 2297–2303.

Zhuo, Z., Y. Yu, M. Wang, J. Li, Z. Zhang, J. Liu, X. Wu, A. Lu, G. Zhang and B. Zhang (2017) Recent advances in SELEX technology and aptamer applications in biomedicine. *J. Mol. Sci* 18(10): 2142.

Zhou, N., F. Su, Z. Li, X. Yan, C. Zhang, B. Hu, L. He, M. Wang and Z. Zhang (2019) Gold nanoparticles conjugated to bimetallic manganese (II) and iron (II) Prussian Blue analogues for aptamer-based impedimetric determination of the human epidermal growth factor receptor-2 and living MCF-7 cells. *Microchim. Acta* 186: 1–10.

Zhou, F., Y. Yao, J. Luo, X. Zhang, Y. Zhang, D. Yin, F. Gao and P. Wang (2017) Proximity hybridization-regulated catalytic DNA hairpin assembly for electrochemical immunoassay based on in situ DNA template-synthesized Pd nanoparticles. *Anal. Chim. Acta* 969: 8–17.

5 Aptamer-based point-of-care diagnostic devices for infectious diseases

Kalpesh V. Bhavsar, Hardik S. Churi, and Uday P. Jagtap

5.1 INTRODUCTION

The world's rising population is strongly affected by an increasing resistance of infectious organisms to various medications. Infectious diseases have the potential to create pandemic situations. Over the past decades, many emerging viruses and pathogenic microorganisms have caused illness and death which affect the world population. Thus, diagnosis and treatment of such life-threatening diseases are important. Infectious diseases are spread rapidly therefore, the diagnosis technique of such diseases should be rapid and ultrasensitive. Traditionally antibodies were used for the detection of infectious agents in various immunoassays (Peruski and Peruski, 2003). Antibodies can bind with different types of biological molecules such as antigens, antibodies, proteins, enzymes, metals, and nucleic acids. The antibodies act as a capture molecule in different types of techniques like immuno-assay, Enzyme-Linked ImmunoSorbent Assay (ELISA), chromatography, immuno-chromatography, biosensor, and immuno-sensors (Tomita and Tsumoto, 2011). A drastic increase in contagious diseases over the last few decades focuses on the development of in vitro diagnostic tools with Point of Care (POC) technology for rapid, specific, and accurate diagnosis of diseases. These POC techniques are inexpensive and easy.

Biomarkers act as indicators, which are made up of biological material produced inside the biological system responding to any biological and pathogenic condition. Biomarker levels are abnormal in patients' body fluids, blood, cells, and tissues during infection. Infected cells or tissues produce different types of molecules which are not produced by normal cells; such molecules can be used for the detection of infected cells. These abnormal molecules are better for the detection of physiological and pathological conditions of any living organism. For the detection of such abnormal constituents, different assay methods are used from which most of the assays use antibodies for the detection of biomarkers. The antibodies are specific for their target molecules but are unable to detect low concentrations of target molecules. Due to mutations, sometimes structural modification alters the structure of target molecules and makes it difficult for antibodies to detect such altered target

DOI: 10.1201/9781003304227-5

molecules. In such conditions, antibodies need to modify however it takes time for the organism naturally to create modifications in antibodies. Immunoassay is used as a diagnostic tool for the diagnosis of different diseases by using antigens as target molecules and antibodies as detecting agents. ELISA is specifically used for biomarker detection using immobilized antibodies (Perez et al., 2002). Body fluids are directly analyzed for the detection of microbial infections by using Gas-Liquid Chromatography (GLC). Abnormal metabolic constituents are detected using GLC for rapid and early diagnosis of infectious diseases. Immunochromatography is an advanced technology in which immunoassay and chromatography are used in combination with the sandwich immunoassay method which is used for the detection of viral or pathogenic antigens (Nagata et al., 1999). Rapid early diagnosis of infectious diseases is possible with the help of biosensors. Advanced technologies in biosensors have the potential for POC diagnosis (Sin et al., 2014). Rapid POC techniques with the help of in vitro detection methods give accurate results for the sample analysis. In antibodies-based assay methods, different errors are possible such as cross-reactivity, complexity, high cost, and poor reproducibility. Early detection of cancer cells is difficult due to a lack of specific, accurate, and sensitive antibodies. Therefore, the synthesis of specific affinity agents is important for the effective and efficient detection of target molecules. The in vitro synthesis of antibodies is important for such mutated target biomarkers.

Aptamers are oligonucleotides also termed chemical antibodies. Aptamers are small biomolecules made up of 40–80 nucleotides having three-dimensional structures that help them to bind with any target molecules (Tuerk and Gold, 1990). The aptamer is a word acquired from the Latin language 'apta' means 'to fit' (Ellington and Szostak, 1990). The synthesis of the aptamer is mainly dependent on the types of the target molecule. Traditionally nucleic acid aptamers were used widely for the detection of elements, organic dyes, proteins, nucleic acids, antibiotics, biomolecules, and various synthetic proteins or enzymes. Aptamers are also used in the diagnosis of viral material, pathogens, cancer cells, and other toxic chemicals. The chemical approach used for the synthesis of oligonucleotides is known as the systematic evolution of ligands by exponential enrichment (SELEX). SELEX is an in vitro method that allows the synthesis of any type of oligonucleotide sequence. SELEX helps for the synthesis of oligonucleotide sequences with higher affinity towards the target molecule and also allows any modification in aptamer molecule according to the target sequence. Development of the aptamer library is possible by using SELEX technology. The size of the aptamer molecule is very small and can be changed by using the SELEX modification technique which helps the aptamer to enter any target site (Stoltenburg et al., 2007). SOMAScan is becoming a powerful tool that helps with biomarker discovery. SOMAScan is a proteomic platform used for the modification of aptamers that enhance the sensitivity and specificity of an aptamer to target a molecule. SOMAScan assay minimizes cross-reaction and non-specific binding of aptamers. Advancement in SOMAScan uses a two-step capture technique to avoid low sensitivity in Mass Spectrophotometry and multiplex immunoassay. Advanced techniques like CELL-SELEX and SOMAlogic help in the identification and discovery of various biomarkers from different samples with high sensitivity and affinity (Huang et al., 2021).

This chapter provides information on advanced technology for aptamer-based biomarkers and POC testing (POCT) discovery for various infectious diseases. Aptamer-based POC devices are very useful for the early and accurate diagnosis of infectious diseases. Biosensors play a significant part in POC diagnostic equipment, and advancements such as non-invasive biosensor approaches are more advantageous for the detection of many infectious illnesses.

5.2 APTAMER-BASED TECHNOLOGIES

The concept of single-stranded oligonucleotides was discovered in 1990 which can bind with various target compounds (Ilgu et al., 2019). Aptamers are short sequences of nucleic acid. The small sequence of nucleotides is termed an oligonucleotide. Aptamers are made up of oligonucleotides that contain 15–60 nucleotides. Single-stranded RNA can fold into any form of tertiary structure. RNA aptamers are specifically used because they have the potential to fold into a vast group of tertiary structures that can easily bind with any target molecule. The tertiary structure of aptamer acts similarly to a protein molecule such as antibodies which can bind with different types of target molecules.

Aptamer structure has the backbone of phosphate molecules due to which aptamers possess a negative charge. Aptamer molecules prefer interaction with positively charged molecules of target proteins due to a negative charge backbone. The tertiary structure of aptamer easily binds with target molecules with the help of electrostatic force (Adachi and Nakamura, 2019). The patient's body fluids contain different abnormal constituents like proteins, enzymes, antigens, antibodies, biomolecules, viral particles, and infectious agents. Patients with pathogenic infections produce high levels of IgG1 antibodies. Aptamer containing 23 nucleotides binds with the hFc1 region of the IgG1 antibody (Miyakawa et al., 2008). The bonding between the aptamer and hFc1 region of the antibody is non-electrostatic because the surface of the hFc1 of the IgG1 antibody region lacks a positive charge (Deisenhofer, 1981). Some aptamer-proteins have neutral interactions due to which multiple weak bonds such as hydrophobic interactions and hydrogen bonds are formed (Nomura et al., 2010). Depending on the specificity of the aptamer and target molecule, aptamers are modified by changing the nucleotide sequence, length of the sequence, and chemical stability of the nucleotide sequence.

Aptamer synthesis begins with the oligonucleotide library and the selection of specific nucleotide sequences is done by scanning random sequences of the oligonucleotide library. SELEX is the best process to obtain nucleotide sequences by enriching the target molecule directly into the oligonucleotide sequence. This enrichment will allow the binding of sequences from the library to target molecules with high affinity. Then such sequences with a higher affinity toward target molecules are amplified with PCR or RT-PCR technique. For the synthesis of DNA, aptamer PCR is used while for the synthesis of RNA, aptamer RT-PCR is used. Generally, primers of 20 nucleotides are used for the PCR. SELEX technique primarily starts with the synthesis of a small oligonucleotide sequence library which approximately consists of 10^{12} to 10^{15} different sequences (Stoltenburg et al., 2007). For the development of the RNA library, T7 RNA polymerase is used for in vitro transcription of oligonucleotide sequences from the DNA library. The primary structure of aptamer consists of a simple straight chain of 15–60 nucleotides. The secondary structure contains helical turns with single-stranded loops. The tertiary structure has some special folding patterns with loops and bulges of a single sequence that allow aptamer molecules to bind with the target molecule by stacking aromatic rings, and various non-covalent interactions (Hermann et al., 2000). The main focus of the SELEX is to minimize the size of the library pool which only contains sequences with a higher affinity toward target molecules. This involves repetitive enrichment cycles of library sequences with target motifs for the selection of higher affinity and specificity sequences, refer Figure 5.1.

This process has four steps,

1. Synthesis of random oligonucleotide sequence library.
2. Enrichment of oligonucleotide sequence and target motifs to remove unbound molecules.
3. Amplification of selected oligonucleotide sequences by using PCR or RT-PCR.
4. Repetitive enrichment for characterization and selection of higher affinity and specificity aptamers.

The advanced SELEX method not only shortened the time but also reduced the number of cycles required for the completion of the SELEX method. CELL-SELEX is an advanced method that directly screens aptamer molecules with the whole cell. This is an advanced technique that helps to select aptamer which easily distinguishes between normal and disease cells. CELL-SELEX technique helps to develop new biomarkers from disease cells and also identify the aptamers having the potential to

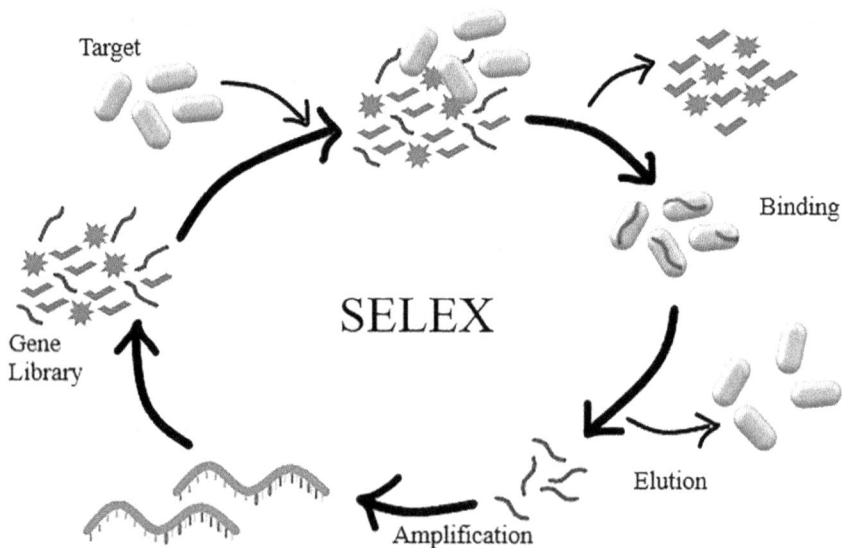

FIGURE 5.1   SELEX (Systematic evolution of ligands by exponential enrichment) technique.

bind with purified proteins and crude proteins present in native form. In this technique, the target cell is enriched in an ssDNA or RNA oligonucleotide library. This step allows the binding of aptamer sequences to target molecules and the unbound molecules removed by repetitive washing. These bound oligonucleotides are enriched with control cells for negative selection and the oligonucleotides which recognize target cells are unable to recognize control cells, therefore, unbound oligonucleotide sequences in the negative selection are eluted and possess high affinity toward target cells. Oligonucleotides that remain unbound and eluted are amplified with PCR and further screening is carried out through the flow cytometry technique. Some selected aptamers have the potential to differentiate normal cell lines, tumour cells, cancerous cells, and infected cells.

SOMAscan is an advanced technique used for the synthesis of biomarkers from patients' body fluids with the help of a proteomics assay. This is a multiplexed proteomic assay method that helps in the synthesis of slow Off-Rate Modified Aptamer (SOMAmers) (Huang et al., 2021). SOMAmers are small oligonucleotides that bind with high specificity towards the target molecule due to chemical modification. SOMAScan assay helps to minimize the cross-reactivity and non-specific binding of oligonucleotides to target molecules. Advanced techniques like CELL-SELEX, SOMAScan, Aptabid, and Microfluidic SELEX (M-SELEX) are beneficial for POC technologies to discover specific biomarkers and aptamers for the early detection of various infectious diseases.

5.3 INTRODUCTION TO POC TECHNOLOGY

The goal of this review is to bring attention to POCT as another clinical field. The clinical staff is gradually employing POCT technologies to shorten remedial completion time, i.e. therapeutic turnaround time, the time between requesting and executing a test to treat the patient. POCT has the potential to deliver test results quickly and precisely which reduces the cost of medical services for the general public.

POCT improves patient happiness by an increase in health benefits and product cost-effectiveness. POCT has become standard in the United States and other high-gross-product countries where a quick reaction is essential. In this age of health care industry expansion, POC practice follows a trend, which depends on natural disasters, terrorism, and serious illnesses. In the evolution of POC, a rich theoretical foundation and practical expertise have developed to validate its implementation as a new discipline. This method is practiced since it reflects current medical trends and brings medical treatment closer to patients' homes and workplaces.

5.3.1 DISCOVERY OF POCT

In 1955, haematology testing manuals reported the consideration raised in England (Kost, 1977). Dr. Kost began research on biosensors and measuring pH changes in vivo in the presence of cardiovascular stress and trauma in 1972. In innovative visual logistics depicting clinical pathophysiology, he conceived the emerging area of patient-centred testing. Then, in the mid-1980s, during the research on biosensor-based sequential estimations of ionized calcium in the blood of a patient undergoing a liver transplant, Dr. Kost introduced the phrase "point of care testing" (England et al., 1995). Dr. Kost did a comprehensive blood study right next to the patient in the operating room and swiftly informed the anaesthesiology and surgical teams, who subsequently followed up. He showed that by utilizing multiparameter adjustment equations or real-time POC trends in the operating room, the ionized calcium could not be consistently estimated. It has to be directly and quickly quantified in whole blood using biosensor-based Ca^{2+} (Na^+ and K^+) devices. As a result of the shortened turnaround time, the anesthesiology-surgery team was in a position to respond to data swiftly supporting the patient's cardiovascular function. POC's quick response has proven to be critical in providing appropriate evidence-based treatment during patient emergencies to this day.

As a new and multidisciplinary profession, POC must effectively collaborate with health care specialists, gynaecology, obstetricians, cardiologists, surgeons, emergency medical responders, and other aspects of current practice. In order to provide patients with timely economic benefits through POC testing, epidemiology, pathology, laboratory procedures, illness diagnosis, and therapy must be integrated. Future applications must also incorporate point-of-careology management, informatics, and public health implications, for example, employing POCT to identify urine lipoarabinomannan can help Human Immunodeficiency Virus (HIV)-positive patients with TB treatment decisions. POC lipoarabinomannan testing may be really beneficial in hospitals having limited diagnostic facilities, as well as in patients who are immunocompromised or unable to cough up sputum. For example, it has been proposed that troponin T or troponin I POCT is essential in the diagnosis of patients with acute coronary syndromes. In Canada, the detection of cardiac troponin POC lowered the test cost and time. This integrated strategy benefits the emergency rooms, hospitals, and non-urban health care centres Table 5.1.

5.3.2 NEED FOR POC DIAGNOSTIC TECHNOLOGIES

POCT improved diagnostic capability for various diseases. POC diagnostic devices provide a significant economic advantage, as a big portion of India's population cannot afford traditional tests. POC tests are appropriate for ongoing analyte monitoring or to track therapy progress by repeating the testing. POCT reduces the time it takes to diagnose and treat serious illnesses like heart disease. Low turnaround time is especially beneficial for patients travelling from a distance for clinical diagnosis since it avoids further travel expenses through one-time visit diagnosis. In the case of infectious conditions, the diagnosis is also done in one visit, lowering the chance of further infection spreading across the community. POC analysis also assists in the regular health check-ups of people living in rural areas which lack facilities. POC equipment such as blood pressure monitors, glucose monitoring systems, and oxygen level measuring devices employ high-end digital platforms to relieve the load on nurses and other front-line healthcare workers. The device's automated multiplex analytical tools handle the result interpretation, which eliminates the need for an experienced technician (Konwar and Borse, 2020). POC test results may be saved in a clinical system shared with healthcare professionals through a cloud service by connecting it with the appropriate software, which benefits both the patient and the physician.

TABLE 5.1

Difference between laboratory technique and the POC technique

	Distinguish in the laboratory technique and the POC technique	
	The general laboratory technique	The POC technique
Detection principle	Biochip technology, immunoelectrophoresis, electrophoretic analysis reaction, electrochemical and chemical sensors, emission spectrometric analysis, gas chromatograph–mass spectrometer	Biosensor technique, membrane carrier enzyme immunoassay, biochip technology, multiplex PCR technique, non-nucleic acid hybridization, multiplex molecular testing for infection diseases, amperometry, conductometry, dot immunogold filtration assay, dot immunochromatographic assay, spread spectrum radio frequency, microfluidic chip
The type of instruments	Designed not to be moved	Blood, microscale evolving to nanoscale in the future; urine, 1 mL
The sample volume	Blood, generally 3 mL; urine, several millilitres	Blood, generally 3 mL; urine, several millilitres
Turnaround time	Several hours to several days	5–30 min
Detection range	Examining physiological and pathological signs of health and illness from afar; cost savings associated with bigger mainframe devices and automation; high operational vulnerability during epidemics, crises, or disasters	Patient specimens are examined on-site for disease markers and pathogens; rapid response diagnosis, monitoring, and therapeutic decision-making; isolation units are located near patients for testing highly infectious disease specimens; and evidence-based results are connected for health care management
Results	Laboratory diagnostic	POC diagnostic, bed sit diagnostic

The POC diagnostic plays an important role in the detection of blood sugar and heart disease sectors. POC diagnostic technology for blood glucose monitoring has been considered one of the most important aids in diabetes control and treatment (Rajendran and Rayman, 2014). The usefulness of POC diagnostic systems has boosted management assurance through quick analysis, as well as promoted POC diagnostic device penetration in the Indian market and at home. Seasonal infectious illnesses including influenza, dengue fever, malaria, and others have added to the other existing hazardous disorders like thyroid dysfunction, tuberculosis (TB), urinary tract infection, and pneumonia.

As a result, current diagnostic procedures, such as laboratory-based systems, must be replaced by POC tests which are quick, convenient, and cost-effective. The healthcare industry's increased demand for speedy diagnosis has inspired the creation of a host of POC testing equipment and techniques. Researchers from across the world are exploring and reporting on emerging methodologies that might be turned into POC diagnostic equipment. Apart from blood glucose and cardiac biomarker sensing, the POC approach for infectious illness diagnosis is in high demand in underdeveloped countries (St John and Price, 2014). In this discipline, the development and deployment of POC diagnostics is crucial for infection prevention and treatment. Biosensors, microfluidics, biomedical systems, lab-on-a-chip devices, and smartphone-based diagnostic devices are being developed by researchers all over the world for application in POC medical diagnostics (Vashist, 2017, Khan and Song, 2020).

5.4 POC DIAGNOSTICS TOOLS AND DEVICES

In recent years, improper waste disposal and shortage of freshwater have increased due to the rapid rise in population which creates a major impact on healthcare workers. Due to unhygienic activities, various endemic and pandemic situations are rising. For accurate and sensitive diagnosis of such diseases, POC devices are important and a variety of techniques are commercially available for on-site detection. Recent advances in POC devices include aptamers that help for accurate diagnosis and detection of infectious diseases. The Aptamer-Linked Immobilised Sorbent Assay (ALISA) is one of the best POC techniques for the detection of various infectious diseases such as tularemia, and tuberculosis. The gold nanoparticles are conjugated with an aptamer that detects single-cell *Staphylococcus aureus* within 1.5 hours (Chang et al., 2013). Gold nanoparticles with ssDNA are used for the detection of *Staphylococcal enterotoxin* B by using a colorimeter (Liu et al., 2013). *S. enterotoxin* B is the most common bacteria that causes food poisoning. The plasmodium lactate dehydrogenase (pLDH) enzyme is used as a biomarker for the detection of malaria by aptasensors attached to gold nanoparticles (Jeon et al., 2013). The red-to-blue colour change is the indication of positive detection of plasmodium.

5.4.1 TYPES OF POC DEVICES

The adoption of POC diagnostic instruments to monitor blood pressure, temperature, oxygen levels, and ECG has greatly benefited the clinical and customized healthcare sector. Several novel POC diagnostic gadgets for various purposes have been developed as a result of technological breakthroughs. Degradable kits, like fast assay dipsticks, glucose monitoring kits, reusable devices, and multipurpose table-top equipment, which are usually used in labs, are among the devices utilized in POC settings. The POC diagnostic devices range in complexity from simple to complicated and are capable of multiplex operation. Depending on the application and sensitivity, POC diagnostic devices can produce qualitative, semi-quantitative, or quantitative data. Some POC diagnostic instruments, such as fast test pads and dipsticks, are relatively simple and require a single sample application to receive a comprehensive result. Colorimetry, potentiometry, fluorimetry, electrochemistry, and microfluidics techniques are used in these devices. The taxonomy of POC diagnostic equipment is depicted in Figure 5.2.

In most POC diagnostic devices, biosensors are the most critical component. A biosensor detects an analyte and turns it into a readable signal using a detector (Mahato et al., 2018). Nanotechnology includes a variety of nanomaterials like magnetic nanoparticles, quantum dots, carbon dots, and gold and silver nanomaterials

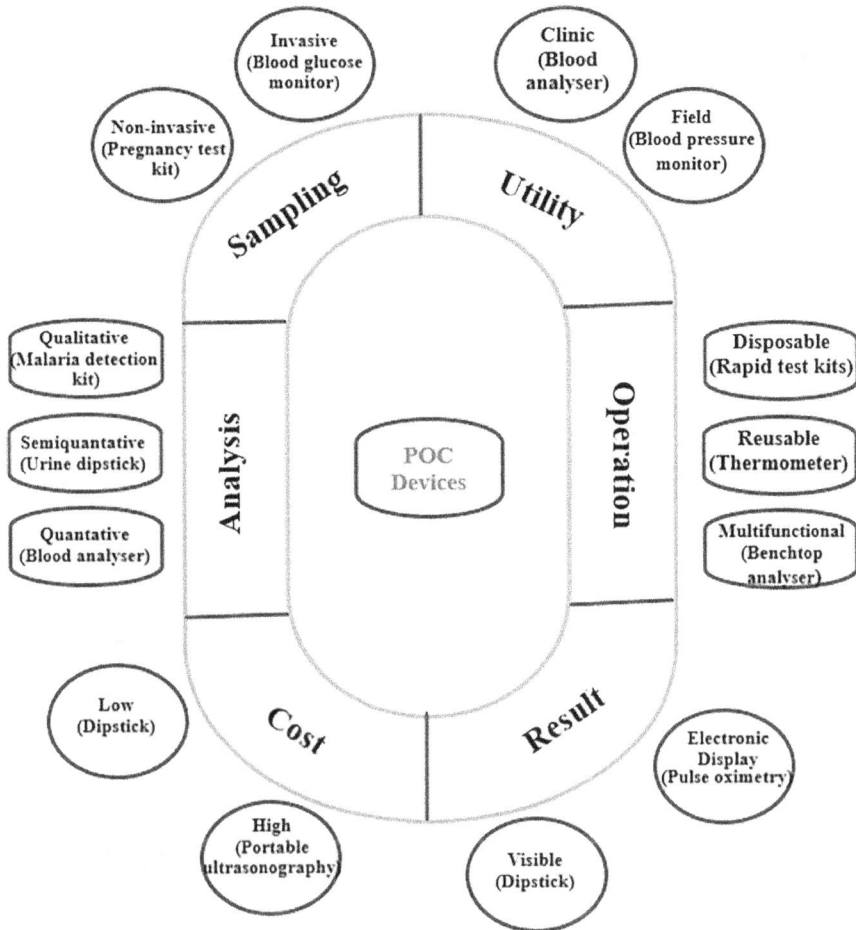

FIGURE 5.2 Types of POC devices.

which revolutionized POCT, and a range of other nanomaterials have been employed in biosensor design. In the last few years, nanotechnology-enabled biosensing used in two major ways: first, by amplification methods through a variety of nanomaterials, and second, by conjugating bio-recognition components with nano-surfaces (Mahato et al., 2016).

POC devices are employed in a variety of contexts, including clinics, hospitals, laboratories, and also at home (Pai et al., 2012).

5.4.2 POC DEVICES IN THE MEDICAL INDUSTRY

Advanced gadgets have been created in response to industrial demands and world-wide situations since, the creation of the stethoscope. The impact of the COVID-19 pandemic, for example, has prompted diagnostic device manufacturers to develop small and portable devices that can quickly detect SARS-CoV-2 infections. The portable equipment used to check a patient during a consultation is known as point-of-care testing (POCT), which is also termed 'near-patient testing'. POC devices can deliver immediate findings and allow healthcare providers to provide prompt patient treatment. Doctors and patients no longer have to wait for lab findings before making an accurate diagnosis. Medical POC devices are widely available in clinics and hospitals, allowing doctors to obtain quick and reliable findings on therapy and patient care (Banerjee et al., 2019).

The big advantage of POC devices is the delivery of lab-quality testing at near-patient diagnosis Table 5.2.

TABLE 5.2
Aptamer-based POC devices for disease diagnosis

Sr. no.	Type of disease/infection	Aptamer-based POC devices	References
1	*Escherichia coli* infection	MBSpinChip	Wei et al. (2018)
2	Tularemia	ALISA and dot blot	Vivekananda and Kiel (2006)
3	*Salmonella* infection	APT-FMNPs	Liao et al. (2018)
4	*Staphylococcus* aureus infection	SEM	Chang et al. (2013)
5	*Staphylococcal* enterotoxin infection	Colorimetric device	Liu et al. (2013)
6	Cholera	Lateral flow assay	Frohnmeyer et al. (2019)
7	Tuberculosis	ALISA and electrochemical sensor	Zhou et al. (2017)
		Aptamer-based sandwich electrochemical assay	Chen et al. (2019)
		Dot blot assay	L. Li et al. (2018a, 2018b)
		Graphene oxide-based assay	Thakur et al. (2017)
8	Anthrax	ELISA	Kim et al. (2013)
		Fluorescent assay	
9	*L. monocytogenes* infection	Double-site binding sandwich technique	Suh et al. (2018)
10	Chagas	PCR	Nagarkatti et al. (2012)
11	Malaria	Aptasensors and colorimetric method	Jeon et al. (2013)
12	Leishmania infection	DNA-based aptamer-magnetic bead sandwich technique with a fluorometer	Bruno et al. (2014)
13	Schistosomiasis	Binding assay	Long et al. (2016)
14	Influenza	Paper-based lateral flow immunoassay	Kang et al. (2019)
15	AIDS	Fluorescent lateral flow assay	Deng et al. (2018)
		Spectral ellipsometry	Caglayan and Üstündağ (2020)
16	Hepatitis	Electrochemical assay	Ghanbari and Roushani (2018)

POC devices have different functions like Pregnancy test kits, faecal immuno-chemical assays, blood glucose analyzers, and haemoglobin analyzers as point-of-care equipment. The bulk of POC devices rely on chemiluminescence and boronate affinity fluorescence quenching by inbuild camera integration is becoming more common in the field. Compact, user-friendly POC devices with sophisticated vision systems can provide substantial benefits to the medical industry. The camera in the POC device analyzes sample contents to generate visual data for software process-ing, which allows doctors to perform tests outside of the laboratory. This testing by clinicians acquires lab-quality results, which allow faster and more accurate diagno-sis of serious and deadly diseases (Balaji et al., 2021).

The advent of POC technologies for quick, automated testing of patients for a rou-tine clinical diagnostics approach is one of the best developments of the century for medical diagnostics. The broad availability of low-cost testing, as well as the capabil-ity of long-distance data transmission and analysis, is projected to give rise to a new era of global and real-time public health activities. Aptasensors are one of the most promising possibilities to help accelerate the conversion of traditional benchtop med-ical diagnostics into POC testing in the digitized and individualized era of medicine. Aptamers are single-stranded nucleic acids that have 3D folded structures which selectively attach to target molecules. Aptamers have been extensively explored for POC diagnostics, which has shown worldwide health benefits in the last decade due to, these features some of the inventions have been directly converted into com-mercial products. SOMAscan®, a SomaLogic-developed aptamer-based proteomics assay, can identify 1,305 human protein analytes in 50 mL of some body fluids with excellent accuracy and precision (Huang et al., 2021).

5.5 POC DEVICES FOR INFECTIOUS DISEASES

Infectious diseases are increasing day by day in the world by common causative agents like bacteria, viruses, parasites, and fungi. Contagious diseases spread in the world rapidly, having the potential to create a pandemic situation. In such cases, a rapid accurate diagnosis of the infectious agent is important to provide accurate treatment and medication to the patient. POC devices are peculiarly used for detect-ing infectious pathogens on-site. Below are some major examples of POC equip-ment for infectious disease detection that are commercially available and utilized by healthcare professionals Figure 5.3a.

5.5.1 BACTERIAL INFECTIONS

A bacterial infection develops when a group of bacteria enters the body, multiplies, and causes a reaction in the body. Viruses can enter the body through airways, as with bacterial pneumonia, or through an opening in your skin. We describe two types of aptamers here: (A) predefined antigens or virulence factors found on bac-terial cell surfaces; and (B) entire cells containing known or unknown molecular targets.

Escherichia coli is such a common infection, that it's critical to develop a quick, easy, and accurate diagnostic approach. The MBSpinChip is a portable multifunction

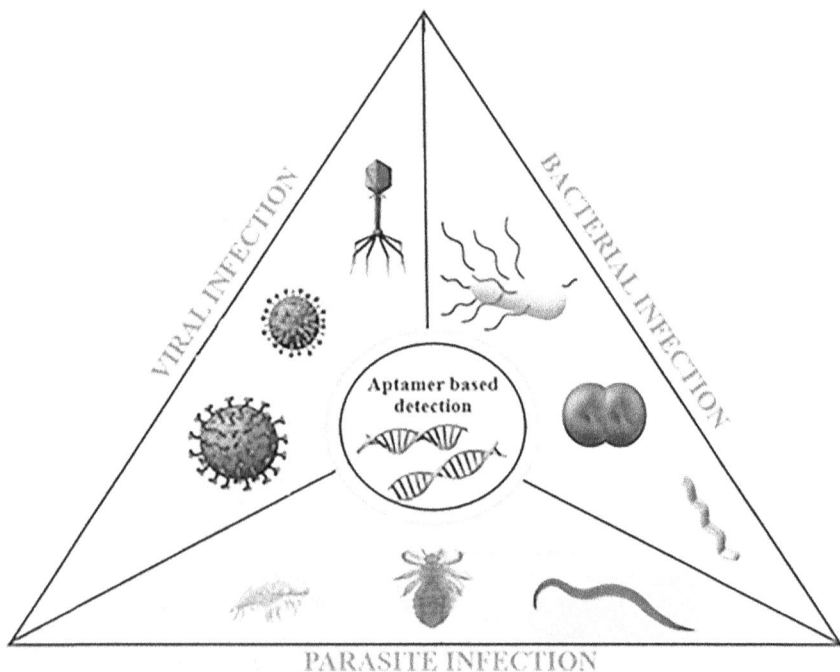

FIGURE 5.3   Aptamer-based detection of infectious agents.

bar graph rotation chip that was designed for the quantitative diagnosis of a variety of medical conditions using magnetic sensors made from nanoparticles (Wei et al., 2018). For sensitive POCT, this multiplexed SpinChip combines pressure amplification catalyzed by nanoparticles with aptamer-specific identification. This MBSpinChip delivers a visually measurable output through a bar chart, can identify many pathogens at once, and shows broad area applications in pathogen screening, environmental monitoring, and food safety (Li et al., 2020).

Tularemia is a rare type of bacterial infectious disease caused by *Francisella tularensis* that infects macrophages and attacks the skin, lymph nodes, eyes, and lungs. Vivekananda and Kiel (2006) identified 25 different unique DNA sequences and used them as aptamers against *F. tularensis*. They tested these aptamer molecules with the help of ALISA and Dot Blot analysis showed promising results for the detection of some tularensis species (Vivekananda and Kiel 2006).

Salmonella infects thousands of individuals each year as a result of contaminated food. As a result, finding Salmonella in tainted food is an important public health precaution. The LA80, an ssDNA aptamer have the ability to bind to (lipopolysaccharides) LPS from four separate source materials, further, development helps to reduce the number of nucleotide in aptamer and is labelled as LA27 which is used for the identification of Lipopolysaccharide from *Salmonella typhimurium* (Ye et al., 2019). Based on magnetic multifunctional nanoprobes with aptamer modifications (APT-FMNPs), a magnetic and quantitative fluorescence technology was created to concurrently distinguish various pathogens to enhance bacterial isolation and collection procedures.

S. aureus is a gram-positive facultative anaerobic pathogen that causes various infections in humans. A fluorescent assay was utilized to identify *S. aureus* in biological materials using ssDNA aptamers against *S. enterotoxin* (SES) (Cai et al., 2019). The chimaera sequence is made up of complementary and aptamer sequences against *S. aureus*. Target recovery depending on chain displacement was used to increase the sensitivity and strength of the signals. This approach was used for the detection of *S. aureus* from various water samples because of its great recovery and reproducibility (Chang et al., 2013). The detection of *S. aureus* with the POC devices was done by using aptamer-conjugated gold nanoparticles. The SELEX method was used for aptamer synthesis and the scanning electron microscopy (SEM) technique detected *S. aureus* in 1.5 hours (Chang et al., 2013). *S. enterotoxin* causes food poison that can be detected by using gold nanoparticles conjugated with ssDNA with the help of a simple colorimetric device (Liu et al., 2013).

Cholera is caused by *Vibrio cholera* creating an epidemic situation specifically in the South Asia region (Kaper et al., 1995). This bacteria can easily spread through contaminated water and release toxins that cause acidosis, diarrhoea, and death if not treated early. Cholera toxins (CT) are specifically selected for the detection of cholera infection. CT can be detected with the help of aptamers by using colorimetric and electrochemical assays (Bruno and Kiel 2002). A recent study found that CT916 DNA aptamer can easily detect CT (Frohnmeyer et al., 2019). Gold nanoparticles conjugated with DNA aptamers are used for CT detection. Lateral Flow Assay (LFA) developed by Fischer detects CT produced by cholera (Frohnmeyer et al., 2019).

Tuberculosis (TB) is still one of the world's top causes of mortality. It is still incurable and the mortality rate is very high. Traditional methods for the diagnosis of TB are available but they are less sensible (Martin et al., 2021). The ultrasensitive detection of *Mycobacterium tuberculosis* (M. TB) is important. In order to acquire rapid and secure ways for early detection of TB, two diagnostic procedures were developed based on DNA aptamers; one is aptamer ALISA (aptamer connection fixation adsorption analysis), and another is based on biomarker HspX detection electrochemical sensor (ECS) (Zhou et al., 2017). DNA aptamers have the potential to detect biomarkers from sputum with the help of an electrochemical sensor. Lavania et al., in 2018 used a H63SL2-M6 aptamer for the detection of HspX biomarker present in sputum samples of TB patients (Lavania et al., 2018). The *Mycobacterium tuberculosis* produces different peptides that possess pathogenic properties from which MPT64 is detected by using an aptamer-based sandwich electrochemical assay (Chen et al., 2019).

The MPT64 secretory protein, a highly pathogenic and immunogenic factor of *Mycobacterium tuberculosis*, was detected by synthetic aptamers with a reference range of 81 pMol in the patient's blood specimen (Sypabekova et al., 2019). MPT64 was also determined using a one-of-a-kind sandwich electrochemical body-fitted sensor. The H37R is a type of *Mycobacterium tuberculosis* that can be detected by a POC device dot blot assay (L. Li et al., 2018a, 2018b). The *Mycobacterium tuberculosis* coupled with gold nanoparticles was detected by using an electrochemical aptasensor and due to high sensitivity, these aptasensors are peculiarly used in the early diagnosis. Carbon Nanotubes with graphene oxide-based assay is widely applied for profiling of M.TB (Thakur et al., 2017).

Anthrax is spread by spores forming the bacterium bacillus anthracis that cause epizootic diseases. This bacterium infects animals and exposure of humans to such infected animals can cause serious issues like skin, and lung infections. The bacillus anthracis produces different lethal factors (LF), protective antigens (PA), and toxins that can be used as biomarkers for diagnosis (Lahousse et al., 2018). Kim used a DNA aptamer to detect LF by using an ELISA assay. The fluorescent assay shows promising results for the detection of PA. The AuNPs conjugated with aptamer are also used for the detection of PA (Kim et al., 2013).

The *L. monocytogenes*, a bacterial infection prevalent in food, causes listeriosis, a fatal condition. In ready-to-eat food, both the European Medicines Agency and the US FDA show a policy of no-tolerance for *L. monocytogenes*, motivating extensive development into extremely sensitive biosensors for detecting foodborne pathogens. A unique single-strand DNA aptamer was used to identify the pathogen using a double-site binding sandwich technique (Suh et al., 2018). The *L. monocytogenes* are captured using antibody-immobilised immunomagnetic beads, which are subsequently exposed to aptamer probes. PCR amplification and aptamer were used to detect the virus and the detection limit is 5 CFU/mL. The first inoculation dose of 1–2 log10 CFU per 25 g produced favourable results when this sandwich technique was applied to cooked turkey flesh. Because of its low detection limit, the method can be used to identify *L. monocytogenes* in food and environmental samples.

5.5.2 PARASITIC INFECTION

Hundreds of millions of individuals worldwide are affected by protozoa parasitic infections, and they continue to be a serious public health issue globally. Insect vectors or potentially contaminated edibles are the most common routes for parasitic diseases to spread; because their increased rate is interconnected to inadequate sanitation and immunodeficiency. The emerging microscopic detection of infections in clinical samples, and immunological identification of parasitic proteins and pathogenic genomes with the help of PCR are currently the most used diagnostic procedures. These therapies have significant drawbacks since they require a lot of time and need cryogenic storage facilities as well as specialized instruments, both of which are scarce in rural regions. A lot of research has gone into finding new parasite targets. Aptamer has shown to be an appealing technique for generating alternative diagnostic tools in this scenario.

The *T. evansi* is a parasite that causes Chagas disease. *T. evansi* genome was detected by using PCR-based technologies in the blood of affected people (Singhal et al., 2021). However, the level of parasites in the blood is low during the early stages of a natural infection, as well as during the chronic phase of illness. Therefore serum-stable RNA aptamers which get attached to active *T. cruzi trypomastigotes* have been created using the whole-cell SELEX technique (Nagarkatti et al., 2012). To enhance PCR detection, paramagnetic beads coated with Apt68 were used to attract parasites present in the samples having a low amount of parasites. These aptamers show a strong affinity and specificity for parasites, which are exclusively found in *T. cruzi trypomastigotes*.

From both the genotypes, Apt68 effectively gathered and aggregated trypanosomes from different parasitic isolates. These studies revealed that aptamers are pathogen-specific ligands and have the ability to detection and identification of *T. cruzi* from blood samples (Nagarkatti et al., 2012).

Malaria is a parasitic infection caused by plasmodium. There is a high demand for reliable malaria diagnosis. SELEX method was used to create aptamers for different cationic polymers (Jeon et al., 2013). Plasmodium produces different polymeric substances such as polydiallyl-dimethyl-ammonium chloride, lactate dehydrogenase, and poly allyl-amine hydrochloride. These polymers aggregate with gold nanoparticles (AuNPs) to form a complex that helps to increase the sensitivity of this POC aptasensor. PDDH and PAH complex aptasensors are conjugated with gold nanoparticles that can easily detect the minute amount of lactate dehydrogenase produced by plasmodium parasites which shows colour change (i.e. red to blue) and detected by a simple colorimetric method. The detection limit for *plasmodium vivax* is 74 parasites/µL for PAH and 80 parasites/µL for PDDH (Jeon et al., 2013). Resazurin dye was converted into Resorufin dye (pink, 570 nm) in a substrate-dependent reaction; we then recognized the parasite PLDH and PFGDH enzymes with fluorescence intensity and absorbance ratio (570/605 nm) as well as a colour change of resorcinol from blue to pink at 660 nm. Hence, based on the shades and pixel intensity, the plasmodium biomarkers were qualitatively and quantitatively detected (Dirkzwager et al., 2016).

A DNA-based aptamer-magnetic bead sandwich technique which was coupled with fluorescent peroxidase has been developed to identify soluble proteins from leishmania major pro flagellates (Bruno et al., 2014). In this study, quantum dots and nanoparticles were attached to Amplex Ultra Red for fluorescence detection. Many sensitive versions are available but AUR-based versions exhibit the least amount of inter-sample variability. Using this rechargeable fluorometer connected to an onboard computer, the minute amounts of leishmania proflagellate protein extract in sand fly homogenate detected in rural locations, and can map the geographic distribution of parasites in wild sand fly populations.

Another parasitic infection schistosomiasis is caused by *Schistosoma* that affects the urogenital tract, mesentery, and liver of an infected person. There are different species of *Schistosoma* are present from which *Schistosoma haematoidin, Schistosoma japonica, and Schistosoma mansoni* mostly cause infection in humans. *Schistosoma* releases eggs into the patient's body which can be directly used as biomarkers for the diagnosis of parasitic infection (Long et al., 2016). Long et al. developed two ssDNA egg-based aptamers LC6 and LC15 for the detection of *Schistosoma japonica* eggs.

5.5.3 VIRAL INFECTIONS

Viruses are sub-microscopic infectious pathogens that infect people and animals (Dhiman et al., 2017). In 1898, thousands of viral species were discovered in the environment, indicating a variety of biological activity (Virus Taxonomy, 2019). Many illnesses, including influenza, hepatitis, AIDS, and developing viral diseases like lung infections caused by SARS-CoV infection, and Ebola, are caused by viral infection, resulting in severe sickness, and death, as well as substantial economic and societal implications (González et al., 2016). Around 11,000 years ago, smallpox was amongst the worst and most fatal viral epidemics in Indian agricultural communities, and it was the first pandemic in history. Furthermore, from 1918 to 1919 H1N1 virus caused an influenza pandemic and infected nearly 500 million individuals. The death toll was extremely high, at 100 million people, and the epidemic was the deadliest in human history (Johnson and Mueller, 2002).

Aptamers have recently been revealed to have useful applications in the detection of infectious viral illnesses such as influenza, HIV, hepatitis, SARS-COV-2, and COVID-19 (Kumar Kulabhusan et al., 2020). One of the most critical components of avoiding extensive transmission and treating infected persons is identifying viral infections quickly and safely.

Influenza is often regarded as the most common infectious illness in humans. In the twentieth century, three significant pandemics were triggered by new influenza viruses (González et al., 2016). In reality, the Spanish flu virus is thought to have killed 25 million people worldwide (Taubenberger et al., 2012). Because influenza viruses are highly contagious and undergo frequent mutations, as a result, new strains, diseases, and even pandemics have emerged, and hence, early detection and categorization of these viruses are critical. Paper-based lateral flow immunoassays (LFIA) using conventional sandwich immunoassays are commonly used in medical diagnostic techniques. In LFIA, gold nanoparticles fail to bind the target molecules and therefore cannot achieve sensitivity in low concentrations for the detection of biomarkers and infectious agents in samples. Researchers developed an ssDNA-binding protein that serves as a sandwich detection probe with capture antibodies and aptamers included in LFIA to solve this problem (Kang et al., 2019). In Li et. al. (2020) linked the AuNPs to each aptamer, which increases the signal intensity in the detection system. The goal of this approach was to find the cardiac troponin I (CTnI) and influenza nucleoprotein (NP). Gold nanoparticles had detection limits of 0.23 and 0.26 pg/mL, in cardiac troponin I in serum and human nasal fluid respectively. This approach has a far better sensitivity than traditional techniques utilizing antibody binding to AuNPs, which are extensively employed in LFIA (Lara et al., 2020). These findings demonstrate that the suggested approach may be used to identify extremely sensitive chemicals in the field of POC for early detection.

AIDS is caused by the HIV that spreads worldwide. AIDS is treatable in the early stage by using a combination of antiretroviral therapy (cART) but the early diagnosis of HIV infection is important for better treatment of AIDS. The structure of HIV contains different types of surface proteins from which the P24 antigen is the major part of the viral component and is unusually used for detection. Liao identifies two P24 antigen aptamers made up of ssDNA using agarose beads as carriers (Zeng et al., 2017). HIV produces different enzymes from which RNase H is an important enzyme required for the life cycle of HIV. For detection of HIV RNase H plays a key role as a marker. Traditionally Polyacrylamide gel electrophoresis (PAGE) was used for the detection of RNase H but recently RNA aptamers made up of 3,5-difluoro-4-hydroxybenzylidene imidazolinone (DFHBI) can attach with a green fluorescent protein (GFP) that enhances the sensitivity of the assay (Zhang et al., 2019). The binding of the GFP molecule to DFHBI helps for on-site accurate and quick detection of HIV. The HIV-DNA was successfully detected by Deng et al. (2018) from the serum sample of the patient by using a fluorescent LFA combined with a quantum dot. The detection range of the assay is 1 pM to 10 nM. Xie et al. discovered a probe that binds with a GFP-DFHBI RNA aptamer that easily detects RNase H from a single cell (Zhang et al., 2019). To enhance the quality of the diagnosis, the trans-transcriptional activator (HIV-TAT) protein-specific RNA aptamer (Anti-Tat), and spectral ellipsometry are recommended. The protein utilizing both SE and surface plasmon resonance-enhanced total internal reflection ellipsometry was detected by Anti-Tat aptamers (Caglayan and Üstündağ, 2020).

Hepatitis is a viral infection caused by 5 main types of hepatitis species such as A, B, C, D, and E (Prasidthrathsint and Stapleton, 2019). Hepatitis B and C are the most common causes of hepatitis infection. The hepatitis B e antigen is used for the diagnosis of hepatitis B by using a fluorescence-based aptasensor. This assay is accurate and completed in 2 minutes (Huang et al., 2016). Hepatitis B surface antigen is the greatest distinguishing feature of HBV viral protein (HBsAg). A new chemi-luminescent aptamer-sensor based on quick magnetic separation and bifunctional gold nanoparticles was developed using an HBsAg-specific aptamer (Xi et al., 2018). When detecting HBsAg in HBV-positive blood, the ultrasensitive sensor recognizes magnetic separation. Hepatitis C is a single-stranded positive RNA virus that synthe-sizes different proteins from which core antigen molecules are used for ultrasensitive detection by using graphene quantum dots (Ghanbari et al., 2017). For ultrasensi-tive detection of DNA aptamers, the GOD (Glucose Oxidase) based electrochemi-cal assay was used. Multi-wall carbon nanotubes (MWCNT) based electrochemical assay was used by Ghanbari and Roushani (2018). DNA aptamers were used to detect the hepatitis C virus core antigen ultra-sensitively using several detection methods. At each stage of the chemical alteration, these approaches were employed to check the surface changes. The range of 10–70 and 70–400 pg/mL of linear concentration and 3.3 pg/mL detection limit of EIS is a viable alternative technique for detecting the core antigen. Furthermore, the core antigens are the sensor points present in human blood samples thus, the core antigen is detected quickly, accurately, and sen-sitively by these nucleic acid sensors in clinical diagnosis.

SARS-CoV-2, unlike other viruses, has a far wider worldwide distribution and infects far more people than MERS and SARS. The Coronaviridae family includes SARS-CoV-2. There are seven strains of the human SARS-CoV virus, four of which induce mild symptoms akin to a common cold (Hilgenfeld and Peiris, 2013;). Researchers found that the SARS-CoV-2 virus is comparable to prior human coro-naviruses. SARS-COV is a coronavirus-related severe acute respiratory disease (SARS). Although time-consuming and expensive, many diagnostic kits based on RT-PCR techniques for SARS-nCoV-2 detection are now in use and serve as gold standards for quantitative detection; (Woo et al., 2005). Due to expensive diag-nosis and the scarcity of test kits, community transmission handling is difficult. Mylab, India, created the first indigenous RT-PCR diagnostic kits, whereas Roche Diagnostics was one of the first to receive FDA clearance for their RT-PCR diag-nostic test kits. Furthermore, more POC equipment is needed in hotspots to expand diagnostic capabilities in asymptomatic patients. On-site testing will be facilitated by quick and simple instruments (Koteswara Rao, 2021).

Currently, there are no commercial solutions available for aptamer technology-based COVID-19 testing. As a result, aptamer-based kits offer novel diagnostic options for detecting human samples with SARS-CoV-2 viruses quickly and accu-rately. The procedure is well-defined and straightforward. The aptamer test is a fluorescence-free alternative to fluorescence-based assays for detecting target proteins, amino acids, nucleotides, antibiotics, peptides, and other compounds (Shafiei et al., 2020). To achieve high binding efficiency, the targeted proteins with ssDNA oligonucleotides obtained from the library are incubated in the Ni-NTA column. As a result, repeated washing removes unbound oligonucleotides. The oligonucleotides linked are then eluted and utilized as PCR templates. M-fold software tools are used to anticipate secondary structures in positive clones with greater target specificity. The aptamer target proteins' binding efficiency may be assessed using Fluorescence Resonance Energy Transfer (FRET)/SPR/RT-PCR. The aptamers have potential and are used in various assays and fluorescence techniques for the development of COVID-19 POC tools that are rapid, inexpensive, sensitive, and easy to use (Simpson et al., 2020a). The AptaDx (APT diagnostics) is a global leader in aptamer selection for nucleic acids, providing aptamer solutions, aptamer therapies, and aptamer diagnostics across a variety of platforms.

5.6   ADDITIONAL APTAMER-BASED DETECTION METHODS

To diagnose viral infections, researchers use tissue culture virus isolation, and different immunological and molecular techniques (Long et al., 2016). These approaches, on the other hand, have a number of disadvantages: they are expensive and require technicians, and may give false results, whereas an aptamer-based assay shows promising results in viral detection (Vidic et al., 2017). Biosensors combine a bioreceptor with a transducer to perform analytical tasks. With great sensitivity and selectivity, the bioreceptor detects and binds the target (Huang et al., 2021). Following that, the transducer transforms and sends signals generated by the analyte-bioreceptor interaction. An aptamer-based biosensor, known as aptasensor, uses aptamer-based bioreceptors known for capture probes and transducers known for their signal probes. Depending on the kind of transducer, aptasensors are categorized as optical and electronic aptasensor.

Optical aptasensors: Aptamers are used as a detection element in optical aptasensors, and other optical techniques are used as a signal transduction element. Optical aptasensors are categorized on the basis of changes in luminescence found as a result of interactions with various analytes. Based on these optical principles employed for material identification, viral optical aptasensors are divided into six types, including Surface-Enhanced Raman Scattering (SERS), Colorimetric, Chemiluminescence (CL), Fluorescence, Surface Plasmon Resonance (SPR), and Interferometry aptasensors.

Electrical aptasensors: These are used to detect an electrical signal created or altered when the aptamer attaches to the target. The sensing technique of these aptasensors determines whether they are electrochemical aptasensors or piezoelectric transducers.

5.6.1   APTAMER CHEMILUMINESCENCE IMMUNOSORBENT ASSAY

Other immunoassays that combine chemiluminescence technology with immunochemical reactions, such as ELISA, Fluorescent Immunoassays (FIA), and

Radioimmunoassay (RIA), which are comparable to aptamer immunosorbent chemiluminescence assay. The distinction is that instead of a particular antibody, there is an aptamer coating. These short RNA oligonucleotide sequences are specific to the target proteins (Jin et al., 2020). The aptamer hybrid immuno-chemiluminescence test detects minute amounts of viral protein. These RNA aptamers are ultrasensitive and accurately bind to the target.

SPR is a very sensitive method for identifying viruses that includes immobilizing an aptamer on SPR chips and measuring the aptamer's binding affinity to viral proteins, which shows the metal's free electrons resonance. The conjugation of gold nanoparticles (AuNP) with an aptamer forms a complex, and the viral protein attaches to the complex creating a fraction change in refractive index shift which is measured by polarised light intensity (Kumar et al., 2018; Zou et al., 2019). Because the equipment required for this method is expensive, this assay will not be transformed into a POC diagnostic kit.

5.6.2 NANOARRAY APTAMER-BASED CHIP ASSAY

An approach for identifying viral infections on a nanoscale is the nanoarray aptamer chip test. Dip-pen nanolithography is a technique for drawing patterns on a glass plate using an atomic force microscope (AFM) tip. Dip-pen nanolithography modification in the designs, a special aptamer is put on the surface (Ahn et al., 2009). Because this is a nanotechnology-based method, viral protein identification only takes a few microliters of sample. Antibodies are added to the aptamer and a viral protein complex is generated. This Ag-Ab combination is labelled with a fluorescence probe detected by a fluorescent microscope (Zon, 2022). This nanodevice is highly sensitive, and only a small sample volume is required.

5.6.3 APTAMER TECHNIQUE BASED ON FLUORESCENCE ENERGY TRANSFER

The FRET technique helps in biological research and medication development. FRET works by transferring energy across a distance from a donor molecule to an acceptor molecule where chromophore is the donor molecule. The fluorescence intensity and excited-state longevity of the donor are reduced as a result of the energy transfer, while the emission intensity of the acceptor rises. The combinations of nanomaterial, target, and ssDNA/RNA are combined to provide a fluorescence quenching detection platform that is sensitive and selective. The reduced graphene oxide (GO) reacts with nucleotides in rGOSELEX to improve its selection. This method does not need immobilization, it takes less time. The capture-SELEX method includes immobilizing nucleotide sequences, which results in the precise selection of single-stranded DNA for a specific target molecule. The linked aptamer to a fluorophore and the signal is quenched by FRET using a quencher. Because graphene is an energy acceptor, it is commonly used as a quencher. The fluorescence signal strength fluctuates when the interaction takes place, which may be used to quantify and maintain the target concentration. For multiplex tests employing FRET detection, the created new aptamer is tagged with biotin or fluorescein amidite (FAM) (Lee et al., 2017). The binding produces a conformational change in the reporter molecules, and as an increase in the distance between them, biotin-labelled aptamer shows promising results for multiplex detection through FRET. The complementary oligonucleotide release increases by the conformational shift in the aptamer, which turns on fluorescence in a fast quantitative gain of a signal after interaction with the target (Loeffelholz and Tang, 2020). The fluorescence may be measured using portable devices, and this assay can be used as a POC diagnostic tool.

5.7 NANOTECHNOLOGY IN DIAGNOSIS

In recent decades, nanotechnology has received considerable attention, because it provides a unique potential for developing the next generation of sensing instruments. POC devices that use modified nanoparticles to selectively detect biomolecules are a major focus of diagnostic research (Dai et al., 2016). The purpose of this article is to offer an outline of how POC-related nanotechnology works in identifying antibodies, nucleic acids, proteins, and pathogens. Future nanoparticle integrations with potential biomarkers will allow for quick therapeutic intervention against dangerous diseases by targeting particular microbes.

Nanoparticles (NPs) that are super paramagnetic and have a strong magnetic dipole–dipole attraction and ferromagnetic activity, such as some metal oxides, and quantum dots, have generated a lot of interest (Gonzalez-Rodriguez et al., 2019). Biosensors, medication, medical diagnostic instruments, pathogen detection, and extraction all employ nanoparticles (Ni et al., 2020). As a result of their high sensitivity, accuracy, selectivity, and cost-effectiveness, they are used to detect DNAs, and RNAs (Campos et al., 2020; Zhou et al., 2020).

The nucleotides in rGO-SELEX attach to the reduced GO nanoparticles, which contribute to the selection process. Immobilizing nucleotide sequences in the capture-SELEX method enables precise ssDNA selection against the specific target. In Immuno-SELEX, antibodies are developed against antigens, and the concepts of ELISA are utilized to increase efficiency. Quantum dots can be used in a variety of diagnostic systems. FRET-based nanosensors are capable of detecting a variety of tiny chemicals, and pathogens, including the H5N1 avian influenza virus (Bhalla et al., 2020; Zou et al., 2019).

Cadmium telluride quantum dots (QDs) were coupled with silica nanoparticles to magnify ECM signals. This technique was created to identify LMP-1 (latent membrane protein 1) generated from the Epstein-Barr virus (Chen et al., 2010). The nano-sized carriers provide a huge surface that allows a large number of QDs to be immobilized. Square wave voltammetry is beneficial for measuring the amplification of ECM signals. As a result, the LOD has been lowered to 1 pg/mL. The consistent efficacy of the QDs immobilization method shows high assay repeatability.

The illness rate in India is very high, so researchers focused on cancer diagnostic research. Nanobiosensors have been identified as a promising material for ultrasensitive POC cancer detection. In comparison to traditional diagnostic approaches, it allows for the creation of superior and sophisticated diagnostic techniques (Chandra et al., 2017). Singh et al. (2018) created a graphene-based biosensor with remarkable sensitivity for assessing the cancer biomarker carcinoembryonic antigen (CEA).

Antigen-12 was detected using a multi-walled carbon nanotube with a zinc oxide nanowire as a sensing device (Paul et al., 2017).

Many researchers and groups have created and employed EC aptasensors for CTC detection (Shangguan et al., 2006). The CCRF-CEM (leukaemia) cells were detected using a cell-SELEX–derived EC aptasensor, and Ramos (human Burkitt's lymphoma) cells were used as experimental controls. The nanomaterials enhance sensor performance by improving electron transfer activity, so the label-free EC impedance spectroscopy containing AS1411 aptamer functionalized graphene was successfully constructed to identify HeLa cells (Feng et al., 2011). In the fabrication of EC aptasensors, other nanomaterials have been employed as signal amplification probes (Tian et al., 2017). In addition, QDs were used as an electroactive species to enhance signals, researchers created a super sandwich EC cytosensor that recognized leukaemia CTCs with a LOD of 50 cells/mL. The electrical signal is used in the real-time aptasensor for detecting HIV-1. Nanopores resistive-pulse method and an RNA aptamer (affinity for HIV-1 nucleocapsid protein 7) were employed in this investigation. The ionic current passes through the nanopores after applying a voltage across a silicon nitride membrane. The current was interrupted and replaced with a translocation event signal as the aptamer-protein combination passed the membrane.

5.8 CONCLUSION AND FUTURE SCOPE

In consideration of emergency situations and the associated general health impacts, this review focused on current diagnostic tools and techniques. Several serological diagnostic techniques are available but, these techniques may result in false positives or negatives, the major health issue prerequisites more cheap and efficient POC techniques nowadays.

Point-of-careology is a new profession that will allow on-site diagnostics and evidence-based medicine for patients. This profession provides high-quality point-of-need medical care with some advantages like low-cost testing, high nursing standards, and strong patient interaction with improved outcomes. The idea of point-of-careology incorporates a number of important aspects of POC systems, which include, increasing patient access to primary care, increasing the economic productivity of testing, reducing response time in medical crises, and simplifying speedy testing of novel modalities.

POC technology has revolutionized the medical industry thanks to recent improvements in epidermal electronics and portable diagnostic equipment. Miniature wearables are emerging and sophisticated technologies that allow, continuous and real-time data acquisition for processing and clinical understanding. AI-powered POC devices continue to break new ground in the medical field. Modern POC devices use critical biological data from patients' places by using cameras, and cutting-edge AI technology. These future technologies can also be used to alert medical personnel about patient quick assistance. Medical practitioners are rapidly opting for POC devices due to their availability and sensitivity. This review will aid in the creation of new information for researchers working on diagnostic platforms based on nano-biotechnology to tackle a variety of infectious illnesses.

ACKNOWLEDGEMENT

Kalpesh V. Bhavsar; Uday P. Jagtap and Hardik S. Churi gratefully acknowledge the support provided by the National Centre for Nanosciences and Nanotechnology, University of Mumbai, India, and Sonopant Dandekar Shikshan Mandali's (SDSM) College, Palghar, India.

REFERENCES

Adachi, T. and Nakamura, Y., 2019. Aptamers: A review of their chemical properties and modifications for therapeutic application. *Molecules, 24*(23), p. 4229.

Ahn, D. G., Jeon, I. J., Kim, J. D., Song, M. S., Han, S. R., Lee, S. W., et al., 2009. RNA aptamer-based sensitive detection of SARS coronavirus nucleocapsid protein. *Analyst, 134*(9), pp. 1896–1901.

Banerjee, S. and Nilsen-Hamilton, M., 2019. Aptamers for infectious disease diagnosis. In *E. coli Infections-Importance of Early Diagnosis and Efficient Treatment*. IntechOpen.

Bhalla, N., Pan, Y., Yang, Z. and Payam, A. F., 2020. Opportunities and challenges for biosensors and nanoscale analytical tools for pandemics: COVID-19. *ACS Nano, 14*(7), pp. 7783–7807.

Bruno, J. G. and Kiel, J. L., 2002. Use of magnetic beads in selection and detection of biotoxin aptamers by electrochemiluminescence and enzymatic methods. *BioTechniques, 32*(1), pp. 178–183.

Bruno, J. G., Richarte, A. M., Phillips, T., Savage, A. A., Sivils, J. C., Greis, A. and Mayo, M. W., 2014. Development of a fluorescent enzyme-linked DNA aptamer-magnetic bead sandwich assay and portable fluorometer for sensitive and rapid leishmania detection in sandflies. *Journal of Fluorescence, 24*(1), pp. 267–277.

Caglayan, M. O. and Üstündağ, Z., 2020. Spectrophotometric ellipsometry based Tat-protein RNA-aptasensor for HIV-1 diagnosis. *Spectrochimica Acta Part A: Molecular and Biomolecular Spectroscopy, 227*, p. 117748.

Cai, R., Yin, F., Zhang, Z., Tian, Y. and Zhou, N., 2019. Functional chimera aptamer and molecular beacon based fluorescent detection of *Staphylococcus aureus* with strand displacement-target recycling amplification. *Analytica Chimica Acta, 1075*, pp. 128–136.

Campos, S., Salazar, R., Arancibia-Miranda, N., Rubio, M. A., Aranda, M., García, A., Sepúlveda, P. and Espinoza, L. C., 2020. Nafcillin degradation by heterogeneous electro-Fenton process using Fe, Cu and Fe/Cu nanoparticles. *Chemosphere, 247*, p. 125813.

Chandra, P., Tan, Y. N. and Singh, S. P. eds., 2017. *Next Generation Point-of-Care Biomedical Sensors Technologies for Cancer Diagnosis* (Vol. 10, pp. 978–981). Singapore: Springer Singapore.

Chang, Y. C., Yang, C. Y., Sun, R. L., Cheng, Y. F., Kao, W. C. and Yang, P. C., 2013. Rapid single cell detection of *Staphylococcus aureus* by aptamer-conjugated gold nanoparticles. *Scientific Reports, 3*(1), pp. 1–7.

Chen, Y., Chen, Z., He, Y., Lin, H., Sheng, P., Liu, C., Luo, S. and Cai, Q., 2010. L-cysteine-capped CdTe QD-based sensor for simple and selective detection of trinitrotoluene. *Nanotechnology, 21*(12), p. 125502.

Chen, Y., Liu, X., Guo, S., Cao, J., Zhou, J., Zuo, J. and Bai, L., 2019. A sandwich-type electrochemical aptasensor for Mycobacterium tuberculosis MPT64 antigen detection using C60NPs decorated N-CNTs/GO nanocomposite coupled with conductive PEI-functionalized metal-organic framework. *Biomaterials, 216*, p. 119253.

Dai, T. N. T., Wang, H., Sugiarto, S., Li, T., Ang, W. H., Lee, C. and Pastorin, G., 2016. Advances in nanomaterials and their applications in point of care (POC) devices for the diagnosis of infectious diseases. *Biotechnolgy Advances, 34*(8), pp. 1275–1288.

Deisenhofer, J., 1981. Crystallographic refinement and atomic models of a human Fc fragment and its complex with fragment B of protein A from *Staphylococcus aureus* at 2.9-and 2.8-.ANG. resolution. *Biochemistry, 20*(9), pp. 2361–2370.

Deng, X., Wang, C., Gao, Y., Li, J., Wen, W., Zhang, X. and Wang, S., 2018. Applying strand displacement amplification to quantum dots-based fluorescent lateral flow assay strips for HIV-DNA detection. *Biosensors and Bioelectronics, 105*, pp. 211–217.

Dhiman, A., Kalra, P., Bansal, V., Bruno, J. G. and Sharma, T. K., 2017. Aptamer-based point-of-care diagnostic platforms. *Sensors and Actuators B: Chemical, 246*, pp. 535–553.

Dirkzwager, R. M., Liang, S. and Tanner, J. A., 2016. Development of aptamer-based point-of-care diagnostic devices for malaria using three-dimensional printing rapid prototyping. *ACS Sensors, 1*(4), pp. 420–426.

Ellington, A. D. and Szostak, J. W., 1990. In vitro selection of RNA molecules that bind specific ligands. *Nature, 346*(6287), pp. 818–822.

England, J. M., Hyde, K., Lewis, S. M., Mackie, I. J., Rowan, R. M., Rowan, R. M., Bain, B. J., England, J. M., Hyde, K., Lewis, S. M. and Matutes, E. M., 1995. Guidelines for near patient testing: Haematology. *Clinical & Laboratory Haematology, 17*(4), pp. 301–310.

Feng, L., Chen, Y., Ren, J. and Qu, X., 2011. A graphene functionalized electrochemical aptasensor for selective label-free detection of cancer cells. *Biomaterials, 32*, pp. 2930–2937.

Frohnmeyer, E., Tuschel, N., Sitz, T., Hermann, C., Dahl, G. T., Schulz, F., Baeumner, A. J. and Fischer, M., 2019. Aptamer lateral flow assays for rapid and sensitive detection of cholera toxin. *Analyst, 144*(5), pp. 1840–1849.

Ghanbari, K. and Roushani, M., 2018. A nanohybrid probe based on double recognition of an aptamer MIP grafted onto a MWCNTs-Chit nanocomposite for sensing hepatitis C virus core antigen. *Sensors and Actuators B: Chemical, 258*, pp. 1066–1071.

Ghanbari, K., Roushani, M. and Azadbakht, A., 2017. Ultra-sensitive aptasensor based on a GQD nanocomposite for detection of hepatitis C virus core antigen. *Analytical Biochemistry, 534*, pp. 64–69.

González, V. M., Martín, M. E., Fernández, G. and García-Sacristán, A., 2016. Use of aptamers as diagnostics tools and antiviral agents for human viruses. *Pharmaceuticals, 9*(4), p. 78.

Gonzalez-Rodriguez, R., Campbell, E. and Naumov, A., 2019. Multifunctional graphene oxide/iron oxide nanoparticles for magnetic targeted drug delivery dual magnetic resonance/fluorescence imaging and cancer sensing. *PLoS One, 14*(6), p. e0217072.

Hermann, T. and Patel, D.J., 2000. Adaptive recognition by nucleic acid aptamers. *Science, 287*(5454), pp. 820–825.

Hilgenfeld, R. and Peiris, M., 2013. From SARS to MERS: 10 years of research on highly pathogenic human coronaviruses. *Antiviral Research, 100*(1), pp. 286–295.

Huang, J., Chen, X., Fu, X., Li, Z., Huang, Y. and Liang, C., 2021. Advances in aptamer-based biomarker discovery. *Frontiers in Cell and Developmental Biology, 9*, p. 571.

Huang, R., Xi, Z., Deng, Y. and He, N., 2016. Fluorescence based aptasensors for the determination of hepatitis B virus e antigen. *Scientific Reports, 6*(1), pp. 1–7.

Ilgu, M., Fazlioglu, R., Ozturk, M., Ozsurekci, Y. and Nilsen-Hamilton, M., 2019. Aptamers for diagnostics with applications for infectious diseases. In Ince, M. and Ince, O. K. (eds.), *Recent Advances in Analytical Chemistry* (pp. 1–32). IntechOpen.

Jarczewska, M., Górski, Ł. and Malinowska, E., 2016. Electrochemical aptamer-based biosensors as potential tools for clinical diagnostics. *Analytical Methods, 8*(19), pp. 3861–3877.

Jeon, W., Lee, S., Manjunatha, D. H. and Ban, C., 2013. A colorimetric aptasensor for the diagnosis of malaria based on cationic polymers and gold nanoparticles. *Analytical Biochemistry, 439*(1), pp. 11–16.

Jin, J. M., Bai, P., He, W., Wu, F., Liu, X. F., Han, D. M., et al., 2020. Gender differences in patients with COVID-19: Focus on severity and mortality. *Frontiers in Public Health, 8*, p. 152.

Johnson, N. P. and Mueller, J., 2002. Updating the accounts: global mortality of the 1918-1920" Spanish" influenza pandemic. *Bulletin of the History of Medicine*, pp. 105–115.

Kang, J., Yeom, G., Jang, H., Oh, J., Park, C. J. and Kim, M. G., 2019. Development of replication protein A-conjugated gold nanoparticles for highly sensitive detection of disease biomarkers. *Analytical Chemistry, 91*(15), pp. 10001–10007.

Kaper, J., Morris, J. G. and Levine, M., 1995. Cholera. *Clinical Microbiology Review, 8*(1), pp. 48–86.

Khan, N. I. and Song, E., 2020. Lab-on-a-chip systems for aptamer-based biosensing. *Micromachines, 11*(2), p. 220.

Kim, D. J., Park, H. C., Sohn, I. Y., Jung, J. H., Yoon, O. J., Park, J. S., Yoon, M. Y. and Lee, N. E., 2013. Electrical graphene aptasensor for ultra-sensitive detection of anthrax toxin with amplified signal transduction. *Small, 9*(19), pp. 3352–3360.

Konwar, A. N. and Borse, V., 2020. Current status of point-of-care diagnostic devices in the Indian healthcare system with an update on COVID-19 pandemic. *Sensors International, 1*, p. 100015.

Kost, G. J., 1977. Utilization of surface pH electrodes to establish a new relationship for muscle surface pH, venous pH, and arterial pH. In *Proceedings of the San Diego Biomedical Symposium* (Vol. 16, pp. 25–33). San Diego Biomedical Symposium.

Kumar, A. R., Mudili, V., and Poda, S. (2018). Development of a FRET-based fluorescence aptasensor for the detection of aflatoxin B1 in contaminated food grain samples. *RSC Advances, 8*(19), pp. 10465–10473.

Kumar Kulabhusan, P., Hussain, B. and Yüce, M., 2020. Current perspectives on aptamers as diagnostic tools and therapeutic agents. *Pharmaceutics, 12*(7), p. 646.

Kwon, O. S., Ahn, S. R., Park, S. J., Song, H. S., Lee, S. H., Lee, J. S., Hong, J. Y., Lee, J. S., You, S. A., Yoon, H. and Park, T. H., 2012. Ultrasensitive and selective recognition of peptide hormone using close-packed arrays of hPTHR-conjugated polymer nanoparticles. *ACS Nano, 6*(6), pp. 5549–5558.

Lahousse, M., Park, H. C., Lee, S. C., Ha, N. R., Jung, I. P., Schlesinger, S. R., Shackelford, K., Yoon, M. Y. and Kim, S. K., 2018. Inhibition of anthrax lethal factor by ssDNA aptamers. *Archives of Biochemistry and Biophysics, 646*, pp. 16–23.

Lara, P., Palma-Florez, S., Salas-Huenuleo, E., Polakovicova, I., Guerrero, S., Lobos-Gonzalez, L., Campos, A., Muñoz, L., Jorquera-Cordero, C., Varas-Godoy, M. and Cancino, J., 2020. Gold nanoparticle based double-labeling of melanoma extracellular vesicles to determine the specificity of uptake by cells and preferential accumulation in small metastatic lung tumors. *Journal of Nanobiotechnology, 18*(1), pp. 1–17.

Lavania, S., Das, R., Dhiman, A., Myneedu, V. P., Verma, A., Singh, N., Sharma, T. K. and Tyagi, J. S., 2018. Aptamer-based TB antigen tests for the rapid diagnosis of pulmonary tuberculosis: Potential utility in screening for tuberculosis. *ACS Infectious Diseases, 4*(12), pp. 1718–1726.

Lee, J., Jung, J., Ko, T., Kim, S., Kim, S. I., Nah, J., et al., 2017. Catalytic synergy effect of MoS2/reduced graphene oxide hybrids for a highly efficient hydrogen evolution reaction. *RSC Advances, 7*(9), pp. 5480–5487.

Li, H. Y., Jia, W. N., Li, X. Y., Zhang, L., Liu, C. and Wu, J., 2020. Advances in detection of infectious agents by aptamer-based technologies. *Emerging Microbes & Infections, 9*(1), pp. 1671–1681.

Li, L., Li, Q., Liao, Z., Sun, Y., Cheng, Q., Song, Y., Song, E. and Tan, W., 2018a. Magnetism-resolved separation and fluorescence quantification for near-simultaneous detection of multiple pathogens. *Analytical Chemistry, 90*(15), pp. 9621–9628.

Li, L., Liu, Z., Zhang, H., Yue, W., Li, C. W. and Yi, C., 2018b. A point-of-need enzyme linked aptamer assay for *Mycobacterium tuberculosis* detection using a smartphone. *Sensors and Actuators B: Chemical*, *254*, pp. 337–346.

Liu, A., Zhang, Y., Chen, W., Wang, X. and Chen, F., 2013. Gold nanoparticle-based colorimetric detection of *Staphylococcal enterotoxin* B using ssDNA aptamers. *European Food Research and Technology*, *237*(3), pp. 323–329.

Loeffelholz, M. J., and Tang, Y. W., 2020. Laboratory diagnosis of emerging human coronavirus infections—the state of the art. *Emerging Microbes & Infections, 9*(1), pp. 747–756.

Long, Y., Qin, Z., Duan, M., Li, S., Wu, X., Lin, W., Li, J., Zhao, Z., Liu, J., Xiong, D. and Huang, Y., 2016. Screening and identification of DNA aptamers toward Schistosoma japonicum eggs via SELEX. *Scientific Reports*, *6*(1), pp. 1–9.

Mahato, K., Maurya, P. K. and Chandra, P., 2018. Fundamentals and commercial aspects of nanobiosensors in point-of-care clinical diagnostics. *3 Biotech*, *8*(3), pp. 1–14.

Mahato, K., Prasad, A., Maurya, P. and Chandra, P., 2016. Nanobiosensors: Next generation point-of-care biomedical devices for personalized diagnosis. *Journal of Analytical & Bioanalytical Techniques*, *7*, p. e125.

Martin, D. R., Sibuyi, N. R., Dube, P., Fadaka, A. O., Cloete, R., Onani, M., Madiehe, A. M. and Meyer, M., 2021. Aptamer-based diagnostic systems for the rapid screening of TB at the point-of-care. *Diagnostics, 11*, p. 1352.

McKay, P. F., Hu, K., Blakney, A. K., Samnuan, K., Brown, J. C., Penn, R., Zhou, J., Bouton, C. R., Rogers, P., Polra, K. and Lin, P. J., 2020. Self-amplifying RNA SARS-CoV-2 lipid nanoparticle vaccine candidate induces high neutralizing antibody titers in mice. *Nature Communications*, *11*(1), pp. 1–7.

Miyakawa, S., Nomura, Y., Sakamoto, T., Yamaguchi, Y., Kato, K., Yamazaki, S. and Nakamura, Y., 2008. Structural and molecular basis for hyperspecificity of RNA aptamer to human immunoglobulin G. *RNA, 14*(6), pp. 1154–1163.

Nagarkatti, R., Bist, V., Sun, S., Fortes de Araujo, F., Nakhasi, H. L. and Debrabant, A., 2012. Development of an aptamer-based concentration method for the detection of *Trypanosoma cruzi* in blood. *PLoS One*. https://doi.org/10.1371/journal.pone.0043533

Nagata, S., Tsutsumi, T., Yoshida, F. and Ueno, Y., 1999. A new type sandwich immunoassay for microcystin: production of monoclonal antibodies specific to the immune complex formed by microcystin and an anti-microcystin monoclonal antibody. *Natural Toxins*, *7*(2), pp. 49–55.

Ni, L., Ye, F., Cheng, M.L., Feng, Y., Deng, Y.Q., Zhao, H., Wei, P., Ge, J., Gou, M., Li, X. and Sun, L., 2020. Detection of SARS-CoV-2-specific humoral and cellular immunity in COVID-19 convalescent individuals. *Immunity, 52*(6), pp. 971–977.

Nomura, Y., Sugiyama, S., Sakamoto, T., Miyakawa, S., Adachi, H., Takano, K., Murakami, S., Inoue, T., Mori, Y., Nakamura, Y. and Matsumura, H., 2010. Conformational plasticity of RNA for target recognition as revealed by the 2.15 Å crystal structure of a human IgG–aptamer complex. *Nucleic Acids Research*, *38*(21), pp. 7822–7829.

Pai, N. P., Vadnais, C., Denkinger, C., Engel, N. and Pai, M., 2012. Point-of-care testing for infectious diseases: Diversity, complexity, and barriers in low-and middle-income countries. *PLoS Medicine*. https://doi.org/10.1371/journal.pmed.1001306

Park, K. S., 2018. Nucleic acid aptamer-based methods for diagnosis of infections. *Biosensors and Bioelectronics*, *102*, pp. 179–188.

Paul, K. B., Singh, V., Vanjari, S. R. K. and Singh, S. G., 2017. One step biofunctionalized electrospun multiwalled carbon nanotubes embedded zinc oxide nanowire interface for highly sensitive detection of carcinoma antigen-125. *Biosensors and Bioelectronics*, *88*, pp. 144–152.

Perez, C., 2003. *Technological revolutions and financial capital.* Cheltenham: Edward Elgar Publishing.

Perez, J. M., O'Loughin, T., Simeone, F. J., Weissleder, R. and Josephson, L., 2002. DNA-based magnetic nanoparticle assembly acts as a magnetic relaxation nanoswitch allowing screening of DNA-cleaving agents. *Journal of the American Chemical Society, 124*(12), pp. 2856–2857.

Peruski, A. H. and Peruski Jr, L. F., 2003. Immunological methods for detection and identification of infectious disease and biological warfare agents. *Clinical and Vaccine Immunology, 10*(4), pp. 506–513.

Prasidthrathsint, K. and Stapleton, J. T., 2019. Laboratory diagnosis and monitoring of viral hepatitis. *Gastroenterology Clinics, 48*(2), pp. 259–279.

Rajendran, R. and Rayman, G., 2014. Point-of-care blood glucose testing for diabetes care in hospitalized patients: An evidence-based review. *Journal of Diabetes Science and Technology, 8*(6), pp. 1081–1090.

Raptis, C. A., Hammer, M. M., Short, R. G., Shah, A., Bhalla, S., Bierhals, A. J., Filev, P. D., Hope, M. D., Jeudy, J., Kligerman, S. J. and Henry, T. S., 2020. Chest CT and coronavirus disease (COVID-19): A critical review of the literature to date. *AJR American Journal of Roentgenology, 215*(4), pp. 839–842.

Röthlisberger, P. and Hollenstein, M., 2018. Aptamer chemistry. *Advanced Drug Delivery Reviews, 134*, pp. 3–21.

Santosh, B. and Yadava, P. K., 2014. Nucleic acid aptamers: Research tools in disease diagnostics and therapeutics. *BioMed Research International, 2014*, p. 540451.

Shafiei, G., Markello, R. D., De Wael, R. V., Bernhardt, B. C., Fulcher, B. D. and Misic, B., 2020. Topographic gradients of intrinsic dynamics across neocortex. *Elife, 9*, p. e62116.

Shangguan, D., Li, Y., Tang, Z., Cao, Z. C., Chen, H. W., et al., 2006. Aptamers evolved from live cells as effective molecular probes for cancer study. *PNAS, 103*, pp. 11838–11843.

Shigdar, S., 2019. Aptamer-based diagnostics and therapeutics. *Pharmaceuticals, 12*(1), p. 6.

Shukla, S., Haldorai, Y., Khan, I., Kang, S. M., Kwak, C. H., Gandhi, S., Bajpai, V. K., Huh, Y. S. and Han, Y. K., 2020. Bioreceptor-free, sensitive and rapid electrochemical detection of patulin fungal toxin, using a reduced graphene oxide@ SnO_2 nanocomposite. *Materials Science and Engineering: C, 113*, p. 110916.

Simpson, S., Kay, F. U., Abbara, S., Bhalla, S., Chung, J. H., Chung, M., Henry, T. S., Kanne, J. P., Kligerman, S., Ko, J. P. and Litt, H., 2020a. Radiological Society of North America expert consensus statement on reporting chest CT findings related to COVID-19. Endorsed by the Society of Thoracic Radiology, the American College of Radiology, and RSNA. *Journal of Thoracic Imaging, 35*(4), pp. 219–227.

Sin, M. L., Mach, K. E., Wong, P. K. and Liao, J. C., 2014. Advances and challenges in biosensor-based diagnosis of infectious diseases. *Expert Review of Molecular Diagnostics, 14*(2), pp. 225–244.

Singh, N. K., Ray, P., Carlin, A. F., Magallanes, C., Morgan, S. C., Laurent, L. C., Aronoff-Spencer, E. S. and Hall, D. A., 2021. Hitting the diagnostic sweet spot: Point-of-care SARS-CoV-2 salivary antigen testing with an off-the-shelf glucometer. *Biosensors and Bioelectronics, 180*, p. 113111.

Singh, V. K., Kumar, S., Pandey, S. K., Srivastava, S., Mishra, M., Gupta, G., Malhotra, B. D., Tiwari, R. S. and Srivastava, A., 2018. Fabrication of sensitive bioelectrode based on atomically thin CVD grown graphene for cancer biomarker detection. *Biosensors and Bioelectronics, 105*, pp. 173–181.

Singhal, C., Bruno, J. G., Kaushal, A. and Sharma, T. K., 2021. Recent advances and a road-map to aptamer-based sensors for bloodstream infections. *ACS Applied Bio Materials*, *4*(5), pp. 3962–3984.

St John, A. and Price, C. P., 2014. Existing and emerging technologies for point-of-care testing. *The Clinical Biochemist Reviews*, *35*(3), p. 155.

Stoltenburg, R., Reinemann, C. and Strehlitz, B., 2007. SELEX—a (r) evolutionary method to generate high-affinity nucleic acid ligands. *Biomolecular Engineering*, *24*(4), pp. 381–403.

Suh, S. H., Choi, S. J., Dwivedi, H. P., Moore, M. D., Escudero-Abarca, B. I. and Jaykus, L. A., 2018. Use of DNA aptamer for sandwich type detection of Listeria monocytogenes. *Analytical Biochemistry*, *557*, pp. 27–33.

Sypabekova, M., Jolly, P., Estrela, P. and Kanayeva, D., 2019. Electrochemical aptasensor using optimized surface chemistry for the detection of *Mycobacterium tuberculosis* secreted protein MPT64 in human serum. *Biosensors and Bioelectronics*, *123*, pp. 141–151.

Taubenberger, J. K., Baltimore, D., Doherty, P. C., Markel, H., Morens, D. M., Webster, R. G. and Wilson, I. A., 2012. Reconstruction of the 1918 influenza virus: Unexpected rewards from the past. *MBio*, *3*(5), pp. e00201-12.

Thakur, H., Kaur, N., Sareen, D. and Prabhakar, N., 2017. Electrochemical determination of *M. tuberculosis* antigen based on poly(3,4-ethylenedioxythiophene) and functionalized carbon nanotubes hybrid platform. *Talanta*, *171*, pp. 115–123.

Tian, L., Qi, J., Qian, K., Oderinde, O., Liu, Q., et al., 2017. Copper (II) oxide nanozyme based electrochemical cytosensor for high sensitive detection of circulating tumor cells in breast cancer. *Journal of Electroanalytical Chemistry*, *812*, pp. 1–9.

Tomita, M. and Tsumoto, K., 2011. Hybridoma technologies for antibody production. *Immunotherapy*, *3*(3), pp. 371–380.

Tuerk, C. and Gold, L., 1990. Systematic evolution of ligands by exponential enrichment: RNA ligands to bacteriophage T4 DNA polymerase. *Science*, *249*(4968), pp. 505–510.

Vashist, S. K., 2017. Point-of-care diagnostics: Recent advances and trends. *Biosensors*, *7*(4), p. 62.

Vidic, J., Manzano, M., Chang, C. M. and Jaffrezic-Renault, N., 2017. Advanced biosensors for detection of pathogens related to livestock and poultry. *Veterinary Research*, *48*(1), pp. 1–22.

Vivekananda, J. and Kiel, J. L., 2006. Anti-*Francisella tularensis* DNA aptamers detect tula-remia antigen from different subspecies by aptamer-linked immobilized sorbent assay. *Laboratory Investigation*, *86*(6), pp. 610–618.

Wei, X., Zhou, W., Sanjay, S. T., Zhang, J., Jin, Q., Xu, F., Dominguez, D. C. and Li, X., 2018. Multiplexed instrument-free bar-chart spinchip integrated with nanoparticle-mediated magnetic aptasensors for visual quantitative detection of multiple pathogens. *Analytical Chemistry*, *90*(16), pp. 9888–9896.

Woo, P. C., Lau, S. K., Chu, C. M., Chan, K. H., Tsoi, H. W., Huang, Y., Wong, B. H., Poon, R. W., Cai, J. J., Luk, W. K. and Poon, L. L., 2005. Characterization and complete genome sequence of a novel coronavirus, coronavirus HKU1, from patients with pneumonia. *Journal of Virology*, *79*(2), pp. 884–895.

Xi, Z., Gong, Q., Wang, C. and Zheng, B., 2018. Highly sensitive chemiluminescent apta-sensor for detecting HBV infection based on rapid magnetic separation and double-functionalized gold nanoparticles. *Scientific Reports*, *8*(1), pp. 1–7.

Ye, H., Duan, N., Gu, H., Wang, H. and Wang, Z., 2019. Fluorometric determination of lipo-polysaccharides via changes of the graphene oxide-enhanced fluorescence polarization caused by truncated aptamers. *Microchimica Acta*, *186*(3), pp. 1–8.

Zeng, J., Li, X., Yuan, H., Ma, M., Li, D., Ma, J. and Liao, S., 2017. Screening ssDNA aptamers against HIV P24 antigen using agarose beads as carriers. In *BIO Web of Conferences* (Vol. 8, p. 03009). EDP Sciences.

Zhang, K., Yang, Q., Huang, W., Wang, K., Zhu, X. and Xie, M., 2019. Detection of HIV-1 ribonuclease H activity in single-cell by using RNA mimics green fluorescent protein based biosensor. *Sensors and Actuators B: Chemical*, *281*, pp. 439–444.

Zhou, B., Qiu, Y., Wen, Q., Zhu, M. and Yang, P., 2017. Dual electrochemiluminescence signal system for in situ and simultaneous evaluation of multiple cell-surface receptors. *ACS Applied Materials & Interfaces*, *9*(3), pp. 2074–2082.

Zon, G., 2022. Recent advances in aptamer applications for analytical biochemistry. *Analytical Biochemistry, 644*, 113894.

Zou, X., Wu, J., Gu, J., Shen, L., and Mao, L., 2019. Application of aptamers in virus detection and antiviral therapy. *Frontiers in Microbiology, 10*, 1462.

6 Aptamer-based colorimetric biosensor

Yasmin Bano and Sadhana Chaturvedi

6.1 INTRODUCTION

Since the genetic material discovered, a common thought has been come into existence that nucleic acids (DNA and RNA) are the genetic blueprint of everyone's life because they carry the information of an organism's life about their growth, development, and replication (Lander et al. 2001, Venter et al. 2001). Furthermore, scientific studies revealed that these molecules can also form complex 3D shapes (ribozymes or DNAzymes etc.) that catalyse reactions (Doudna and Cech 2002), communicate cellular responses (Zovoilis et al. 2016), gene regulations (Sonenberg and Hinnebusch 2009) and protein regulations (Moore and Steitz 2002). Not only, the biological importance of folded RNA has been recognized long before but the non-biological functions were also achieved with the *in vitro* evolution of these molecules, this happened only when producing bulks of degenerate oligonucleotides by solid-phase synthesis and PCR (polymerase chain reaction) amplify every solo molecule (Caruthers 1985, Saiki et al. 1988). Through several technologies, functionally active oligonucleotides can easily be isolated and enabled to bind with a respective target and/or catalyze a chemical reaction (Wilson and Szostak 1999). These DNA or RNA-based affinity molecules or reagents are referred to as aptamers, the word aptamers is derived from a linguistic chimera composed of the Latin word 'aptus' (-to fit) and the Greek suffix 'meros' or 'mer' (-part) (Ellington and Szostak 1990, Tuerk and Gold 1990). Aptamers are a newly emerged class of oligonucleotide-based molecular recognition elements that rival antibody-based methods. Aptamers can be synthesized according to the need to bind to a wide range of chemical and biological targets from small molecules to whole cells (Dunn et al. 2017). On the other hand, colorimetric analysis is a technique to detect coloured compounds in the medium generated during the analysis assay. Colorimetric assay employing sensitivity and convenience to detect even pico-molar concentration of target molecule that can be readily detectable with the naked eye. Biosensors are analytical devices able to detect specific analytes and work even when challenged with complex sample matrices such as whole blood or blood serum. Thus, aptamers have been extensively used for target recognition in the development of biosensors (McConnell et al. 2020, Röthlisberger and Hollenstein 2018, Yu et al. 2021, Zhou and Tang 2020). Herein, basically, this chapter focused on the techniques relay upon the aptamer-based colorimetric biosensing assays and discussed the construction and working methodology of colorimetric aptasensors. These devices and designs are used in various fields for the betterment

DOI: 10.1201/9781003304227-6

of human life (especially medical diagnostics and therapeutics) and environmental health. Furthermore, this endeavor not only highlights recent advances in aptamer-based screening methods but also describes their analytical application.

6.2 TRENDS IN APTAMERS-BASED TECHNIQUES

The SELEX (systematic evolution of ligands by exponential enrichment) process called as *in vitro* selection is the selection process of aptamers from large random-sequence libraries (Ellington and Szostak 1990, Robertson and Joyce 1990, Tuerk and Gold 1990). Once the oligonucleotide molecules bound to their respective target are separated from the unbound pool, further to be amplified to generate a new population of molecules that share a common parental functional property (Levine and Nilsen-Hamilton 2007). Selecting sensitivity further increased firstly by performing the counter selection, a process of adding similar molecular structure to the analyte, and second by removing extra base-pair are bound to the non-targeted targets (Prante et al. 2020). Nucleic acids are suitable candidates that can fold into 3D structures with a defined sequence (genotypes) and function (phenotypes) and *in vitro* replication capability to make thousands of progenies with similar parental characteristics (Wilson and Szostak 1999). Optimizing their functions by directed evolution makes nucleic acid ideal and distinguished from the other organic molecules which cannot replicate due to lack of a genotype-phenotype connections (Joyce 1994, Szostak 1992). The selection process and backbone chemistry influenced the properties which an aptamer inherent with minimal possibility of not determining the approached target (Wilson and Szostak 1999, Wu et al. 2019a). Consequently, studies support that selection of the way of development tends to favour targets that are used successfully and that are considered to be highly aptagenic for example VEGF (vascular endothelial growth factor), human α-thrombin, and influenza haemagglutinin having clear implications for aptamer therapeutics (Keefe et al. 2010). While, some took advantage of selection protocols that implement directly to produce aptamers after little selective amplification cycles like ATP (Adenosine 5′-triphosphate) and streptavidin (Sassanfar and Szostak 1993, Wilson et al. 2001).

Aptamers are single-stranded nucleic acid (ssRNA or ssDNA) molecules, on folding mimic like antibodies that bind to the specific targets. As aptamer production is a chemical rather than a biological process i.e., can be engineered or synthetically generated *in vitro* with the least viral or bacterial contamination. Some aptamers exist naturally like ligand-binding elements of riboswitches, or can be tailored for defined specific targets (Weinberg et al. 2017). Because of their ease of synthesis, inexpensive production, small size, regeneration, low batch-to-batch variability, labelling, reversible folding properties, high target binding affinity, and less immunogenicity preferred aptamers over antibodies (Arshavsky-Graham et al. 2020, Keefe et al. 2010, Zhao et al. 2022). However, the true value of aptamers lies in the simplicity by which these molecules can be engineered into sensors, actuators, and other devices that are often central to emerging technologies. Ongoing research approved that aptamers have the capability to bind a wide variety of target molecules like simple inorganic molecules, protein complexes, etc. with great affinity and specificity (Alkhamis et al. 2019, Ruscito and DeRosa 2016). Initially, studies were focused

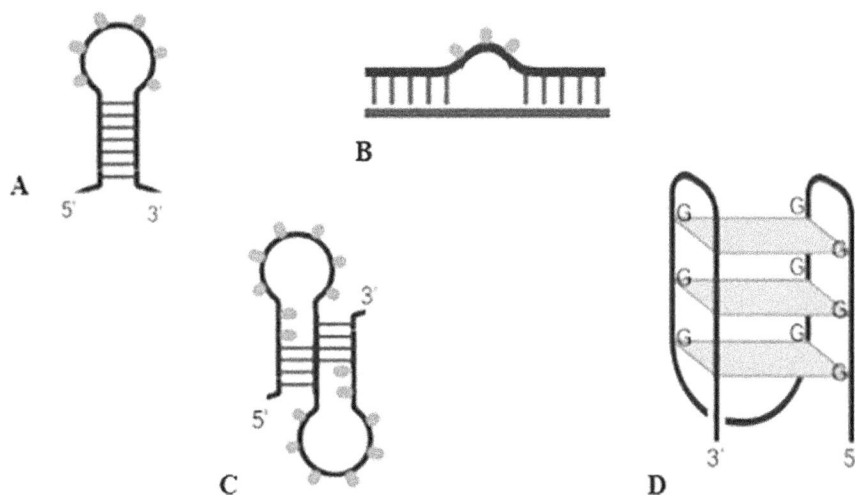

FIGURE 6.1 Aptamer's 2D structures. (a) Stem loop. (b) K-turn loop. (c) Pseudoknot. (d) 3D G-quadruplex.

only on protein targets, but now expanded to an extensive range of target molecules such as low-molecular weight inorganic and organic compounds, amino acids, peptides, proteins, nucleotides molecules drugs, antibiotics, or metabolites are the hot spot research areas with the aim to develop a rapid and simple analytical methods supports in the fields of medical diagnostics, environmental monitoring, food safety and national defence against targets including chemical warfare.

Aptamers are unique in recognizing specific targets and form non-covalent interactions, sometimes able to bind their target analytes through changing coil structures to rigid tertiary structures like hairpin or G-quadruplex (Figure 6.1) (Lönne et al. 2014). Most aptamer-based biosensors are created on the basis of target-binding responsive conformational changes of aptamers (Komarova et al. 2018, Pan et al. 2013). One of the crucial characteristics is that they are more vigorous at ambient temperatures, unfolding at higher temperatures but this thermal denaturation is reversible. Therefore, thermal renaturation restores their properties and increases shelf life (Thiviyanathan and Gorenstein 2012). Prolonged storage at extensive temperatures may cause deformation but can refold into a functional state via simple annealing cycles of heating and cooling in an appropriate buffer (Dunn et al. 2017). Aptasensor-based diagnosis is handling of chemical modification, attachment of needed functional groups, and labelling of oligonucleotides with $-NH_2$, $-SH$, and biotin, facilitating the immobilization compatibility with a number of sensing platforms (Chen and Yang 2015).

6.3 APTAMER-TARGET CONFIGURATIONS

Aptamers on time of binding transduce bio-recognition events, and can adopt various configurations to combine with their targeted targets. The design for biosensors depends on the recognition pattern of each and every aptamer-target complex

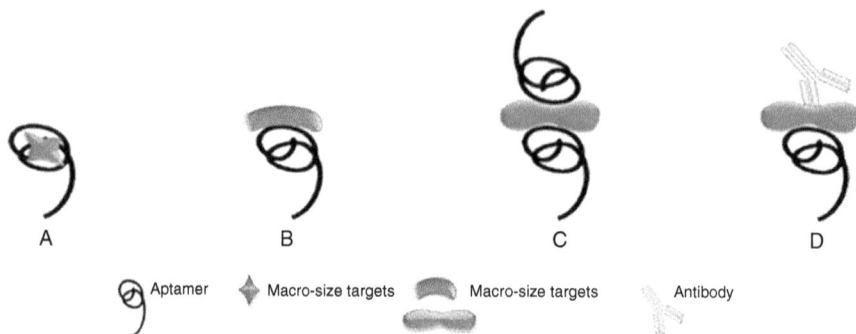

FIGURE 6.2 Aptamer configuration-based assay format of micro and macro-size molecules. (a) small-size molecule targets fit within the pockets of aptamer. (b) single-site format for macro-size molecule. (c) dual-site binding format with two aptamers. (d) sandwich binding format with an aptamer and an antibody.

(Hermann and Patel 2000) discussed further in the chapter. In literatures, various configurations have been illustrated that can be broadly divided into two basic categories – (1) single-site binding and (2) dual-site binding (sandwich assay). Thus, the target can be categorized as an embedded group and an outside-binding group. Small molecules such as ATP (Han et al. 2009), cocaine (Liu and Lu 2006), K^+ (Zhao et al. 2008), and theophylline (Ferapontova et al. 2008), are considered targets of embedded groups. NMR (nuclear magnetic resonance) clearly reveals that small molecular (single-site binding configuration) targets entrap within the formed aptamers pockets and reduce the possibility of binding with another interacting molecule (Figure 6.2a). Proteins or whole cell-like macro-molecular targets are complicated in structure (stacking, shape complementarity) and hold various intramolecular non-covalent interactions assayed both type binding configurations – single-site (Figure 6.2b) and dual-site (Figure 6.2c and d). Neves et al. (2017) detected cocaine by using a dual-site ligand-binding format. Additionally, dual-binding side molecules form a sandwich-like complexes where the targeted molecule sandwiches between two recognizing molecules, and enhances the specificity and sensitivity of the model (Seo and Gu 2017).

6.4 CONSTRUCTION OF APTAMER-BASED BIOSENSORS

Till now, plenty of research works concerned with the fabrication of aptamer-based biosensors have been accounted for. Varieties of methodology have been put forward for assembling biosensors including optical biosensors. The basic assembly of these biosensors has multifaceted analogical elements. In order to make it comprehensible, these can be categorized (Han et al. 2010) into the following modes.

6.4.1 TARGET-INDUCED STRUCTURE SWITCHING (TISS) MODE

Structure-switching (or binding-induced conformational changes) is the process of switching of aptasensor's structure upon target binding. Upon binding, disrupted hybridization equilibrium (stated between aptamer and labelled targets) produced sensible changes depending on target-analyte concentration, offering a powerful and challenging strategy for molecular detection (Lackey et al. 2020). TISS promises more efficient results by rejecting false positives as the majority of aptasensors are operated by this mode. This mode involves direct binding of the target to its respective aptamers, followed by conformational switching of aptamers to specific patterns instead of random structures that eventually embark on changes of detectable characters, such as (a) signal moieties which are linked covalently to the end of aptamers or adsorbed on the aptamers through electrostatic force, stacking, hydrogen bond, undergoes changes in terms of position, quantity or status, (b) formation of aptamer-target complexes along with changes in the size or weight of the same, (c) apart from these changes, other properties may also be affected such as ability to stabilize gold nanoparticles (AuNPs). Each progression suggests a difference in signals and chance for the plan of aptamer-based biosensors (Feagin et al. 2018, Mir et al. 2008, Radi et al. 2006, Rangel et al. 2020, Zuo et al. 2007). Structure-switching concept (Figure 6.3) was primarily established to fabricate an anti-ATP and anti-thrombin aptamer (Nutiu and Li 2003) then further was cast-off for other targets including arginine, cocaine, GTP, PDGF (platelet-derived growth factor) lysozyme, Hg^{2+}, cathepsin, K^+, IgE, quinine, oxytetracycline (OTC) and L-tyrosinamide (Lau and Li 2013, Liu and Lu 2006, Null and Lu 2010, Nutiu and Li 2005, Swensen et al. 2009, Yang et al. 2007). Consequential research has also expanded the use of structure-switching aptamers in secondary applications to facilitate high-throughput screening, monitor enzymatic reactions, and develop nano-devices and solid-phase assays (Elowe et al. 2006, Nutiu and Li 2005, Nutiu et al. 2004, Rupcich et al. 2005, 2006).

Ligand-binding RNA aptamers as an element of riboswitches regulate gene expression in cells. Only a few research articles explore RNA aptamers as biosensors because of their less chemical stability and high degradation susceptibility (Fowler et al. 2008, Huang et al. 2010, Wang et al. 2008). Based on the previous records of DNA structure-switching, Lau et al. (2010) approached stabilizing RNA aptamers as biosensors and hypothesized a general strategy to create structure-switching from existing RNA aptamers. The newly amended design makes utilization of the capability of RNA aptamers to assemble both an aptamer-target complex as well as an RNA–DNA duplex with a complementary sequence (Lau and Li 2013, Lau et al.

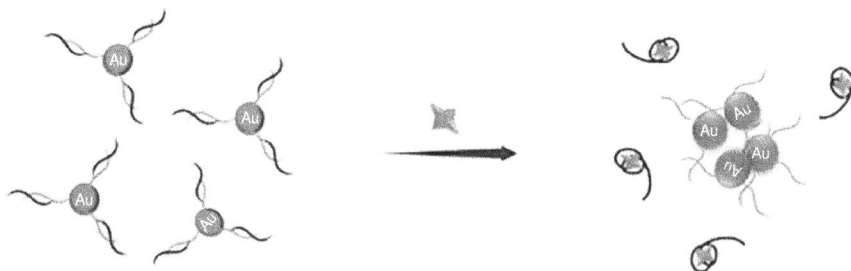

FIGURE 6.3 The general strategy of AuNP-based structural switching of aptamer induced by targets.

2010). In addition, DNA sequence with a single RNA molecule linkage served as cross-linkers when a Pb^{2+} sensing assay is performed that aggregates complementary DNA (cDNA)-attached AuNPs into the environment (Liu and Lu 2005).

The high coefficient of extinction and size-dependent colouration property (based on surface plasmon reverberation) makes AuNPs a perfect material for structure-switching designs based on colorimetric analysis (Zhang et al. 2008). In addition, numerous researches confirmed the adsorption of ssDNA on AuNPs can effectively stabilize the colloid against salt-induced aggregation while dsDNA has no such function (Li and Rothberg 2004a), this property being led to the synthesis of colorimetric aptamer-based biosensors (Li and Rothberg 2004b, Wang et al. 2007). In dispersed form, AuNPs absorb 520 nm wavelength light and appear in red colour which on aggregation turns into purple colour and can be read by the naked eye without trouble. For instance, a colorimetric biosensor was developed for the measure of ATP or K^+, as per this target-actuated structure exchanging of the aptamer altered on a superficial level of AuNPs (Zhao et al. 2008). In the absence of a target, ATP amalgamates with its cDNA and results in the formation of a rigid duplex that fails to resist AuNPs from aggregating as salt-added into the system. If ATP exists, the condition will favour the formation of the ATP-aptamer complex together with the release of its cDNA, which is capable of stabilizing AuNPs and conferring high resistance to salt-induced aggregation. The progress could be clearly observed in terms of changes in solution colour. A new technical concept was added by Chen et al., who developed a nano-sensor based on structure-switching aptamer for the detection of salicylic acid from solution and plant extract, which can detect salicylic acid as low as 0.1 μM (Chen et al. 2019).

6.4.2 SANDWICH OR SANDWICH-LIKE MODE

Apparently, this mode of assay needed one pair of aptamers to bind different targets of a protein so analyte protein gets situated between a pair of aptamers like a sandwich. Of them, one is a capture probe usually immobilized onto compact surfaces like NPs (nanoparticles), micro-particles, electrodes, or glass chips, etc. Another one is the reporter probe able to conjugate with signalling moieties (usually bind with redox markers like POX/peroxidase, methylene blue, and ferrocene or can bind with fluorophores or enzymes) to produce signals. In common both probes share different nucleotide sequences, nevertheless, identification assay of a few proteins based on sandwich conformation format comprises single type aptamer only if the protein possesses two identical sites. Evidently, it is worthwhile to identify numerous aptamers for a solo target (Radi and Abd-Ellatief 2021, Neupane and Stine 2021, Song et al. 2008). The necessity of two aptamers for two different epitopes places this mode in the least interested mode for the fabrication of aptasensors. In the majority, the target of interest not possessing two identical or overlapped binding sites shared by two aptamers in those cases either antibody can be used as the second 'aptamer' or can be bound to the second aptamer (Figure 6.2c and d). Thus, basically two formats i.e., aptamer-target-aptamer and antibody-target-aptamer fabricated models used at different platforms (Tabrizi et al., 2017, Ikebukuro et al. 2005). Additionally, based on ELISA (enzyme-linked immunosorbent assay), enzyme-linked aptamer antibody

(ELAA) sandwich assay antibodies can be tagged with enzymes. This affinity-based assay combines with explicit recognition ability of aptamer and dignified catalytic virtue of enzymes and chromogenic substrate (like TMB/3,3′,5,5′-tetramethylbenzidine, H_2O_2, and ABTS/2,2′-azinobis (3-ethylbenzothiazoline-6-sulfonic acid)) capable to make eye realizable product by catalyze the reaction and confirmed the presence of target and ultimately provide a sensitive, cheap, rapid, and attractive aptameric biosensor. But the manufacture of aptabiosensors based on sandwich mode or other modes for small molecules is complicated due to limited structural motifs.

6.4.3 TARGET-INDUCED DISSOCIATION/DISPLACEMENT (TID) MODE

TID mode is distinguished from TISS mode and the sandwich mode on being utilizing a structure-independent strategy (Han et al. 2009). As every aptamer does not have the ability to undergo appropriate conformational changes, Fan's group to omit this difficulty introduced a displacement-based technique to develop the visual aptabiosensors (Wang et al. 2007). In this strategy, complementary sequences of aptamer are used to hybridize the aptamer instead of aptamers themselves as anchors to limit the aptamers. In addition to target molecules, aptamer released from the duplex and interaction formed target-aptamer complex and finally marked changes can easily be detected. For instance, the detached complementary molecule as ssDNA from duplex stabilizes AuNPs from aggregation and dispersed AuNPs set the solution's colour in red. This general approach can be applied to the form of any kind of aptamer and after TISS this mode is used to operate aptasensors. TID offers less structural data of the used aptamer to recognize the analyte attachment site and area of strong conformational modifies. With this small knowledge and trial and error approach, can be design complementary aptamer sequence which can be liberated into the medium after aptamer-target binding, thus it bids as an effective substitute (Prante et al. 2020). In addition, oligonucleotide can be labelled if their displacement is not monitored to intensify transduction methods. For colorimetric measure, the presence of adenosine instigated the separation of aptamer from dsDNA changed AuNPs and the remained ssDNA adjusted AuNPs would total, which could be seen by the unaided eye (Zhao et al. 2007). Ochratoxin-A (OTA) point of care (POC) monitoring (Zhou et al. 2016) and 25-HydroxyvitaminD3 from human serum samples are TID-based detection. Modified and unmodified AuNPs and salt concentration-assisted analysis are also the models of TID mode-based aptamer sensing, examples are discussed later in the chapter.

6.4.4 COMPETITIVE REPLACEMENT (CR) MODE

As aptamers are called chemically synthesized antibodies that shares the various characteristics, can take the advantage of developing detection methods for aptamer-based analysis. For example, immuno-techniques of small molecules examination relying on CR of surface-bound antibodies by analyte, the same thought was applied to aptamer-based assay in early 2000 (Lee and Walt 2000) and emerged a new mode of biosensor construction named CR mode (Hua et al. 2010). In CR-based aptasensor mode, aptamer bound to labelled target molecules immobilized on the surface (immobilization of targets on the surface that bound to the aptamer can also be possible) and non-labelled or free target molecules compete with immobilized ones resulting in the displacement of bound targets because binding of the non-labelled molecules is preferred if targets present. In context, to detection of small-size analytes, this approach has been used, for instance, chloramphenicol (CAP) can be detected up to 451 pM (LOD/limit of detection) concentration, by immobilizing on the surface and CAP aptamer labelled with biotin was pierced. If free CAP was absent, the CAP-aptamer ligated the immobilized CAP, and transduction was executed via streptavidin-modified AuNPs. However, the availability of free CAP led to the formation of CAP-aptamer duplex, and thereby sandwich-like assembly could not be made (Abnous et al. 2016). CR mode required the designing and synthesis of profuse signal-modified target molecules. To magnify the recognition signal of aptamer a cationic surfactant named CTAB (hexadecyl-trimethyl-ammonium-bromide) was introduced. Positively charged ions promote the clumping of AuNPs having a negative charge, consequently inhibiting the POX-like activity of AuNPs. But the AuNPs can gain their catalytic power by incorporation of negatively charged RNA aptamer against malachite green (MG), binding of cation and negatively charged aptamer prevent the aggregation of AuNPs thus catalysis of TMB by H_2O_2 make solution dark blue when MG is absent. In the presence, negatively charged aptamer competitively binds to the MG target, and the solution appeared in like blue colour due to inhibition of catalytic activity. The presented concept was also validated by the detection of an adequate amount of MG in aquatic water (Zhao et al. 2019). Wang and Zhao developed CR mode-based detection of small antibiotic molecule AFB1 (aflatoxin B1) with a 0.5 nM to 1 µM detection limit (Wang and Zhao 2019).

6.4.5 TARGET-INDUCED REASSEMBLY (TIR) MODE

Apart from the above sensor-making concepts Johanna-Gabriela-Walter introduced another sensor-constructing principle that worked on target-induced rearrangement of aptamer by utilizing aptamer's structural properties (Walter et al. 2012). TIR mode offers an alternative to sandwich-like mode. Fan's group foremost developed this method by dividing a DNA aptamer into two pieces (Figure 6.4). Anti-adenosine

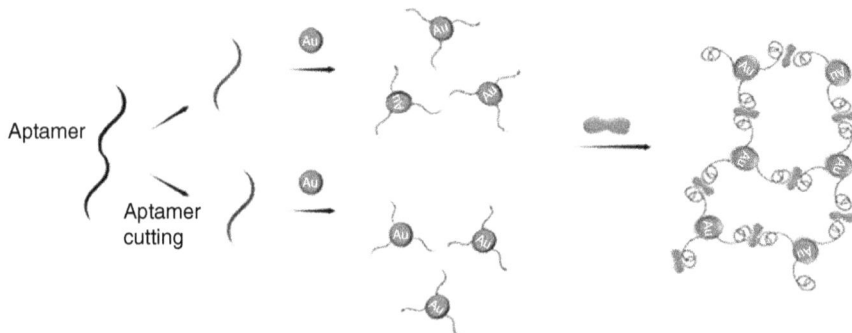

FIGURE 6.4 Schematic illustration of TIR mode-based apta-biosensing of macro-size molecules.

aptamer fragments were immobilized on different AuNPs and mixed into the medium in the presence of the target, and fragments of aptamer were reunited into the precisely assembled triplet with adenosine. The change in colour on agglomeration of the micro-molar level of adenosine particles was easily read by the naked eye and quantified by simple UV-spectroscopy. Moreover, the principle of TIR mode was successfully employed to demonstrate the detection of cocaine. Two aptamer fragments are assembled with silver nanoclusters, where an increased in fluorescence showed the lowering in distances of silver nanoclusters (Zhou et al. 2011).

6.5 MATERIAL-BASED COLORIMETRIC BIOSENSORS

A variety of nano-engineered structures combined with aptamers emphasize lots of unique properties that are suited for sensing applications. To fabricate them can be use nanoparticles, quantum dots, graphene, carbon nanotubes, etc. Nobel metal nanomaterials, specifically, AuNPs and AgNPs (silver nanoparticles), are phenomenal sign transducers for colorimetric investigation because of their critical optical properties related to their molecule size, size circulation, and shape (Jeon et al. 2019, Zhuang et al. 2019). In other words, biosensors can be developed extensively through aptamer coating on gold nanoparticles. The characteristic SPR (surface plasmon resonance) properties of AuNPs and together with AgNPs contribute to colorimetric signal generation (Chang et al. 2016). A summary of various colorimetric aptasensors are listed in Table 6.1 based on different material used for plenty of targets.

6.5.1 GOLD NANOMATERIALS-BASED COLORIMETRIC BIOSENSORS

DNA/RNA does not absorb any light in the wavelength of visible region, therefore coupling aptamers to a colour-producing molecule is required to generate a colour transformation upon target binding. It has been reported that AuNPs undergoes characteristic spectroscopic changes during target-induced aggregation or dispersion and hence can find suitable application in the design of optical biosensor. As the optical phenomenon of SPR persists, the colour of AuNPs reversibly changes from red (dispersed state) to blue (aggregated state) in an aqueous solution. Because the AuNPs are utilized as nano assembly units can be functionalized simply to immobilize desired DNA sequences, allowing the tunability of changing colour by target-aptamer interactions. The diameter of AuNPs is the uttermost essential factor in all described protocols (mostly methods used of size in the range of 10–27 nm diameter). For developing a colorimetric aptasensor, AuNPs on account of their novel highlights, including basic amalgamation and one-of-a-kind optical, warm conductivity, and electronic properties (Jeon and Lee 2019, Lucas et al. 2013, Sunil et al. 2020).

Gopinath along with his team coupled above describes properties with the ease of chemisorption to their surfaces via free thiols to design a striking format of AuNPs for the development of colorimetric sensors (Gopinath et al. 2014). In another example, Smith et al. (2014) procreate a simpler and robust device by combining AuNPs with anti-cocaine DNA aptamers to use at ground level. In one configuration, a complex of cocaine and aptamers combined with the AuNPs then aggregation was induced via charge shielding by adding NaCl and finally, this reaction induced colour shifting

TABLE 6.1

Summary of different colorimetric aptasensors based on used materials, the target of aptamer, limit of detection, mode of detection, and analytical applications

Aptasensor and materials	Detection type	Target/analyte molecule	Linear range	LOD	Colour change	Time for detection (excluding preparation time)	Applications	References
CD63 aptamer-gC$_3$N$_4$ NSs[a]	Colorimetric	Differential expression of CD63 by MCF-7[b] cells and MCF-10A[c]	0.19×10^7–3.38×10^7 particles/µL	13.52×10^5 particles/mL	Blue (control) and Less-intense-blue (sample)	~30 min	Method is useful in clinical diagnosis using liquid biopsy for breast cancer diagnosis	Wang et al. (2017a)
Anti CD63, HER2, integrin αvβ6 aptamers and CD63 aptamer–biotin	Colorimetric	CD63 cells HER2,[d] integrin αvβ6	7.7×10^3 part/mL		Colourless-to-brown-black	10 min	Detect common exosomal marker CD63, disease markers HER2 and integrin αvβ6. Can be used in biomarker cancer discovery and early cancer detection (specially breast cancer)	Xu et al. (2020)
CD63 aptamer-DNA-capped SWCNTs	Label-free colorimetric	MCF-7 cells	1.84×10^6–2.21×10^7 particles/µL	5.2×10^5 particles/µL	Deep-blue-to-moderate	40 min	Useful diagnostic method of MCF-7 exosomes from breast cancer patient's serum for cancer diagnosis	Xia et al. (2017)
PSA-polyA aptamer	Novel label-free colorimetric	PSA[e]-biomarker	0.1–100 ng/mL	20 pg/mL	Red-to-purple	~60 min	Method is applicable to rapid screening of PSA in real samples and cancer diagnosis	Shayesteh and Ghavami (2020)

(Continued)

TABLE 6.1 (Continued)

Summary of different colorimetric aptasensors based on used materials, the target of aptamer, limit of detection, mode of detection, and analytical applications

Aptasensor and materials	Detection type	Target/analyte molecule	Linear range	LOD	Colour change	Time for detection (excluding preparation time)	Applications	References
BG2-MNPs aptamer - MNPs aptamer	Colorimetric (based on magnetic isolation and signal amplification)	IAP-PLAP heterodimer proteins on CTRMs[f] (especially LoVo[g])	0.31–5.00 μg		Yellow		Suggesting great potential for colorectal cancer diagnosis and therapeutic monitoring	Shen et al. (2020)
VEGF aptamer–biotin	Label-free colorimetric	VEGF$_{165}$[h] biomarker	100–1 × 10^5 pg/mL	10 pg/mL	Blue-to-faint blue	~5 hr	Detection of VEGF$_{165}$ in human serum could take the advantage in clinical research and cancer diagnosis	Dong et al. (2020)
P1 (EpCAM)-Fe$_3$O$_4$-SiO$_2$ with Gel/mDNA	Colorimetric	Circulating tumour cells	10–500 cells/mL	10 cells/mL	Green colour cells	~60 min	CTCs is quantified in 12 clinical tumour patients from their peripheral blood samples, and showed remarkable potential in cancer diagnostics	Zhu et al. (2021b)
Cocaine aptamer- MoS$_2$-AuNPs	Novel colorimetric	Cocaine (cancer diagnosis)	0–1 μM	7.49 nM	Red-to-blue	10 min	Cocaine is an addictive drug that blocks the reuptake of the neurotransmitter dopamine. This technique can be applied in biomedical fields	Gao et al. (2020)

(Continued)

TABLE 6.1 (Continued)

Summary of different colorimetric aptasensors based on used materials, the target of aptamer, limit of detection, mode of detection, and analytical applications

Aptasensor and materials	Detection type	Target/analyte molecule	Linear range	LOD	Colour change	Time for detection (excluding preparation time)	Applications	References
AuNPs-IL-6 aptamer	Colorimetry	Interleukin-6	3.3–125 µg/mL	1.95 µg/mL	Red-to-pink	5 min	IL-6 is a key marker of acute inflammation from clinical perspective	Giorgi-Coll et al. (2020)
p-tau231 aptamer-Cu-enhanced-Au aptablot	Colorimetric aptablot	p-tau231[i]	1–1,000 ng/mL	4.71 pg/mL		140 min	Alzheimer's disease causes dementia as its primary symptom. Aptablot can be a potential diagnostic tool for early diagnosis of AD worldwide	Phan and Cho (2022)
CRP-binding aptamer-citrate capped-AuNPs	Colorimetric	CRP	0.889–20.7 µg/mL	1.2 µg/mL	Red-wine to blue-purple	5 min	Well-known biomarkers of inflammation in several diseases such as the cardiovascular, thrombosi, fibrinogen, atherosclerosis	António et al. (2020)
AuNPs-Bruno 69-mer aptamer or the 56-mer Lee aptamer	Colorimetry	Vitamin-D3	1–1,000 nM	10 µM	Red-to-blue	>10 min	Vitamin D3 presence can be diagnosed in blood samples. Can fulfil the need for POC determination	Alsager et al. (2018)
Azlocillin DNA aptamer-AuNPs	Colorimetric (salt-induced aggregation)	Azlocillin	50–500 nM,	11.6 nM	Red-to-blue		Azlocillin antibiotic can detected rapidly in milk and tap water samples	Xiao et al. (2022)

(Continued)

TABLE 6.1 (*Continued*)

Summary of different colorimetric aptasensors based on used materials, the target of aptamer, limit of detection, mode of detection, and analytical applications

Aptasensor and materials	Detection type	Target/analyte molecule	Linear range	LOD	Colour change	Time for detection (excluding preparation time)	Applications	References
STR aptamer-cDNA-SYBR Green-I	Colorimetric with fluorescence (smartphone based)	STR	0.1–100 μM	94 nM	Dark green-to-light green	10 min	Antibiotic residue detection for foodstuff safety at POC level	Lin et al. (2018)
AuNPs -multifunctional aptamer	Label-free colorimetric (smartphone based)	CAP TET (Tetracycline)	0.05–1.8 μM 0.05–3.0 μM	7.0 nM 32.9 nM	Red-to-purple Red-to-blue	<10 min	On-site detection of multiplex antibiotics in the field of food safety	Wu et al. (2020)
Fe-MOF-aptamer-CAP@ AuNP-aptamer	Colorimetric	CAP (including AMP, TET, OTC)	50–200 nM	8.1 ng/mL	Colourless to blue		Strongly selective and sensitive for chloramphenicol detection and can also be analyzed AMP, TET, and OTC	Li et al. (2019)
Truncated aptamer- AuNPs	Colorimetric based on lateral flow assay	OTC	0.245 ± 1.62 ng/mL	5 ng/mL	Two red bands	10 min	It can be anticipated POC detection of OTC in diary samples from field level to plant-based platforms	Birader et al. (2021)
Unmodifiled OFL-specific aptamer-AuNPs with NaCl	Colorimetric	Ofloxacin (OFL)	20–400 nM	3.4 nM	Red-to-blue		OFL antibiotic detection in environmental and biological samples in aqueous solutions	Zhou et al. (2018)

(Continued)

TABLE 6.1 (Continued)

Summary of different colorimetric aptasensors based on used materials, the target of aptamer, limit of detection, mode of detection, and analytical applications

Aptasensor and materials	Detection type	Target/analyte molecule	Linear range	LOD	Colour change	Time for detection (excluding preparation time)	Applications	References
TOB aptamer-AuNPs with ssDNA	Label-free colorimetric	Tobramycin (TOB)	40–200 nM	23.3 nM	Red-to-purple		Harmful levels of TOB antibiotics can be successfully detected in milk and chicken eggs	Ma et al. (2018)
Thiolated aptamer-AuNPs and non-thiolated polyA aptamer – AuNPs	Colorimetric	AMP (Ampicillin)	1–600 nM and 1–400 nM	0.1 nM and 0.49 nM	Red-to-purple		Non-thiolated polyA Aptamer can be used in place of thiolated-aptamer	Shayesteh and Ghavami (2019)
NFMs-KMC aptamer	Colorimetric biosensor strips	Kanamycin (KMC)	2.5–80 nM	60 nM	Pink-to-white	10 min	Real sample analysis of water and milk can be done by test strips beneficial in food safety control	Abedalwafa et al. (2020)
Gentamicin aptamer-AuNPs	Paper biosensor-based colorimetric	Gentamicin	100–1,000 nM	300 nM	Blue colour at the centre of paper-flower	2 min	Gentamicin antibiotics are rapidly detected from spiked milk samples on paper biosensors to be used in field	Ramalingam et al. (2021)
AFM1 aptamer/CS (dsDNA)-modified-SNPs	Colorimetric (salt-induced aggregation based)	Aflatoxin M1 (AFM1)	300–75,000 ng/L	30 ng/L	Purple-to-red		Determine the AFM1 in milk samples. Can be applied further to other biological samples	Jalalian et al. (2021)

(Continued)

TABLE 6.1 (Continued)

Summary of different colorimetric aptasensors based on used materials, the target of aptamer, limit of detection, mode of detection, and analytical applications

Aptasensor and materials	Detection type	Target/analyte molecule	Linear range	LOD	Colour change	Time for detection (excluding preparation time)	Applications	References
AFM1 aptamer _CRISPR-Cas12a-(T4 DNA ligase - phi29 DNA polymerase)	Colorimetric	AFM1	0.2–300 ng/L	0.05 ng/L	Coluorless to yellow		Detect AFM1 successfully in spiked milk samples. Can apply to identify other mycotoxins from real samples by using compatible aptamer	Abnous et al. (2021)
Enzyme-linked aptamer	ssDNA-biotin cDNA biotin-colorimetry	AFB1	1–80 ng/mL	0.36 ng/mL	Blue-to-yellow	>2 hr	Method may be used to detect AFB1 in foodstuff	Xie et al. (2019)
Cationic perylene probe-AuNPs	Label-free colorimetry	AFB1	1–6 ng/mL	0.36* and 0.18** ng/mL	Red-to-blue	<5 min	Determination of AFB1 (toxins exhibit high toxicity to humans and animal) in rice* and peanut** samples was carried out	Lerdsri et al. (2020)
bIngenious hairpin DNA probe-Exonuclease-III	Label-free colorimetric (Wash-free)	AFB1	1 pM–100 nM	1 pM	Blue		This type of biosensor has the potential to detect AFB1 in fields	Wu et al. (2019b)
Sulfadimethoxine (SDM) aptamer – nanoarticle Gr/ Ni@Pd	Label-free colorimetric	Sulfadimethoxine (SDM)	1–500 ng/mL	0.7 ng/mL	Colourless to deep blue	600 sec	Detect the SDM level in lake water	Wang et al. (2017b)

(Continued)

TABLE 6.1 (*Continued*)

Summary of different colorimetric aptasensors based on used materials, the target of aptamer, limit of detection, mode of detection, and analytical applications

Aptasensor and materials	Detection type	Target/analyte molecule	Linear range	LOD	Colour change	Time for detection (excluding preparation time)	Applications	References
Aptamers@ papain@AuNCs	Colorimetric	*E. coli* O157:H7	39 cfu/mL		Red-to-blue		Detect foodborne bacteria in foods to prevent outbreaks of illness	Song et al. (2022)
MNP aptamer-AuNPs aptamer	Sandwich structure based colorimetric	*V. parahaemolyticus*	10–106 cfu/mL	2.4 cfu/mL	Red-wine to-colourless		Seafood-borne bacterium detected from spiked raw shrimp samples and can be applied to detect other foodborne bacteria	Sadsri et al. (2020)
g-C$_3$N$_4$ nanosheets - Cu$_2$O	Label-free colorimetric	*S. typhimurium*	1.5×10^1 to 1.5×10^5 CFU/mL	15 CFU/mL	Blue colour intensity increased	6 min (paper-based-device)	Analysis method have promising potential, sensitive, rapid for *S. typhimurium* detection from spiked milk samples in medium as well as on paper	Tarokh et al. (2021)
Aptamer-hammerhead ribozyme, and GQ-EXPAR reaction	Colorimetric	Theophylline and its chemical analogue caffeine	0.5–1,000 μM	0.5 μM	Clear to blue	5–10 min	3-stage detection includes aptamer, ribozyme, and GQ-EXPAR reaction approach can engineered a medical diagnostic system for targeted analytes	Liao et al. (2018)

(Continued)

TABLE 6.1 (Continued)

Summary of different colorimetric aptasensors based on used materials, the target of aptamer, limit of detection, mode of detection, and analytical applications

Aptasensor and materials	Detection type	Target/analyte molecule	Linear range	LOD	Colour change	Time for detection (excluding preparation time)	Applications	References
Anatoxin-a DNA aptamer-AuNPs	Colorimetric based (salt-induced aggregation)	Anatoxin-a	10 pM–200 nM	4.45 pM	Red-to-blue		Provide an alternative method of anatoxin detection from water bodies	Nguyen and Jang (2021)
SEB aptamer-AuNPs	Colorimetry	Staphylococcal enterotoxin-B	50 µg/mL to 0.5 ng/mL	50 ng/mL	Red-to-purple	15 min	Important design for food security purpose. Detection performed on artificially spiked milk and naturally contaminated samples	Mondal et al. (2018)
Terminal-fixed DSPs aptamer-AuNPs@Fe²⁺ nanozyme	Label-free colorimetric	Three-DSPsj (Okadaic acid, dinophysistoxin-1 and dinophysistoxin-2)	0.47–7.5 nM	86.28 pM	Turn into blue		Analyzed and detected three types of DSPs in seawater	Li et al. (2022)
PCB-77 binding aptamer-AuNPs probes	Label-free colorimetry	Polychlorinated biphenyls (PCB-77)	0.5–900 nM	0.05 nM	Wine-red-to-purple blue	10 min	PCB-77 (an organic toxic pollutant) can be detected from complex environmental water samples	Cheng et al. (2018)

(Continued)

TABLE 6.1 (Continued)

Summary of different colorimetric aptasensors based on used materials, the target of aptamer, limit of detection, mode of detection, and analytical applications

Aptasensor and materials	Detection type	Target/analyte molecule	Linear range	LOD	Colour change	Time for detection (excluding preparation time)	Applications	References
Label-free T-2 specific aptamer-AuNPs	Colorimetry	T-2 toxin	0.21–10,717.5 nM)	0.124 nM	Red-to-purple-blue		Potentially useful in food detection. As T-2 is a potent inhibitor of DNA, RNA, protein synthesis and mitochondrial function can be found in many kinds of cereal grains and cereal-based products	Zhang et al. (2021)
Acetamiprid aptamer – three DNA hairpin probes (HP, HA1 and HA2)	Colorimetric with HCR-assay	*Acetamiprid*	1–140 μM	1.74 μM	Pinkish-purplish-to blue-purple	—	Portable and unexpansive method useful for on-site detection of acetamiprid pesticide	Xu et al. (2022)
MG-RNA aptamer	Label-free colorimetric	MG	20–300 nM	15.95 nM	Red-to-blue		Method successfully used to determine MG (can be teratogenic, carcinogenic, and mutagenic in humans) in actual fish samples	Jia et al. (2018)

(Continued)

TABLE 6.1 (Continued)

Summary of different colorimetric aptasensors based on used materials, the target of aptamer, limit of detection, mode of detection, and analytical applications

Aptasensor and materials	Detection type	Target/analyte molecule	Linear range	LOD	Colour change	Time for detection (excluding preparation time)	Applications	References
RNA aptamer- AuNPs-CTAB	Colorimetric	MG	10–500 nM/L	1.8 nM/L	Dark blue to light blue		Extremely precise and accurate methods can detect MG from natural aquaculture water	Zhao et al. (2019)
A3 (bispecific)-aptamer -AuNPs	Label-free colorimetric (NaCl-induced-aggregation)	MG and Leucomalachite green (LMG)	0–17.5μM/L	6.93 nM/L (MG) and 6.38 nM/L (LMG)	Red-to-blue	~60 min	Easy, fast and sensitive methods can simultaneously determine the presence of MG and LMG in detecting aquatic products	Wu et al. (2020a)
MC-LR aptamer-AuNPs/Grmanohybrids	Label-free colorimetry	Microcystin-LR	0.01–1.0 µg/L	7.14 ng/L	Red-to-deep green		The presence of MC-LR is an indication of eutrophication could be detected by this method from various targets	Tian (2019)
Hg^{2+} aptamer-AuNPs/Grmanohybrids	Label-free colorimetry	Hg^{2+}	0.01–0.5 µM	3.63 nM	Red-to-deep green		Trace amount of Hg causes harm, health of humans, plants, and the environment. Various targets could be detected by this method	Tian (2019)

(Continued)

TABLE 6.1 (*Continued*)

Summary of different colorimetric aptasensors based on used materials, the target of aptamer, limit of detection, mode of detection, and analytical applications

Aptasensor and materials	Detection type	Target/analyte molecule	Linear range	LOD	Colour change	Time for detection (excluding preparation time)	Applications	References
ATP aptamer-H1 and H2 (two hairpin DNA probes)	Label-free colorimetric	ATP	10–600 nM	1.0 nM	Red-to-purple	~150 min	ATP (as a coenzyme) is key factor of cell structure and facilitates cytoskeleton structure. The assay can also be used to detect other small molecules or mycotoxins	Gao et al. (2017)

a Nanosheets.

b Human breast cancer cell line.

c Control cell line.

d Human epidermal growth factor receptor-2.

e Prostate-specific antigen.

f Circulating tumour-related materials.

g Highly metastatic cell line (human colon cancer).

h Factors promote the growth of tumors.

i Alzheimer's disease biomarker.

j Diarrheic shellfish poisons.

from red-to-blue. In the other configuration, cocaine was added after only aptamers were adsorbed onto the surface of AuNPs which reduced the non-specific adsorption by other non-targeted moieties, and thus this would lead to specific aggregation and accuracy of results.

Other workers have also been exploiting similar aggregation techniques to develop state-dependent colorimetric detection sensors for antibiotics (Birader et al. 2021, Xiao et al. 2022), thrombin (Chen et al. 2014), and *S. enterotoxin*-B (Liu et al. 2013a, Mondal et al. 2018). Uropathogenic *Escherichia coli* identified by the synthesized sensor (Liu et al. 2013b) synchronized with hybridization chain reaction/HCR (Dirks and Pierce 2004). Many other techniques were also invented to amplify the signal, based on the cascading concatenation of DNA and artificially designed specific nucleotides (Bao et al. 2020, Chen et al. 2016, Gao et al. 2017). Simply, AuNPs either can be used as an element to help in colorimetric shift or have been used as a sensor's structural element to employ signal transduction mechanisms. Very recently, acetamiprid pesticide analysis through an HCR-based but instruments-free colorimetric sensor was established. Synthesized three DNA hairpin probes with sticky ends assist AuNPs to restrict the salt-induced aggregation. The aptamer hairpin loop of HP opened because of target identification in the presence of acetamiprid. Consequently, hybridization starts between probes HA-1 & HA-2 which reduced the amount of hairpin probes that triggered the salt-induced aggregation of AuNPs resulting colour shift from pinkish-purplish-to blue-purple (Xu et al. 2022; Figure 6.5).

In a different approach, before the immobilization of two different DNA probes on the surface of AuNPs, hybridization connected AuNPs between these aptamers. Later on, the addition of a target broke this networking, and the dispersion of AuNPs in the solution converted appearance into red (Liu and Lu 2006) as illustrated in

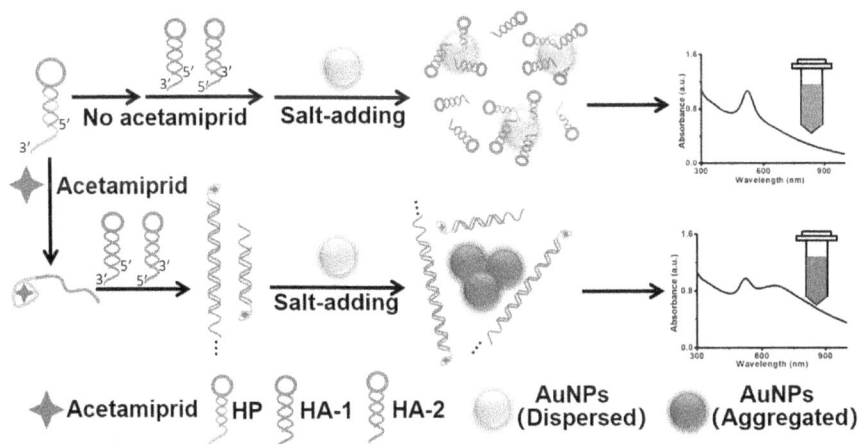

FIGURE 6.5 Diagrammatic representation of acetamiprid detection based on HCR amplified colorimetric aptasensor.

Reprinted from Food Control, with the permission of Xu et al. (2022), Copyright (2022), with permission from Elsevier.

Figure 6.6a. Platelet-derived growth factor and thrombin (Huang et al. 2005) and Hg^{2+} and Ag^+ (Ono et al. 2011) like metal ions can be looked out by target-induced cross-linked aggregation of AuNPs. Thymine/T base pairs captured Hg^{2+} while cysteine base pairs captured Ag^+ and formed highly stable $T-Hg^{2+}-T$ and $C-Ag^+-C$ metallo-base pairs in DNA. Hg^{2+} and Ag^+ lead to the aggregation of AuNPs in solution by the formation of these metallo-base pairs causing the changing of colours from red-to-purple. For colorimetric metal ion detection this phenomenon was successfully adopted by many researchers (Lee et al. 2007, Li et al. 2009, Xu et al. 2012). Around two decades ago, Li and Rothberg suggested using unmodified AuNPs, a more efficient, less time, and money-taking approach (synthesizing thiolated or modified aptamers is costly and takes time to immobilize them on NPs). Adsorbed DNA molecule on unmodified AuNPs averts the aggregation of NPs in a salty solution that screens the repulsive interactions of citrate ions (Li and Rothberg 2004a; Figure 6.6b). This phenomenon inspired researchers (Liu et al. 2008, Kim et al. 2010, 2011, Wang et al. 2006). Wei and his group have developed a Pb^{2+} detection assay by using 17E DNAzyme. In the presence of Pb^{2+}, 17E DNAzyme cleaves its substrate 17DS and released ssDNA is adsorbed onto unmodified AuNPs, inhibiting the aggregation of AuNPs (Wei et al. 2008). From time to time, this simple approach of using unmodified AuNPs or other NP-based colorimetric detection assay has been combined with other approaches like target-induced conformational changes, displaced-based assay has been developed. In addition, literature reported polydiacetylene (PDA) liposomes and coloured polymers for AuNP-based colorimetric aptasensor assay. Primarily, Kim's group assembled PDA liposomes with colorimetric aptasensors, making them highly sensitive and can suddenly change their colour if any external fluctuation like pH, temperature, ligand interaction, or solvent occurred. PDA liposomes conjugate aptamers on their surface and the binding of the aptamer to target molecules persuades the colour transformation of liposomes (Figure 6.6c), K^+ detection is an example of this assay (Lee et al. 2008, 2012). The other material i.e. conjugated polymer was used to detection of Hg^{2+} ions, composed of PMNT (poly(3-(30-N,N,N-triethylamino-10-propyloxy)-4-methyl-2,5-thiophene hydrochloride)) and Hg^{2+} specific T-rich ssDNA. Polythiophene has a very sensitive optical property that can sensitize conformational changes of its backbone very quickly. Straight T-rich ssDNA bind electrostatically with positive charged PMNT in the absence of Hg^{2+} (red colour solution). If Hg^{2+} is present in solution it leads to form a PMNT surrounded stem loop structure of ssDNA because of the binding of Hg^{2+}, resulting in a change of colour from red to yellow (Liu et al. 2007).

Different forms of Au nanomaterials such as Au-nano-cubes, Au-nano-spheres, Au-nano-rods, Au-nano-bipyramids (AuNBPs), and Au-nano-branche have been used since times before an account of first easily tunable in different shapes and secondly flexible localized-SPR peak ranging between visible to near IR spectrum (Chen et al. 2008). AuNBPs have some properties over the remaining gold-nanomaterials like sharp plasmon line width, high extinction cross section, excellent sensitivity towards refractive index, low-frequency wavelength (Liu et al. 2009) place it in the category of an ideal chromogenic structure to designed multicolor biosensor based on colour. Thereby, a variety of target molecules can be assayed by them – CN^- ions (Sasikumar and Ilanchelian 2020), Fe^{2+} ions (He et al. 2020), $C_6H_{12}O_6$

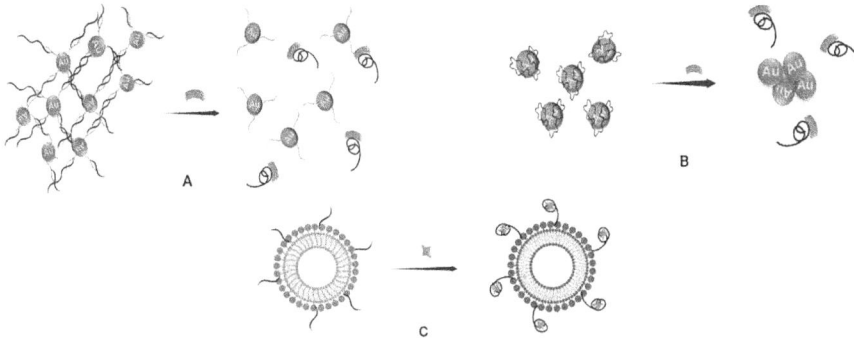

FIGURE 6.6 Different strategy of colorimetric aptasensors: (a) colorimetric assay using dispersion of aptamer and AuNPs. (b) colorimetric aptasensing using unmodified AuNPs. (c) PDA liposome-based colorimetric aptasensing.

(Xu et al. 2019), Ochratoxins (Wei et al. 2019), influenza (Xu et al. 2017) and many more. Unfortunately, the process of synthesis and purification of AuNBPs is intricate, sophisticated, and time-consuming taking around 3–4 days (Qi et al. 2016, Zhu et al. 2016). The answer to this problem has been searched for in recent studies. Wang and coauthors approached an *in situ* growth kinetics, which can harvest extremely uniform AuNBPs by ignoring the purification step (Wang et al. 2019, 2021) and they manufactured an alkaline phosphate (ALP)-mediated *in situ* growth of AuNBPs. Obviously, the change in colour is directly proportional to ALP concentration. This approach significantly enhanced the sensitivity, and affinity of detection, minimize the synthesis periods from 72 hr to 15 min, and the ease in the numeral of operation steps, pronounced it a promising strategy for application in multicolor colorimetric detection assays (Wang et al. 2019).

6.5.2 GRAPHENE (GR) BASED COLORIMETRIC BIOSENSORS

Exclusively, Gr and Graphene oxide (GO) have the adsorption property to detect DNA, RNA, proteins, and peptide biomolecules, even they can differentiate ssDNA from dsDNA.

Detection of protein: The specificity of Gr and Gr-based materials depends on adsorption capacity. Liu's group described that π–π interaction is responsible for the binding of circular aptamer to Gr. Configuration of ring aptamer changed on the addition of protein targets, consequent isothermal amplification or can say on the paper surface circular aptamer generate rolling ring extension, alternatively, magnify the peroxidase (POD) activity (catalytic activity of TMB) resulting colour production indicate the presence of specific proteins (Liu et al. 2014).

Detection of viruses and bacteria: Specific binding patterns of ssDNA aptamer/ antibodies towards targeted bacteria can simply be detectable on GO-based colorimetric sensing platform. For instance, Gupta and co-workers synthesized a sensitive, potent, and tensile method for rapid sensing of *E. coli* via ssDNA aptamers and modified GO-coated AuNPs, because the coating of GO enhances binding of aptamers on Gr. Bacterial absence was confirmed when the solution's colour retained its original colour. In addition, the binding of aptamers with targeted bacterial targets on the surface of the cell and absorbing AuNPs, subsequently switched AuNPs aggregation. Thus, the solution generates a significant observable colour shift (colour turns into blue from red) to accomplish the purpose of *E. coli* presence. This technique is sublimely contributed to controlling related diseases (Gupta et al. 2021). In another report, Wu et al. (2017) designed nanozyme-based method for *Salmonella typhimurium* detection, and synthesized $ZnFe_2O^4$- rGO hybrid nanostructure has been functionalized as peroxidase nanozyme. Later on, Kaushal and colleagues via abetment of specific antibodies develop a GO and AuNP-based acute sensing platform for *E. coli* and *S. typhimurium* (Kaushal et al. 2021). Very recently, Yang's group has assembled a novel aptamers@papain@AuNCs model to detect *E. coli* O157:H7 from different milk samples. Through this model, they enhanced the POX activity by rejoining covalent bonds (Au–S) between thiolated-aptamers and the papain@AuNCs. They are pioneers in the field of using papain as a template for the synthesis of AuNCs (Au-nano-clusters). *E. coli* O157:H7 from the samples caught via aptamers@papain@AuNCs model, enhanced POX activity catalyzes the substrate TMB and thus blue colour product formed (Song et al., 2022).

Detection of small molecules: Small-size biomolecules, drug molecules, and other organic molecules can be detected easily through 2D material-based colorimetric aptasensors. Yuan's group illustrated a method for OTC detection by using OTC aptamer and modified Gr particles hybridized with Au, bestowing regulated POX activity (Yuan et al. 2017). π–π interaction enabled the adsorption of ssDNA on a hybrid of Gr–Au particles, this complex blocked the activity of POX-like hybrid Gr–Au material. In addition to OTC, made a complex with aptamer and displacement of aptamer from the complex revived the peroxidase-like of the hybrid Gr molecules. This incident accelerated the colour change of the medium which fulfil the target of OTC detection.

As the literature suggested and discussed above it can be found that Gr or GO containing other biosensing probes such as aptamers are more suitable platforms for colorimetric biosensors. Conjugation with other nano-scaled probes- nano-metal molecules, nano-metal-oxide particles, and nano cords, enhanced the sensing capacity of graphene of GO-based materials in a manner like improved LOD, specificity, sensitivity, etc (Zhu et al. 2021a).

6.5.3 CARBON DOTS (CDS) AND NANOTUBES-BASED COLORIMETRIC BIOSENSORS

CDs have fascinating qualities as easy to prepare, strong photostable, and biocompatible (Cho and Park 2019, Phan and Cho 2022, Shi et al. 2014). A team of researchers constructed a single-walled carbon nanotube device to detect exosomes (Xia et al. 2017). Exosomes are the biomarkers to predict numerous diseases especially for cancer (Chiu et al. 2016). Xia's group demonstrates a method for exosomes assay by integrating exosome-aptamers and s-SWCNTs (water-soluble single-walled carbon nanotubes). Aptamers (target the specific CD63 transmembrane protein) adsorbed onto s-SWCNTs, complex enhanced POX-like activity can oxidize TMB in H_2O_2 presence which turns medium blue from colourless. However, on adding exosomes, due to conformational changes aptamers left s-SWCNTs and bound to CD63 targets restricting POX activity and resulting in a moderate colour of solution (Xia et al. 2017). Exosome detection is an important tool in terms of public health reporting as a supporting biomarker for tumour diagnosis, anti-tumour immune response, and clinical therapeutics (Chiu et al. 2016, Clark et al. 2015). In addition, recently Tarokh et al. developed a promising device to detect *S. typhimurium* from spiked milk samples and presented a label-free, sensitive, and fast detection technique, while the paper-based model scanned only in 6 min. But, for the colorimetric detection, they used the reverse strategy of above-described method means blue colour intensity had a positive correlation with the concentration of *S. typhimurium*. Level-free aptamer has been combined with a unique composite combination of graphitic carbon nitride (g-C_3N_4) nanosheets and Cu_2O (copper oxide-I) nanocrystals exhibit POX activity and oxidized TMB. In the presence of the bacterium, aptamers targeted their targets, consequently, g-C_3N_4@ Cu_2O activity was increased with respect to the concentration of *S. typhimurium* and produced dark blue colour (Tarokh et al. 2021). Yang and group published research, developed a novel idea of aptasensor via using the arrest of AuNPs-aptamer coupled with departing of multi-walled carbon nanotubes (MWCNT)@ CIP (carbonyl iron powder) probe for rapid monitoring of *E. coli O157:H7* in milk samples. AuNPs-aptamer immobilized on *E. coli* O157:H7. MWCNT@CIP hybridized with a DNA probe. Smart phone-based aptasensor exhibited transformation from 518 to 524 nm in the presence of target molecules (Yang et al. 2021). Quantum dots could be an option for the detection of target molecules, they belong to the class of semiconductor NPs, and their small size consequences quantum confinement and size-dependent fluorescence properties. QDs are a class of semiconductor NPs whose small size results in quantum confinement and size-dependent fluorescence properties, in contrast to small-molecule fluorophores (e.g. dyes). Many researchers have been employing QDs instead of using organic fluorescent dyes to improve their assay performance (Choi et al. 2006, Matea et al. 2017) and to detect drug delivery in cells (Bagalkot et al. 2007, Jing et al. 2021).

6.5.4 2D METAL NANOPLATES

Two-dimensional metal nanoplates unveil good colorimetric qualities. In addition, Bera and colleagues conceptualized the strategy of triangular 2D Ag-nanoplates showing sensitivity to H2O2 and the reaction produced colour can be observed by the naked eye (Bera and Raj 2013). Based on the above concept, Liu's squad formalized a bimetallic Ag@Au hybrid stuff or can say a triangular-nanoplate (Ag@Au core/shell TNLs). POX-like activity of the Au shell oxidizes glucose and mediates change in absorbance because of the etching of Ag core by H_2O_2 and extinct blue colour (Liu et al. 2020). Correspondingly, for the detection of Cu^{2+} based on colorimetric aptasensing Chang et al (2017), develop a device via iodine-mediated Au-triangular-nanoplates. That thought assists in creating another strategy of aptamer-based colorimetric detection of CAP by using modified Au-triangular-nanoplates.

6.5.5 Silica beads and silica nanoparticles (SiNPs)

SiO_2 (Silica oxide) has with few superior qualities as compatibility with biological samples, contracting resistance, broad surface area, and high loading ability. Luan et al. formulated a sensitive probe to detect STR (streptomycin) POC testing by utilizing the porous-SiO_2 microbeads along with enzyme-linked polymer, while for the amplification of signal target recycling was done by exonuclease-I (Luan et al. 2017). Dye-doped SiNPs put forward benefits atop organic dyes. Increased optical intensity forwarded by incorporating different dyes. Furthermore, nanoparticles reduced the photobleaching and the dye is secure from surrounding impacts. Rajagopal and the group developed a colorimetric aptasensor based on the TISS system for thrombin relay on aptamer-modified SiNPs (Babu et al. 2013). In another approach pang et al used SiNPs to identify ATP based on TID (Cai et al. 2011) while Wang and Liu (2009) detect thrombin based on a sandwich-based approach. Colorimetric detection of AFM1 was performed based on target-induced shielding of AuNPs against NaCl-generated aggregation and SiNPs (Jalalian et al. 2021).

6.5.6 Magnetic beads (MBs)

The incorporation of micro- or nano-sized MBs established improved analytical aptasensing methods due to superparamagnetic properties, MBs can be used for coating or immobilization of aptamers, peptides, or antibodies (Modh et al. 2018). Liang et al. stated an interesting aggregation concept for human α-thrombin detection. This aggregation is associated with aptamer-protein binding. Two types of aptamers were immobilized on MB-AuNPs core-shell (called nano-roses-flower-like structure) against thrombin (Liang et al. 2011). Modified MBs parade POX-like activity exploited colorimetric aptasensors. For instance, detection of metal ions (Kim and Jurng 2013), thrombin in plasma (Zhang et al. 2010), Hg(II) detection based on hybridization chain reaction (Wang et al. 2016a), OTA in cereal samples (Wang et al. 2016b) and *Vibrio parahemolyticus* in spiked raw shrimp samples (Sadsri et al. 2020). QDs and AuNPs associated limitations could also be conquered like scattering generated background effect and auto-fluoresence (Bamrungsap et al. 2012). The flexibility in design adored the versatile designing of aptasensors for the qualitative and quantitative determination of targets like allergens, bacterial or viral pathogens, heavy metals ions, toxins or myotoxins, antibiotics, etc. (Ahmadi et al. 2021, Arshavsky-Graham et al. 2020, Jalalian et al. 2018, Khedri et al. 2018, Majdinasab et al. 2018) in foodstuff from food safety point of view.

6.5.7 MOFs (metal-organic framework)

MOFs are a relatively new class of porous material that has properties like adsorption, catalysis, drug delivery, and chemical sensing, promisingly fluorescence analysis (Yang et al. 2013) including unique qualities like nano-size, ease of synthesis, cost-effective, flexible shape, and size, compatible nature, high stability nominate MOFs as proficient lab chip tools (Khoshbin et al. 2022). In addition, MOF-based colorimetrics own themselves to detect H2O2, glucose, or some normal analytes, like to work as artificial nanozymes. To enhance MOF functionalization incorporation of aptamer was done by Wang's team to detect the thrombin based on label-free colorimetric sensing. Initially, a blue colour formed because Fe-MIL-88A can oxidize TMB to make blue TMB. Thrombin aptamer targeted thrombin targets in the mixture and create stable TA@thrombin complex (intramolecular G-quadruplex structure), therefore the surface of Fe-MIL-88A (class of MOFs) got blocked, causing no transfer of e⁻ between Fe-MIL-88A and TMB resulting colourless solution instead of blue (Wang et al. 2016c).

6.5.8 ENZYMES

ELAA grounded sandwich assay set a trend toward emerging optical diagnostic platforms for on-site diagnosis. Natural enzyme utilized to design skilled RNA-based SQ2 aptamer (2′-fluoro modified) to identify marker of pancreatic ductal adenocarcinoma named ALPPL2 (alkaline phosphatase placental-like 2) (Dua et al. 2013) and later this work extended by Shin and group quantified ALPPL2 on extracellular vesicles based on ELAA as shown in Figure 6.7a (Shin et al. 2019). A researcher's group customized a biosensor chip for the rapid diagnosis of C-reactive protein (CRP), an inflammatory, sepsis, and tissue necrotic biomarker based on RNA aptamer-antibody and claimed sandwich assay has greater measuring advantages over antibody-based biosensors (Pultar et al. 2009) and has selectivity advantages over the single use of aptamer (Mo et al. 2022). Utilization of a device of artificial nanozymes (reduced purification and storage difficulty) revealed competency to natural enzymes with aptamer functionalized MBs and took the colorimetric sandwich technique to the next level. The complex can be captured magnetically and a colorimetric signal is produced by catalyzing the reaction by nanozymes (Hu et al. 2014, Wang et al. 2015). Additionally, magnification of catalytic activity done by increasing the active area via coating of AuNPs with gold shells detects factor-1α (hypoxia-inducible factor) on exosomes (Wang et al. 2020). Nanozymes with POX activity have been widely used for exosome detection (Chen et al. 2018, Xia et al. 2017). Meanwhile, DNAzymes are attentive catalysts that manifest heat resistance, expedient synthesis, and easy SELEX selection making them attractive choices for visual bioanalysis (Kosman and Juskowiak 2011, Willner et al. 2008) as its G-quadruplex structure can bind to hemin with expanded POX-like activity (Zhu et al. 2012). Aptamer-based hybridization strategy increases the number of G-quadruplex structures and can lead to specific/sensitive binding with the targeted surface to visualize the presence of the target (Norouzi et al. 2018, Xu et al. 2018). Shahbazi's group visualizes the presence of carcinoembryonic-antigen through split G-quadruplex tactics from saliva with a limit of 5.5 pM. Fragment of DNAzyme attached with the loop formed by folding of split G-quadruples into an intramolecular G-quadruplex. Complementary sequences of aptamer allow the hybridization and loop define the activity of the split molecule, which is controlled by the binding of target and aptamer as represented in Figure 6.7b (Shahbazi et al. 2017). In the absence of a target molecule G-quadruples formation is blocked due to hybridization occurring between aptamer and DNAzyme.

Figure 6.7b visualizes the presence of carcinoembryonic-antigen through split G-quadruplex tactics from saliva. In the figure fragment of DNAzyme attached with

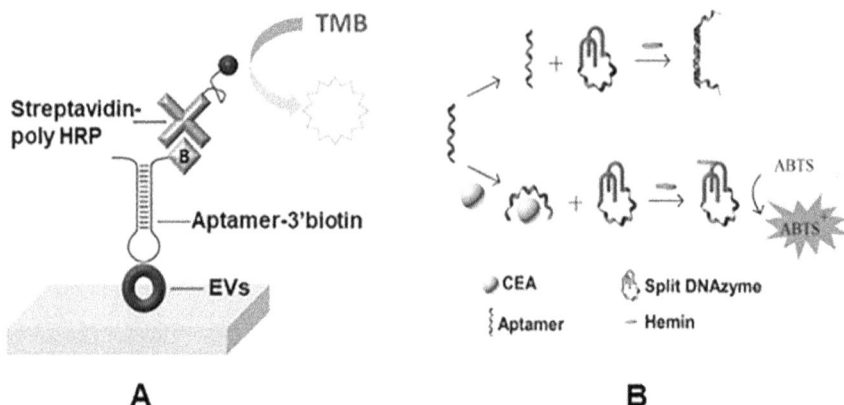

FIGURE 6.7 (a) SQ2 aptamer-based ELAA sandwich assay for extracellular vesicles detection (Shin et al. 2019). (b) Split G-quadruplex coupled aptasensor for colorimetric detection of carcinoembryonic-antigen.

(a) Reprinted from open access article under the CC BY-NC-ND license (http://creativecommons.org/licenses/by-nc-nd/4.0/), Copyright © 2019. (b) Reprinted from Sensors and Actuators B: Chemical, with the permission of Shahbazi et al. (2017), Copyright (2017), with permission from Elsevier.

the loop formed by folding of split G-quadruples into an intramolecular G-quadruplex and complementary sequences of aptamer allow the hybridization and loop define the activity of the split molecule, which is controlled by the binding of target and aptamer.

6.6 COLORIMETRIC BIOSENSING ASSAY AS POC TESTING

Among the accessible assay acknowledgement signals, colorimetric techniques are thought of as straightforward and proficient with an incredible potential for POC diagnostics, as the discovery reactions are essentially visually discerned by the unaided eye. POC testing is a direct, low-expensive, and instrument-free procedure and is further utilized for real-life monitoring through aptasensors. Recent research is recommended for designing, stability, and modification of sensors to enable practical POC testing owing to effortless testing, easy readout, and reproducible outcomes with accuracy. Advanced chromatic detection avails disease screening and diagnosis tools in field and resource-poor areas. Very initially, Stojanovic and Landry (2002) developed the first colorimetric aptasensor for a small molecule i.e. cocaine was synthesized by the method of intermolecular displacement of the dye from an aptamer–dye complex in the presence of the cocaine target. Displacement of dye by cocaine and forming a cocaine aptamer compound, causing an immediate reduction or mitigation of absorbance of relative wavelength and eventual precipitation of the dye. With a similar approach, heavy metal ions (Pb^{2+} and Cu^{2+}) were also detected using DNAzymes (Liu and Lu 2007, Zhang et al. 2008). A range of target molecules can be detected through colorimetric assays are cocaine, ATP, cysteine, homocysteine, melamine, dopamine, glucose, trinitrotoluene, different types of anions (such as oxoanions, F^-, I^-, NO_2^{2-}, CN^-, $PF6^-$) and cations (such as Al^{3+}, As^{3+}, Hg^{2+}, Pb^{2+}, Pt^{2+}, Ca^{2+}) have been detected since years ago (Liu et al. 2011, Sang et al. 2018).

Zhang et al. (2022), discovered exclusive DNA-based MSA52 aptamer that binds to aptamer@HRP immobilized on streptavidin-coated plate, capable of binding wildtype SARS-CoV-2's spike proteins and seven other recent variants of concern. MSA52 likely bound to specific amino acids of the virus and produced a blue colour due to catalyzing of the reaction by TMB. Colorimetric-based POC detection of SARS-CoV-2 also favoured by many scientists during the pandemic generated by COVID-19 (Peinetti et al. 2021, Ventura et al. 2020, Yadav et al. 2021).

Other most known examples are pregnancy tests and HIV test kits based on colorimetric assay assembled with lateral flow assay. For this target, specific NP aggregates and linked with aptamers were loaded onto a device. Such type of antigen-captured assay composites nitrocellulose, nylon, or other paper membrane-bounded with labelled antibodies (Pashchenko et al. 2018). The binding point of the antigen-antibody colour band indicates the presence of the target. For instance, OTA (type of myotoxin) on-site monitored by strip assay in *Astragalus membranaceus*, a common Chinese dietary supplement present in medicine. The strip was constructed with the help of specific AuNPs and aptamer detecting probes. The total number of aptamers chemically displaced from AuNPs using DTT is the quantity of AuNPs aptamer loaded. In an optimized state presence of nano-gram of OTA can be detected (red line) in 15 min (Zhou et al. 2016). Similarly, contamination of KMC in food was detected by the KMC-inspection aptasensor. AgNPs–DNA1–apt-AuNP mixture immobilized on a strip (Liu et al. 2018). Birader et al. (2021) developed a device to detect OTC from milk, for this truncated (27-base-pair long) aptamer was used based on the principle of competitive lateral flow assay by unifying the aptamer@AuNPs and OTC@carrier protein. Aptamer@AuNPs dish out on strip pad whereas OTC-carrier protein immobilized at A-line and biotin-labelled probe (cDNA of aptamer) coated at B-line. Free OTC in the sample preferred to bind with aptamer@AuNPs and formed OTC@aptamer@AuNPs complex. A little amount of free conjugate (aptamer@AuNPs) moved and may drag on OTC to form a red band at A-line (showed the presence of OTC). Conformation of the test was done by presenting of red B-line band due to paring of aptamer with DNA probe (Figure 6.8). POC test strip devices are attractive, instrument-free, rapid, and cheap techniques, which are needed in the present scenario to secure food safety, and human and environmental health. Ruefully, most POC testing is merely qualitative and cannot allude severity of disease or infection.

Smartphone POC testing emerges as a promising platform for rapid quantitative and qualitative assessments of samples (McLeod et al. 2015). It facilitates on-site monitoring, and rapid testing and saves cost of laboratory equipment (Celikbas et al. 2018, Quesada-González and Merkoçi 2017, Zhang et al. 2019). This bioanalysis application composed of high-resolution camera and light sensors (Kurup et al. 2021) finds application in data analysis, obtaining photometric readings as well as data storage and communication, in areas where visual inspection stands unreliable. Detection of cocaine, Hg^{2+}, and arsenic (III) from different sources were analyzed

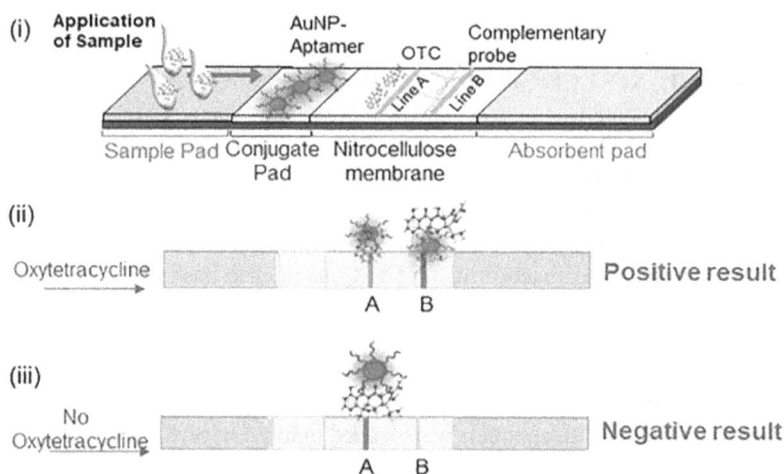

FIGURE 6.8 A strategy for POC testing of oxytetracycline in milk samples worked on colorimetric aptasensor (i) and two red lines/bands at positions A and B anticipated a positive result (ii) while a single red line/band at position B anticipated a negative result (iii).

Reprinted from Food Chemistry, with the permission of Birader et al. (2021), Copyright (2021), with permission from Elsevier.

(Shrivas et al. 2020, Smith et al. 2014, Xiao et al. 2016). Smartphone-based active testing of milk to identify the presence of *E. coli* O157:H7 to prevent epidemics of foodborne infection can be conceivable by utilization of AuNPs@aptasensor-multi-walled carbon nanotubes (Yang et al. 2021).

6.7 CONCLUSION AND FUTURE REMARKS

Aptamer-based colorimetric biosensor offers an extensive advantage in contrast to other aptasensing methods because the major advantage of the colorimetric method is on-site analysis in the area where resources are limited. In addition, aptamers' versatile features of easy and cheap bulk synthesis, long lifespan, biocompatibility, and stability make them suitable not only for the detection of small molecules but large size proteins and whole cells can be detected. Different operational modes of aptamer synthesis like TISS, sandwich-like, TID, CR, and TIR increase the specificity and potential of aptamer, and adding of new strategy makes the sensor more flexible to achieve the aim. But the selection of appropriate aptamer for small-sized targets places the great bottleneck to innovate a novel aptasensor for example fabrication or selection of aptamer for testosterone and/or other hormones dig up the difficulties. Moreover, a review of the literature divulges the fact that aptasensors are majorly tested in buffers rather the directly in complex biological, clinical, or environmental samples like serum and plasma. Occasionally, conformational alterations make aptamer susceptible to noising in compound matrix analysis and confront glitches like cross-reactivity resulting in less specific and false positive signals and lowering the signal-to-noise percentage. The utilization of AuNPs, AgNPs, SiNPs, GO, and MOF pave the strength to aptamer many folds. These modified or unmodified particles not only amplify the signal but also provide a surface for aptamer immobilization which extensively offers a tool for dealing with aptasensor. In terms of dealing with clinical sample handling and environment-assisting approaches POC testing somewhere extend the way for rapid and effective detection. Nonetheless, the need to extend the present quality and characteristics of aptameric biosensors must be translated into the commercialized test kit form. While aptasensors-based smart-mobile technologies might be in the initial phase of development. In a concluding remake, with respect to the number of investigational researches the simplicity and necked eye detection make colorimetric aptasensor a powerful candidate for next-generation biosensing, but still needs to be carried out more work on making portable, lodge able, commercialized environment.

ABBREVIATIONS

3D	3 dimension
TMB	3,3′,5,5′-tetramethylbenzidine
ATP	Adenosine 5′-triphosphate
AFB1	Aflatoxin B1
AFM1	Aflatoxin M1
ALP	Alkaline Phosphatase
CDs	Carbon dots
CIP	Carbonyl iron powder
CAP	Chloramphenicol
CTRMs	Circulating tumour-related materials
Cu^2O	Copper oxide-I
CRP	C-reactive protein
DSPs	Diarrheic shellfish poisons
AuNBPs	Gold nanobipyramids
AuNCs	Gold nanoclusters
AuNPs	Gold nanoparticles
Gr	Graphene
$g\text{-}C_3N_4$	Graphitic carbon nitride
HER2	Human epidermal growth factor receptor 2
HCR	Hybridization chain reaction
KMC	Kanamycin
LOD	Limit of detection
MBs	Magnetic beads
MG	Malachite green
MWCNT	Multi-walled carbon nanotube
NFMs	Nanofibers
NPs	Nanoparticles
OTA	Ochratoxin-A
OFL	Ofloxacin
OTC	Oxytetracycline
POX	Peroxidase
POC	Point of care

PMNT   Poly(3-(30-*N*,*N*,*N*-triethylamino-10-propyloxy)-4-methyl-2,5-thiophene hydrochloride
PCB-77 Polychlorinatedd biphenyls
PDA   Polydiacetylene
PSA   Prostate-specific antigen
AgNPs   Silver nanoparticles
SWCNTs Single-walled carbon nanotubes
SDM   Sulfadimethoxine
SPR   Surface plasmon resonance
TET   Tetracycline
TOB   Tobramycin
VEGF165 Vascular endothelial growth factor$_{165}$

REFERENCES

Abedalwafa, M.A., Tang, Z., Qiao, Y., Mei, Q., Yang, G., Li, Y. and Wang, L., 2020. An aptasensor strip-based colorimetric determination method for kanamycin using cellulose acetate nanofibers decorated DNA–gold nanoparticle bioconjugates. *Microchimica Acta*, 187, pp. 1–9.

Abnous, K., Danesh, N.M., Ramezani, M., Alibolandi, M., Nameghi, M.A., Zavvar, T.S. and Taghdisi, S.M., 2021. A novel colorimetric aptasensor for ultrasensitive detection of aflatoxin M1 based on the combination of CRISPR-Cas12a, rolling circle amplification and catalytic activity of gold nanoparticles. *Analytica Chimica Acta*, 1165, p. 338549.

Abnous, K., Danesh, N.M., Ramezani, M., Emrani, A.S. and Taghdisi, S.M., 2016. A novel colorimetric sandwich aptasensor based on an indirect competitive enzyme-free method for ultrasensitive detection of chloramphenicol. *Biosensors and Bioelectronics*, 78, pp. 80–86.

Ahmadi, M., Ghoorchian, A., Dashtian, K., Kamalabadi, M., Madrakian, T. and Afkhami, A., 2021. Application of magnetic nanomaterials in electroanalytical methods: A review. *Talanta*, 225, p. 121974.

Alkhamis, O., Canoura, J., Yu, H., Liu, Y. and Xiao, Y., 2019. Innovative engineering and sensing strategies for aptamer-based small-molecule detection. *TrAC Trends in Analytical Chemistry*, 121, p. 115699.

Alsager, O.A., Alotaibi, K.M., Alswieleh, A.M. and Alyamani, B.J., 2018. Colorimetric aptasensor of vitamin D3: A novel approach to eliminate residual adhesion between aptamers and gold nanoparticles. *Scientific Reports*, 8(1), pp. 1–12.

António, M., Ferreira, R., Vitorino, R. and Daniel-da-Silva, A.L., 2020. A simple aptamer-based colorimetric assay for rapid detection of C-reactive protein using gold nanoparticles. *Talanta*, 214, p. 120868.

Arshavsky-Graham, S., Urmann, K., Salama, R., Massad-Ivanir, N., Walter, J.G., Scheper, T. and Segal, E., 2020. Aptamers vs. antibodies as capture probes in optical porous silicon biosensors. *Analyst*, 145(14), pp. 4991–5003.

Babu, E., Mareeswaran, P.M. and Rajagopal, S., 2013. Highly sensitive optical biosensor for thrombin based on structure switching aptamer-luminescent silica nanoparticles. *Journal of Fluorescence*, 23(1), pp. 137–146.

Bagalkot, V., Zhang, L., Levy-Nissenbaum, E., Jon, S., Kantoff, P.W., Langer, R. and Farokhzad, O.C. 2007. Quantum dot–aptamer conjugates for synchronous cancer imaging, therapy, and sensing of drug delivery based on Bi-fluorescence resonance energy transfer. *Nano Letters*, 7(10), pp. 3065–3070.

Bamrungsap, S., Chen, T., Shukoor, M.I., Chen, Z., Sefah, K., Chen, Y. and Tan, W., 2012. Pattern recognition of cancer cells using aptamer-conjugated magnetic nanoparticles. *ACS Nano*, 6(5), pp. 3974–3981.

Bao, Y., Jiang, Y., Xiong, E., Tian, T., Zhang, Z., Lv, J., Li, Y. and Zhou, X., 2020. CUT-LAMP: contamination-free loop-mediated isothermal amplification based on the CRISPR/Cas9 cleavage. *ACS Sensors*, 5(4), pp. 1082–1091.

Bera, R.K. and Raj, C.R., 2013. A facile photochemical route for the synthesis of triangular Ag nanoplates and colorimetric sensing of H_2O_2. *Journal of Photochemistry and Photobiology A: Chemistry*, 270, pp. 1–6.

Birader, K., Kumar, P., Tammineni, Y., Barla, J.A., Reddy, S. and Suman, P., 2021. Colorimetric aptasensor for on-site detection of oxytetracycline antibiotic in milk. *Food Chemistry*, 356, p. 129659.

Cai, L., Chen, Z.Z., Dong, X.M., Tang, H.W. and Pang, D.W., 2011. Silica nanoparticles based label-free aptamer hybridization for ATP detection using hoechst33258 as the signal reporter. *Biosensors and Bioelectronics*, 29(1), pp. 46–52.

Caruthers, M.H., 1985. Gene synthesis machines: DNA chemistry and its uses. *Science*, 230(4723), pp. 281–285.

Celikbas, E., Guler Celik, E. and Timur, S., 2018. Paper-based analytical methods for smartphone sensing with functional nanoparticles: Bridges from smart surfaces to global health. *Analytical Chemistry*, 90(21), pp. 12325–12333.

Chang, C.C., Wang, G., Takarada, T. and Maeda, M., 2017. Iodine-mediated etching of triangular gold nanoplates for colorimetric sensing of copper ion and aptasensing of chloramphenicol. *ACS Applied Materials & Interfaces*, 9(39), pp. 34518–34525.

Chang, D., Zakaria, S., Deng, M., Allen, N., Tram, K. and Li, Y., 2016. Integrating deoxyribozymes into colorimetric sensing platforms. *Sensors*, 16(12), p. 2061.

Chen, A. and Yang, S., 2015. Replacing antibodies with aptamers in lateral flow immunoassay. *Biosensors and Bioelectronics*, 71, pp. 230–242.

Chen, C., Feng, S., Zhou, M., Ji, C., Que, L. and Wang, W., 2019. Development of a structure-switching aptamer-based nanosensor for salicylic acid detection. *Biosensors and Bioelectronics*, 140, p. 111342.

Chen, C., Li, N., Lan, J., Ji, X. and He, Z., 2016. A label-free colorimetric platform for DNA via target-catalyzed hairpin assembly and the peroxidase-like catalytic of graphene/Au-NPs hybrids. *Analytica Chimica Acta*, 902, pp. 154–159.

Chen, H., Kou, X., Yang, Z., Ni, W. and Wang, J., 2008. Shape-and size-dependent refractive index sensitivity of gold nanoparticles. *Langmuir*, 24(10), pp. 5233–5237.

Chen, J., Xu, Y., Lu, Y. and Xing, W., 2018. Isolation and visible detection of tumor-derived exosomes from plasma. *Analytical Chemistry*, 90(24), pp. 14207–14215.

Chen, Z., Tan, Y., Zhang, C., Yin, L., Ma, H., Ye, N., Qiang, H. and Lin, Y., 2014. A colorimetric aptamer biosensor based on cationic polymer and gold nanoparticles for the ultrasensitive detection of thrombin. *Biosensors and Bioelectronics*, 56, pp. 46–50.

Cheng, R., Liu, S., Shi, H. and Zhao, G., 2018. A highly sensitive and selective aptamer-based colorimetric sensor for the rapid detection of PCB 77. *Journal of Hazardous Materials*, 341, pp. 373–380.

Chiu, Y.J., Cai, W., Shih, Y.R., Lian, I. and Lo, Y.H., 2016. A single-cell assay for time lapse studies of exosome secretion and cell behaviors. *Small*, 12, pp. 3658–3666.

Cho, M.J. and Park, S.Y., 2019. Carbon-dot-based ratiometric fluorescence glucose biosensor. *Sensors and Actuators B: Chemical*, 282, pp. 719–729.

Choi, J.H., Chen, K.H. and Strano, M.S., 2006. Aptamer-capped nanocrystal quantum dots: a new method for label-free protein detection. *Journal of the American Chemical Society*, 128(49), pp. 15584–15585.

Clark, D.J., Fondrie, W.E., Liao, Z., Hanson, P.I., Fulton, A., Mao, L. and Yang, A.J., 2015. Redefining the breast cancer exosome proteome by tandem mass tag quantitative proteomics and multivariate cluster analysis. *Analytical Chemistry*, 87(20), pp. 10462–10469.

Dirks, R.M. and Pierce, N.A., 2004. Triggered amplification by hybridization chain reaction. *Proceedings of the National Academy of Sciences*, 101(43), pp. 15275–15278.

Dong, J., He, L., Wang, Y., Yu, F., Yu, S., Liu, L., Wang, J., Tian, Y., Qu, L., Han, R. and Wang, Z., 2020. A highly sensitive colorimetric aptasensor for the detection of the vascular endothelial growth factor in human serum. *Spectrochimica Acta Part A: Molecular and Biomolecular Spectroscopy*, 226, p. 117622.

Doudna, J.A. and Cech, T.R., 2002. The chemical repertoire of natural ribozymes. *Nature*, 418(6894), pp. 222–228.

Dua, P., Kang, H.S., Hong, S.M., Tsao, M.S., Kim, S. and Lee, D.K., 2013. Alkaline phosphatase ALPPL-2 is a novel pancreatic carcinoma-associated protein. *Cancer Research*, 73(6), pp. 1934–1945.

Dunn, M.R., Jimenez, R.M. and Chaput, J.C., 2017. Analysis of aptamer discovery and technology. *Nature Reviews Chemistry*, 1(10), pp. 1–16.

Ellington, A.D. and Szostak, J.W., 1990. In vitro selection of RNA molecules that bind specific ligands. *Nature*, 346(6287), pp. 818–822.

Elowe, N.H., Nutiu, R., Allali-Hassani, A., Cechetto, J.D., Hughes, D.W., Li, Y. and Brown, E.D., 2006. Small-molecule screening made simple for a difficult target with a signaling nucleic acid aptamer that reports on deaminase activity. *Angewandte Chemie International Edition*, 45(34), pp. 5648–5652.

Feagin, T.A., Maganzini, N. and Soh, H.T., 2018. Strategies for creating structure-switching aptamers. *ACS Sensors*, 3(9), pp. 1611–1615.

Ferapontova, E.E., Olsen, E.M. and Gothelf, K.V., 2008. An RNA aptamer-based electrochemical biosensor for detection of theophylline in serum. *Journal of the American Chemical Society*, 130(13), pp. 4256–4258.

Fowler, C.C., Navani, N.K., Brown, E.D. and Li, Y., 2008. Aptamers and their potential as recognition elements for the detection of bacteria. In Zourob, M., Elwary, S., Turner, A. (eds) *Principles of Bacterial Detection: Biosensors, Recognition Receptors and Microsystems* (pp. 689–714). Springer, New York, NY.

Gao, L., Xiang, W., Deng, Z., Shi, K., Wang, H. and Shi, H., 2020. Cocaine detection using aptamer and molybdenum disulfide-gold nanoparticle-based sensors. *Nanomedicine*, 15(04), pp. 325–335.

Gao, Z., Qiu, Z., Lu, M., Shu, J. and Tang, D., 2017. Hybridization chain reaction-based colorimetric aptasensor of adenosine 5′-triphosphate on unmodified gold nanoparticles and two label-free hairpin probes. *Biosensors and Bioelectronics*, 89, pp. 1006–1012.

Giorgi-Coll, S., Marín, M.J., Sule, O., Hutchinson, P.J. and Carpenter, K.L., 2020. Aptamer-modified gold nanoparticles for rapid aggregation-based detection of inflammation: an optical assay for interleukin-6. *Microchimica Acta*, 187(1), pp. 1–11.

Gopinath, S.C., Lakshmipriya, T. and Awazu, K., 2014. Colorimetric detection of controlled assembly and disassembly of aptamers on unmodified gold nanoparticles. *Biosensors and Bioelectronics*, 51, pp. 115–123.

Gupta, R., Kumar, A., Kumar, S., Pinnaka, A.K. and Singhal, N.K., 2021. Naked eye colorimetric detection of *Escherichia coli* using aptamer conjugated graphene oxide enclosed Gold nanoparticles. *Sensors and Actuators B: Chemical*, 329, p. 129100.

Han, K., Chen, L., Lin, Z. and Li, G., 2009. Target induced dissociation (TID) strategy for the development of electrochemical aptamer-based biosensor. *Electrochemistry Communications*, 11(1), pp. 157–160.

Han, K., Liang, Z. and Zhou, N., 2010. Design strategies for aptamer-based biosensors. *Sensors*, 10(5), pp. 4541–4557.

He, Z., Zhu, J., Weng, G.J., Li, J.J. and Zhao, J.W., 2020. Detection of ferrous ion by etching-based multi-colorimetric sensing of gold nanobipyramids. *Nanotechnology*, 31(33), p. 335505.

Hermann, T. and Patel, D.J., 2000. Adaptive recognition by nucleic acid aptamers. *Science*, 287(5454), pp. 820–825.

Hu, H., Li, H., Zhao, Y., Dong, S., Li, W., Qiang, W. and Xu, D., 2014. Aptamer-functionalized silver nanoparticles for scanometric detection of platelet-derived growth factor-BB. *Analytica Chimica Acta*, 812, pp. 152–160.

Hua, M., Tao, M., Wang, P., Zhang, Y., Wu, Z., Chang, Y. and Yang, Y., 2010. Label-free electrochemical cocaine aptasensor based on a target-inducing aptamer switching conformation. *Analytical Sciences*, 26(12), pp. 1265–1270.

Huang, C.C., Huang, Y.F., Cao, Z., Tan, W. and Chang, H.T., 2005. Aptamer-modified gold nanoparticles for colorimetric determination of platelet-derived growth factors and their receptors. *Analytical Chemistry*, 77(17), pp. 5735–5741.

Huang, L., Serganov, A. and Patel, D.J., 2010. Structural insights into ligand recognition by a sensing domain of the cooperative glycine riboswitch. *Molecular Cell*, 40(5), pp. 774–786.

Ikebukuro, K., Kiyohara, C. and Sode, K., 2005. Novel electrochemical sensor system for protein using the aptamers in sandwich manner. *Biosensors and Bioelectronics*, 20(10), pp. 2168–2172.

Jalalian, S.H., Karimabadi, N., Ramezani, M., Abnous, K. and Taghdisi, S.M., 2018. Electrochemical and optical aptamer-based sensors for detection of tetracyclines. *Trends in Food Science & Technology*, 73, pp. 45–57.

Jalalian, S.H., Lavaee, P., Ramezani, M., Danesh, N.M., Alibolandi, M., Abnous, K. and Taghdisi, S.M., 2021. An optical aptasensor for aflatoxin M1 detection based on target-induced protection of gold nanoparticles against salt-induced aggregation and silica nanoparticles. *Spectrochimica Acta Part A: Molecular and Biomolecular Spectroscopy*, 246, p. 119062.

Jeon, H. and Lee, K., 2019. Effect of gold nanoparticle morphology on thermal properties of polyimide nanocomposite films. *Colloids and Surfaces A: Physicochemical and Engineering Aspects*, 579, p. 123651

Jeon, H.B., Tsalu, P.V. and Ha, J.W., 2019. Shape effect on the refractive index sensitivity at localized surface plasmon resonance inflection points of single gold nanocubes with vertices. *Scientific Reports*, 9(1), pp. 1–8.

Jia, J., Yan, S., Lai, X., Xu, Y., Liu, T. and Xiang, Y., 2018. Colorimetric aptasensor for detection of malachite green in fish sample based on RNA and gold nanoparticles. *Food Analytical Methods*, 11(6), pp. 1668–1676.

Jing, H., Pálmai, M., Saed, B., George, A., Snee, P.T. and Hu, Y.S., 2021. Cytosolic delivery of membrane-penetrating QDs into T cell lymphocytes: Implications in immunotherapy and drug delivery. *Nanoscale*, 13(10), pp. 5519–5529.

Joyce, G.F., 1994. In vitro evolution of nucleic acids. *Current Opinion in Structural Biology*, 4(3), pp. 331–336.

Kaushal, S., Pinnaka, A.K., Soni, S. and Singhal, N.K., 2021. Antibody assisted graphene oxide coated gold nanoparticles for rapid bacterial detection and near infrared light enhanced antibacterial activity. *Sensors and Actuators B: Chemical*, 329, p. 129141.

Keefe, A.D., Pai, S. and Ellington, A., 2010. Aptamers as therapeutics. *Nature Reviews Drug discovery*, 9(7), pp. 537–550.

Khedri, M., Ramezani, M., Rafatpanah, H. and Abnous, K., 2018. Detection of food-born allergens with aptamer-based biosensors. *TrAC Trends in Analytical Chemistry*, 103, pp. 126–136.

Khoshbin, Z., Davoodian, N., Taghdisi, S.M. and Abnous, K., 2022. Metal organic frameworks as advanced functional materials for aptasensor design. *Spectrochimica Acta Part A: Molecular and Biomolecular Spectroscopy*, 276, p. 121251.

Kim, Y.S. and Jurng, J., 2013. A simple colorimetric assay for the detection of metal ions based on the peroxidase-like activity of magnetic nanoparticles. *Sensors and Actuators B: Chemical*, 176, pp. 253–257.

Kim, Y.S., Kim, J.H., Kim, I.A., Lee, S.J. and Gu, M.B., 2011. The affinity ratio—its pivotal role in gold nanoparticle-based competitive colorimetric aptasensor. *Biosensors and Bioelectronics*, 26(10), pp. 4058–4063.

Kim, Y.S., Kim, J.H., Kim, I.A., Lee, S.J., Jurng, J. and Gu, M.B., 2010. A novel colorimetric aptasensor using gold nanoparticle for a highly sensitive and specific detection of oxytetracycline. *Biosensors and Bioelectronics*, 26(4), pp. 1644–1649.

Komarova, N., Andrianova, M., Glukhov, S. and Kuznetsov, A., 2018. Selection, characterization, and application of ssDNA aptamer against furaneol. *Molecules*, 23(12), p. 3159.

Kosman, J. and Juskowiak, B., 2011. Peroxidase-mimicking DNAzymes for biosensing applications: a review. *Analytica Chimica Acta*, 707(1–2), pp. 7–17.

Kurup, C.P., Tlili, C., Zakaria, S.N.A. and Ahmed, M.U., 2021. Recent trends in design and development of nanomaterial-based aptasensors. *Biointerface Research in Applied Chemistry*, 11, pp. 14057–14077.

Lackey, H.H., Peterson, E.M., Harris, J.M. and Heemstra, J.M., 2020. Probing the mechanism of structure-switching aptamer assembly by super-resolution localization of individual DNA molecules. *Analytical Chemistry*, 92(10), pp. 6909–6917.

Lander, E.S., Linton, L.M., Birren, B., Nusbaum, C., Zody, M.C., Baldwin, J., Devon, K., Dewar, K., Doyle, M., Fitzhugh, W. and Funke, R., 2001. Erratum: Initial sequencing and analysis of the human genome: international human genome sequencing consortium [Nature (2001) 409 (860–921)]. *Nature*, 412(6846), pp. 565–566.

Lau, P.S. and Li, Y., 2014. Exploration of structure-switching in the design of aptamer biosensors. In Gu, M. and Kim, H.S. (eds) *Biosensors Based on Aptamers and Enzymes. Advances in Biochemical Engineering/Biotechnology* (vol. 140). Springer, Berlin, Heidelberg, pp. 69–92.

Lau, P.S., Coombes, B.K. and Li, Y., 2010. A general approach to the construction of structure-switching reporters from RNA aptamers. *Angewandte Chemie International Edition*, 49(43), pp. 7938–7942.

Lee, J., Kim, H.J. and Kim, J., 2008. Polydiacetylene liposome arrays for selective potassium detection. *Journal of the American Chemical Society*, 130(15), pp. 5010–5011.

Lee, J., Seo, S. and Kim, J., 2012. Colorimetric detection of warfare gases by polydiacetylenes toward equipment-free detection. *Advanced Functional Materials*, 22(8), pp. 1632–1638.

Lee, J.S., Han, M.S. and Mirkin, C.A., 2007. Colorimetric detection of mercuric ion (Hg2+) in aqueous media using DNA-functionalized gold nanoparticles. *Angewandte Chemie International Edition*, 46(22), pp. 4093–4096.

Lee, M. and Walt, D.R., 2000. A fiber-optic microarray biosensor using aptamers as receptors. *Analytical Biochemistry*, 282(1), pp. 142–146.

Lerdsri, J., Chananchana, W., Upan, J., Sridara, T. and Jakmunee, J., 2020. Label-free colorimetric aptasensor for rapid detection of aflatoxin B1 by utilizing cationic perylene probe and localized surface plasmon resonance of gold nanoparticles. *Sensors and Actuators B: Chemical*, 320, p. 128356.

Levine, H.A. and Nilsen-Hamilton, M., 2007. A mathematical analysis of SELEX. *Computational Biology and Chemistry*, 31(1), pp. 11–35.

Li, B., Du, Y. and Dong, S., 2009. DNA based gold nanoparticles colorimetric sensors for sensitive and selective detection of Ag (I) ions. *Analytica Chimica Acta*, 644(1–2), pp. 78–82.

Li, H. and Rothberg, L., 2004a. Colorimetric detection of DNA sequences based on electrostatic interactions with unmodified gold nanoparticles. *Proceedings of the National Academy of Sciences*, 101(39), pp. 14036–14039.

Li, H. and Rothberg, L.J., 2004b. Label-free colorimetric detection of specific sequences in genomic DNA amplified by the polymerase chain reaction. *Journal of the American Chemical Society*, 126(35), pp. 10958–10961.

Li, J., Yu, C., Wu, Y.N., Zhu, Y., Xu, J., Wang, Y., Wang, H., Guo, M. and Li, F., 2019. Novel sensing platform based on gold nanoparticle-aptamer and Fe-metal-organic framework for multiple antibiotic detection and signal amplification. *Environment International*, 125, pp. 135–141.

Li, L., Ma, R., Zhao, Y., Wang, L., Wang, S. and Mao, X., 2022. Development of a colorimetric aptasensor fabricated with a group-specific aptamer and AuNPs@ Fe2+ nanozyme for simultaneous detection of multiple diarrheic shellfish poisons. *Talanta*, 246, p. 123534.

Liang, G., Cai, S., Zhang, P., Peng, Y., Chen, H., Zhang, S. and Kong, J., 2011. Magnetic relaxation switch and colorimetric detection of thrombin using aptamer-functionalized gold-coated iron oxide nanoparticles. *Analytica Chimica Acta*, 689(2), pp. 243–249.

Liao, A.M., Pan, W., Benson, J.C., Wong, A.D., Rose, B.J. and Caltagirone, G.T., 2018. A simple colorimetric system for detecting target antigens by a three-stage signal transformation–amplification strategy. *Biochemistry*, 57(34), pp. 5117–5126.

Lin, B., Yu, Y., Cao, Y., Guo, M., Zhu, D., Dai, J. and Zheng, M., 2018. Point-of-care testing for streptomycin based on aptamer recognizing and digital image colorimetry by smartphone. *Biosensors and Bioelectronics*, 100, pp. 482–489.

Liu, A., Li, M., Wang, J., Feng, F., Zhang, Y., Qiu, Z., Chen, Y., Meteku, B.E., Wen, C., Yan, Z. and Zeng, J., 2020. Ag@ Au core/shell triangular nanoplates with dual enzyme-like properties for the colorimetric sensing of glucose. *Chinese Chemical Letters*, 31(5), pp. 1133–1136.

Liu, A., Zhang, Y., Chen, W., Wang, X. and Chen, F., 2013a. Gold nanoparticle-based colorimetric detection of staphylococcal enterotoxin B using ssDNA aptamers. *European Food Research and Technology*, 237(3), pp. 323–329.

Liu, C.W., Hsieh, Y.T., Huang, C.C., Lin, Z.H. and Chang, H.T., 2008. Detection of mercury (II) based on Hg 2+–DNA complexes inducing the aggregation of gold nanoparticles. *Chemical Communications*, (19), pp. 2242–2244.

Liu, D., Wang, Z. and Jiang, X., 2011. Gold nanoparticles for the colorimetric and fluorescent detection of ions and small organic molecules. *Nanoscale*, 3(4), pp. 1421–1433.

Liu, J. and Lu, Y., 2005. Stimuli-responsive disassembly of nanoparticle aggregates for light-up colorimetric sensing. *Journal of the American Chemical Society*, 127(36), pp. 12677–12683.

Liu, J. and Lu, Y., 2006. Fast colorimetric sensing of adenosine and cocaine based on a general sensor design involving aptamers and nanoparticles. *Angewandte Chemie International Edition*, 45(1), pp. 90–94.

Liu, J. and Lu, Y., 2007. A DNAzyme catalytic beacon sensor for paramagnetic Cu2+ ions in aqueous solution with high sensitivity and selectivity. *Journal of the American Chemical Society*, 129(32), pp. 9838–9839.

Liu, J., Zeng, J., Tian, Y. and Zhou, N., 2018. An aptamer and functionalized nanoparticle-based strip biosensor for on-site detection of kanamycin in food samples. *Analyst*, 143(1), pp. 182–189.

Liu, M., Lee, T.W., Gray, S.K., Guyot-Sionnest, P. and Pelton, M., 2009. Excitation of dark plasmons in metal nanoparticles by a localized emitter. *Physical Review Letters*, 102(10), p. 107401.

Liu, M., Song, J., Shuang, S., Dong, C., Brennan, J.D. and Li, Y., 2014. A graphene-based biosensing platform based on the release of DNA probes and rolling circle amplification. *ACS Nano*, 8(6), pp. 5564–5573.

Liu, P., Yang, X., Sun, S., Wang, Q., Wang, K., Huang, J., Liu, J. and He, L., 2013b. Enzyme-free colorimetric detection of DNA by using gold nanoparticles and hybridization chain reaction amplification. *Analytical Chemistry*, 85(16), pp. 7689–7695.

Liu, X., Tang, Y., Wang, L., Zhang, J., Song, S., Fan, C. and Wang, S., 2007. Optical detection of mercury (II) in aqueous solutions by using conjugated polymers and label-free oligonucleotides. *Advanced Materials*, 19(11), pp. 1471–1474.

Lönne, M., Zhu, G., Stahl, F. and Walter, J.G., 2014. Aptamer-modified nanoparticles as biosensors. *Advances in Biochemical Engineering/Biotechnology*, 140, pp. 121–154.

Luan, Q., Miao, Y., Gan, N., Cao, Y., Li, T. and Chen, Y., 2017. A POCT colorimetric aptasensor for streptomycin detection using porous silica beads-enzyme linked polymer aptamer probes and exonuclease-assisted target recycling for signal amplification. *Sensors and Actuators B: Chemical*, 251, pp. 349–358.

Lucas, T.M., Moiseeva, E.V., Zhang, G., Gobin, A.M. and Harnett, C.K., 2013. Thermal properties of infrared absorbent gold nanoparticle coatings for MEMS applications. *Sensors and Actuators A: Physical*, 198, pp. 81–86.

Ma, Q., Wang, Y., Jia, J. and Xiang, Y., 2018. Colorimetric aptasensors for determination of tobramycin in milk and chicken eggs based on DNA and gold nanoparticles. *Food Chemistry*, 249, pp. 98–103.

Majdinasab, M., Hayat, A. and Marty, J.L., 2018. Aptamer-based assays and aptasensors for detection of pathogenic bacteria in food samples. *TrAC Trends in Analytical Chemistry*, 107, pp. 60–77.

Matea, C.T., Mocan, T., Tabaran, F., Pop, T., Mosteanu, O., Puia, C., Iancu, C. and Mocan, L., 2017. Quantum dots in imaging, drug delivery and sensor applications. *International Journal of Nanomedicine*, 12, p. 5421.

McConnell, E.M., Nguyen, J. and Li, Y., 2020. Aptamer-based biosensors for environmental monitoring. *Frontiers in Chemistry*, 8, p. 434.

McLeod, E., Wei, Q. and Ozcan, A., 2015. Democratization of nanoscale imaging and sensing tools using photonics. *Analytical Chemistry*, 87(13), pp. 6434–6445.

Mir, M., Jenkins, A.T.A. and Katakis, I., 2008. Ultrasensitive detection based on an aptamer beacon electron transfer chain. *Electrochemistry Communications*, 10(10), pp. 1533–1536.

Mo, T., Liu, X., Luo, Y., Zhong, L., Zhang, Z., Li, T., Gan, L., Liu, X., Li, L., Wang, H. and Sun, X., 2022. Aptamer-based biosensors and application in tumor theranostics. *Cancer Science*, 113(1), p. 7.

Modh, H., Scheper, T. and Walter, J.G., 2018. Aptamer-modified magnetic beads in biosensing. *Sensors*, 18(4), p. 1041.

Mondal, B., Ramlal, S., Lavu, P.S. and Kingston, J., 2018. Highly sensitive colorimetric biosensor for staphylococcal enterotoxin B by a label-free aptamer and gold nanoparticles. *Frontiers in Microbiology*, 9, p. 179.

Moore, P.B. and Steitz, T.A., 2002. The involvement of RNA in ribosome function. *Nature*, 418(6894), pp. 229–235.

Neupane, D. and Stine, K.J., 2021. Electrochemical sandwich assays for biomarkers incorporating aptamers, antibodies and nanomaterials for detection of specific protein biomarkers. *Applied Sciences*, 11(15), p. 7087.

Neves, M.A., Slavkovic, S., Churcher, Z.R. and Johnson, P.E., 2017. Salt-mediated two-site ligand binding by the cocaine-binding aptamer. *Nucleic Acids Research*, 45(3), pp. 1041–1048.

Nguyen, D.K. and Jang, C.H., 2021. A simple and ultrasensitive colorimetric biosensor for anatoxin-a based on aptamer and gold nanoparticles. *Micromachines*, 12(12), p. 1526.

Norouzi, A., Ravan, H., Mohammadi, A., Hosseinzadeh, E., Norouzi, M. and Fozooni, T., 2018. Aptamer–integrated DNA nanoassembly: a simple and sensitive DNA framework to detect cancer cells. *Analytica Chimica Acta*, 1017, pp. 26–33.

Null, E.L. and Lu, Y., 2010. Rapid determination of enantiomeric ratio using fluorescent DNA or RNA aptamers. *Analyst*, 135(2), pp. 419–422.

Nutiu, R. and Li, Y., 2003. Structure-switching signaling aptamers. *Journal of the American Chemical Society*, 125(16), pp. 4771–4778.

Nutiu, R. and Li, Y., 2005. In vitro selection of structure-switching signaling aptamers. *Angewandte Chemie International Edition*, 44(7), pp. 1061–1065.

Nutiu, R., Yu, J.M. and Li, Y., 2004. Signaling aptamers for monitoring enzymatic activity and for inhibitor screening. *ChemBioChem*, 5(8), pp. 1139–1144.

Ono, A., Torigoe, H., Tanaka, Y. and Okamoto, I., 2011. Binding of metal ions by pyrimidine base pairs in DNA duplexes. *Chemical Society Reviews*, 40(12), pp. 5855–5866.

Pan, L., Huang, Y., Wen, C. and Zhao, S., 2013. Label-free fluorescence probe based on structure-switching aptamer for the detection of interferon gamma. *Analyst*, 138(22), pp. 6811–6816.

Pashchenko, O., Shelby, T., Banerjee, T. and Santra, S., 2018. A comparison of optical, electrochemical, magnetic, and colorimetric point-of-care biosensors for infectious disease diagnosis. *ACS Infectious Diseases*, 4(8), pp. 1162–1178.

Peinetti, A.S., Lake, R.J., Cong, W., Cooper, L., Wu, Y., Ma, Y., Pawel, G.T., Toimil-Molares, M.E., Trautmann, C., Rong, L. and Mariñas, B., 2021. Direct detection of human adenovirus or SARS-CoV-2 with ability to inform infectivity using DNA aptamer-nanopore sensors. *Science Advances*, 7(39), p. eabh2848.

Phan, L.M.T. and Cho, S., 2022. Fluorescent aptasensor and colorimetric Aatablot for p-tau231 detection: Toward early diagnosis of Alzheimer's disease. *Biomedicines*, 10(1), p. 93.

Prante, M., Segal, E., Scheper, T., Bahnemann, J. and Walter, J., 2020. Aptasensors for point-of-care detection of small molecules. *Biosensors*, 10(9), p. 108.

Pultar, J., Sauer, U., Domnanich, P. and Preininger, C., 2009. Aptamer–antibody on-chip sandwich immunoassay for detection of CRP in spiked serum. *Biosensors and Bioelectronics*, 24(5), pp. 1456–1461.

Qi, Y., Zhu, J., Li, J. and Zhao, J., 2016. Highly improved synthesis of gold nanobipyramids by tuning the concentration of hydrochloric acid. *Journal of Nanoparticle Research*, 18(7), pp. 1–16.

Quesada-González, D. and Merkoçi, A., 2017. Mobile phone-based biosensing: An emerging "diagnostic and communication" technology. *Biosensors and Bioelectronics*, 92, pp. 549–562.

Radi, A.E. and Abd-Ellatief, M.R. 2021. Electrochemical aptasensors: Current status and future perspectives. *Diagnostics*, 11, p. 104.

Radi, A.E., Acero Sánchez, J.L., Baldrich, E. and O'Sullivan, C.K., 2006. Reagentless, reusable, ultrasensitive electrochemical molecular beacon aptasensor. *Journal of the American Chemical Society*, 128(1), pp. 117–124.

Ramalingam, S., Collier, C.M. and Singh, A., 2021. A paper-based colorimetric aptasensor for the detection of gentamicin. *Biosensors*, 11(2), p. 29.

Rangel, A.E., Hariri, A.A., Eisenstein, M. and Soh, H.T., 2020. Engineering aptamer switches for multifunctional stimulus-responsive nanosystems. *Advanced Materials*, 32(50), p. 2003704.

Robertson, D.L. and Joyce, G.F., 1990. Selection in vitro of an RNA enzyme that specifically cleaves single-stranded DNA. *Nature*, 344(6265), pp. 467–468.

Röthlisberger, P. and Hollenstein, M., 2018. Aptamer chemistry. *Advanced Drug Delivery Reviews*, 134, pp. 3–21.

Rupcich, N., Nutiu, R., Li, Y. and Brennan, J.D., 2005. Entrapment of fluorescent signaling DNA aptamers in sol– gel-derived silica. *Analytical Chemistry*, 77(14), pp. 4300–4307.

Rupcich, N., Nutiu, R., Li, Y. and Brennan, J.D., 2006. Solid-phase enzyme activity assay utilizing an entrapped fluorescence-signaling DNA aptamer. *Angewandte Chemie International Edition*, 45(20), pp. 3295–3299.

Ruscito, A. and DeRosa, M.C., 2016. Small-molecule binding aptamers: Selection strategies, characterization, and applications. *Frontiers in Chemistry*, 4, p. 14.

Sadsri, V., Trakulsujaritchok, T., Tangwattanachuleeporn, M., Hoven, V.P. and Na Nongkhai, P., 2020. Simple colorimetric assay for Vibrio parahaemolyticus detection using aptamer-functionalized nanoparticles. *ACS Omega*, 5(34), pp. 21437–21442.

Saiki, R.K., Gelfand, D.H., Stoffel, S., Scharf, S.J., Higuchi, R., Horn, G.T., Mullis, K.B. and Erlich, H.A., 1988. Primer-directed enzymatic amplification of DNA with a thermostable DNA polymerase. *Science*, 239(4839), pp. 487–491.

Sang, F., Liu, J., Zhang, X. and Pan, J., 2018. An aptamer-based colorimetric Pt (II) assay based on the use of gold nanoparticles and a cationic polymer. *Microchimica Acta*, 185(5), pp. 1–8.

Sasikumar, T. and Ilanchelian, M., 2020. Colorimetric and visual detection of cyanide ions based on the morphological transformation of gold nanobipyramids into gold nanoparticles. *New Journal of Chemistry*, 44(12), pp. 4713–4718.

Sassanfar, M. and Szostak, J.W., 1993. An RNA motif that binds ATP. *Nature*, 364(6437), pp. 550–553.

Seo, H.B. and Gu, M.B., 2017. Aptamer-based sandwich-type biosensors. *Journal of Biological Engineering*, 11(1), pp. 1–7.

Shahbazi, N., Hosseinkhani, S. and Ranjbar, B., 2017. A facile and rapid aptasensor based on split peroxidase DNAzyme for visual detection of carcinoembryonic antigen in saliva. *Sensors and Actuators B: Chemical*, 253, pp. 794–803.

Shayesteh, O.H. and Ghavami, R., 2019. Two colorimetric ampicillin sensing schemes based on the interaction of aptamers with gold nanoparticles. *Microchimica Acta*, 186(7), pp. 1–10.

Shayesteh, O.H. and Ghavami, R., 2020. A novel label-free colorimetric aptasensor for sensitive determination of PSA biomarker using gold nanoparticles and a cationic polymer in human serum. *Spectrochimica Acta Part A: Molecular and Biomolecular Spectroscopy*, 226, p. 117644.

Shen, L., Jia, K., Bing, T., Zhang, Z., Zhen, X., Liu, X., Zhang, N. and Shangguan, D., 2020. Detection of circulating tumor-related materials by aptamer capturing and endogenous enzyme-signal amplification. *Analytical Chemistry*, 92(7), pp. 5370–5378.

Shi, H., Wei, J., Qiang, L., Chen, X. and Meng, X., 2014. Fluorescent carbon dots for bioimaging and biosensing applications. *Journal of Biomedical Nanotechnology*, 10(10), pp. 2677–2699.

Shin, H.S., Jung, S.B., Park, S., Dua, P. and Ki Lee, D., 2019. Alppl2 is a potential diagnostic biomarker for pancreatic cancer-derived extracellular vesicles. *Molecular Therapy-Methods & Clinical Development*, 15, pp. 204–210.

Shrivas, K., Patel, S., Sinha, D., Thakur, S.S., Patle, T.K., Kant, T., Dewangan, K., Satnami, M.L., Nirmalkar, J. and Kumar, S., 2020. Colorimetric and smartphone-integrated paper device for on-site determination of arsenic (III) using sucrose modified gold nanoparticles as a nanoprobe. *Microchimica Acta*, 187(3), pp. 1–9.

Smith, J.E., Griffin, D.K., Leny, J.K., Hagen, J.A., Chávez, J.L. and Kelley-Loughnane, N., 2014. Colorimetric detection with aptamer-gold nanoparticle conjugates coupled to an android-based color analysis application for use in the field. *Talanta*, 121, pp. 247–255.

Sonenberg, N. and Hinnebusch, A.G., 2009. Regulation of translation initiation in eukaryotes: mechanisms and biological targets. *Cell*, 136(4), pp. 731–745.

Song, S., Wang, L., Li, J., Fan, C. and Zhao, J., 2008. Aptamer-based biosensors. *TrAC Trends in Analytical Chemistry*, 27(2), pp. 108–117.

Song, Y., Wang, L., Zhao, J., Li, H., Yang, X., Fu, S., Qin, X., Chen, Q., Jiang, Y. and Man, C., 2022. A novel colorimetric sensor using aptamers to enhance peroxidase-like property of gold nanoclusters for detection of *Escherichia coli* O157: H7 in milk. *International Dairy Journal*, 128, p. 105318.

Stojanovic, M.N. and Landry, D.W., 2002. Aptamer-based colorimetric probe for cocaine. *Journal of the American Chemical Society*, 124(33), pp. 9678–9679.

Sunil, J., Alex, S., Pravin, A.A., Pooja, M.D. and Ginil, R., 2020. Thermal properties of aqueous silver nanoparticle dispersion. *Materialstoday Proceedings*, 37(2), 80–84.

Swensen, J.S., Xiao, Y., Ferguson, B.S., Lubin, A.A., Lai, R.Y., Heeger, A.J., Plaxco, K.W. and Soh, H.T., 2009. Continuous, real-time monitoring of cocaine in undiluted blood serum via a microfluidic, electrochemical aptamer-based sensor. *Journal of the American Chemical Society*, 131(12), pp. 4262–4266.

Szostak, J.W., 1992. In vitro genetics. *Trends in Biochemical Sciences*, 17(3), pp. 89–93.

Tabrizi, M.A., Shamsipur, M., Saber, R. and Sarkar, S., 2017. Flow injection amperometric sandwich-type aptasensor for the determination of human leukemic lymphoblast cancer cells using MWCNTs-Pdnano/PTCA/aptamer as labeled aptamer for the signal amplification. *Analytica Chimica Acta*, 985, pp. 61–68.

Tarokh, A., Pebdeni, A.B., Othman, H.O., Salehnia, F. and Hosseini, M., 2021. Sensitive colorimetric aptasensor based on g-C_3N_4@ Cu_2O composites for detection of Salmonella typhimurium in food and water. *Microchimica Acta*, 188(3), pp. 1–10.

Thiviyanathan, V. and Gorenstein, D.G., 2012. Aptamers and the next generation of diagnostic reagents. *PROTEOMICS–Clinical Applications*, 6(11–12), pp. 563–573.

Tian, J., 2019. Aptamer-based colorimetric detection of various targets based on catalytic Au NPs/Graphene nanohybrids. *Sensing and Bio-Sensing Research*, 22, p. 100258.

Tuerk, C. and Gold, L., 1990. Systematic evolution of ligands by exponential enrichment: RNA ligands to bacteriophage T4 DNA polymerase. *Science*, 249(4968), pp. 505–510.

Venter, J.C., Adams, M.D., Myers, E.W., Li, P.W., Mural, R.J., Sutton, G.G., Smith, H.O., Yandell, M., Evans, C.A., Holt, R.A. and Gocayne, J.D., 2001. The sequence of the human genome. *Science*, 291(5507), pp. 1304–1351.

Ventura, B.D., Cennamo, M., Minopoli, A., Campanile, R., Censi, S.B., Terracciano, D., Portella, G. and Velotta, R., 2020. Colorimetric test for fast detection of SARS-CoV-2 in nasal and throat swabs. *ACS Sensors*, 5(10), pp. 3043–3048.

Walter, J.G., Heilkenbrinker, A., Austerjost, J., Timur, S., Stahl, F. and Schepe, T., 2012. Aptasensors for small molecule detection. *Zeitschrift für Naturforschung B*, 67(10), pp. 976–986.

Wang, A., Zhao, H., Chen, X., Tan, B., Zhang, Y. and Quan, X., 2017b. A colorimetric aptasensor for sulfadimethoxine detection based on peroxidase-like activity of graphene/ nickel@ palladium hybrids. *Analytical Biochemistry*, 525, pp. 92–99.

Wang, C. and Zhao, Q., 2019. A competitive thrombin-linked aptamer assay for small molecule: Aflatoxin B1. *Analytical and Bioanalytical Chemistry*, 411(25), pp. 6637–6644.

Wang, C., Qian, J., Wang, K., Yang, X., Liu, Q., Hao, N., Wang, C., Dong, X. and Huang, X., 2016b. Colorimetric aptasensing of ochratoxin A using Au@ Fe3O4 nanoparticles as signal indicator and magnetic separator. *Biosensors and Bioelectronics*, 77, pp. 1183–1191.

Wang, H., Wu, T., Li, M. and Tao, Y., 2021. Recent advances in nanomaterials for colorimetric cancer detection. *Journal of Materials Chemistry B*, 9(4), pp. 921–938.

Wang, J., Wang, L., Liu, X., Liang, Z., Song, S., Li, W., Li, G. and Fan, C., 2007. A gold nanoparticle-based aptamer target binding readout for ATP assay. *Advanced Materials*, 19(22), pp. 3943–3946.

Wang, J.X., Lee, E.R., Morales, D.R., Lim, J. and Breaker, R.R., 2008. Riboswitches that sense S-adenosylhomocysteine and activate genes involved in coenzyme recycling. *Molecular Cell*, 29(6), pp. 691–702.

Wang, K., Fan, D., Liu, Y. and Wang, E., 2015. Highly sensitive and specific colorimetric detection of cancer cells via dual-aptamer target binding strategy. *Biosensors and Bioelectronics*, 73, pp. 1–6.

Wang, L., Liu, F., Sui, N., Liu, M. and Yu, W.W., 2016a. A colorimetric assay for Hg (II) based on the use of a magnetic aptamer and a hybridization chain reaction. *Microchimica Acta*, 183(11), pp. 2855–2860.

Wang, L., Liu, X., Hu, X., Song, S. and Fan, C., 2006. Unmodified gold nanoparticles as a colorimetric probe for potassium DNA aptamers. *Chemical Communications*, (36), pp. 3780–3782.

Wang, Q.L., Huang, W.X., Zhang, P.J., Chen, L., Lio, C.K., Zhou, H., Qing, L.S. and Luo, P., 2020. Colorimetric determination of the early biomarker hypoxia-inducible factor-1 alpha (HIF-1α) in circulating exosomes by using a gold seed-coated with aptamer-functionalized Au@ Au core-shell peroxidase mimic. *Microchimica Acta*, 187(1), pp. 1–11.

Wang, Y. and Liu, B., 2009. Conjugated polyelectrolyte-sensitized fluorescent detection of thrombin in blood serum using aptamer-immobilized silica nanoparticles as the platform. *Langmuir*, 25(21), pp. 12787–12793.

Wang, Y., Zhu, Y., Binyam, A., Liu, M., Wu, Y. and Li, F., 2016c. Discovering the enzyme mimetic activity of metal-organic framework (MOF) for label-free and colorimetric sensing of biomolecules. *Biosensors and Bioelectronics*, 86, pp. 432–438.

Wang, Y.M., Liu, J.W., Adkins, G.B., Shen, W., Trinh, M.P., Duan, L.Y., Jiang, J.H. and Zhong, W., 2017a. Enhancement of the intrinsic peroxidase-like activity of graphitic carbon nitride nanosheets by ssDNAs and its application for detection of exosomes. *Analytical Chemistry*, 89(22), pp. 12327–12333.

Wang, Z., Chen, Q., Zhong, Y., Yu, X., Wu, Y. and Fu, F., 2019. A multicolor immunosensor for sensitive visual detection of breast cancer biomarker based on sensitive NADH-ascorbic-acid-mediated growth of gold nanobipyramids. *Analytical Chemistry*, 92(1), pp. 1534–1540.

Wei, H., Li, B., Li, J., Dong, S. and Wang, E., 2008. DNAzyme-based colorimetric sensing of lead (Pb2+) using unmodified gold nanoparticle probes. *Nanotechnology*, 19(9), p. 095501.

Wei, J., Chen, H., Chen, H., Cui, Y., Qileng, A., Qin, W., Liu, W. and Liu, Y., 2019. Multifunctional peroxidase-encapsulated nanoliposomes: Bioetching-induced photoelectrometric and colorimetric immunoassay for broad-spectrum detection of ochratoxins. *ACS Applied Materials & Interfaces*, 11(27), pp. 23832–23839.

Weinberg, Z., Nelson, J.W., Lünse, C.E., Sherlock, M.E. and Breaker, R.R., 2017. Bioinformatic analysis of riboswitch structures uncovers variant classes with altered ligand specificity. *Proceedings of the National Academy of Sciences*, 114(11), pp. E2077–E2085.

Willner, I., Shlyahovsky, B., Zayats, M. and Willner, B., 2008. DNAzymes for sensing, nanobiotechnology and logic gate applications. *Chemical Society Reviews*, 37(6), pp. 1153–1165.

Wilson, D.S. and Szostak, J.W., 1999. In vitro selection of functional nucleic acids. *Annual Review of Biochemistry*, 68(1), pp. 611–647.

Wilson, D.S., Keefe, A.D. and Szostak, J.W., 2001. The use of mRNA display to select high-affinity protein-binding peptides. *Proceedings of the National Academy of Sciences*, 98(7), pp. 3750–3755.

Wu, J., Zeng, L., Li, N., Liu, C. and Chen, J., 2019b. A wash-free and label-free colorimetric biosensor for naked-eye detection of aflatoxin B1 using G-quadruplex as the signal reporter. *Food Chemistry*, 298, p. 125034.

Wu, S., Duan, N., Qiu, Y., Li, J. and Wang, Z., 2017. Colorimetric aptasensor for the detection of Salmonella enterica serovar typhimurium using $ZnFe_2O_4$-reduced graphene oxide nanostructures as an effective peroxidase mimetics. *International Journal of Food Microbiology*, 261, pp. 42–48.

Wu, W., Wang, Y., Liu, K., Li, T. and Yang, Y., 2020a. Simultaneous and rapid determination of malachite green and leucomalachite green by a label-free colorimetric aptasensor. *Se pu= Chinese Journal of Chromatography*, 38(11), pp. 1332–1339.

Wu, Y., Belmonte, I., Sykes, K.S., Xiao, Y. and White, R.J., 2019a. Perspective on the future role of aptamers in analytical chemistry. *Analytical Chemistry*, 91(24), pp. 15335–15344.

Wu, Y.Y., Huang, P. and Wu, F.Y., 2020b. A label-free colorimetric aptasensor based on controllable aggregation of AuNPs for the detection of multiplex antibiotics. *Food Chemistry*, 304, p. 125377.

Xia, Y., Liu, M., Wang, L., Yan, A., He, W., Chen, M., Lan, J., Xu, J., Guan, L. and Chen, J., 2017. A visible and colorimetric aptasensor based on DNA-capped single-walled carbon nanotubes for detection of exosomes. *Biosensors and Bioelectronics*, 92, pp. 8–15.

Xiao, S., Lu, J., Sun, L. and An, S., 2022. A simple and sensitive AuNPs-based colorimetric aptasensor for specific detection of azlocillin. *Spectrochimica Acta Part A: Molecular and Biomolecular Spectroscopy*, 271, p. 120924.

Xiao, W., Xiao, M., Fu, Q., Yu, S., Shen, H., Bian, H. and Tang, Y., 2016. A portable smart-phone readout device for the detection of mercury contamination based on an aptamer-assay nanosensor. *Sensors*, 16(11), p. 1871.

Xie, Y., Ning, M., Ban, J. and Li, Q., 2019. Novel enzyme-linked aptamer assay for the determination of aflatoxin B1 in peanuts. *Analytical Letters*, 52(18), pp. 2961–2973.

Xu, C., Lin, M., Wang, T., Yao, Z., Zhang, W. and Feng, X., 2022. Colorimetric aptasensor for on-site detection of acetamiprid with hybridization chain reaction-assisted amplification and smartphone readout strategy. *Food Control*, 137, p. 108934.

Xu, H., Wang, Y., Huang, X., Li, Y., Zhang, H. and Zhong, X., 2012. Hg^{2+}-mediated aggregation of gold nanoparticles for colorimetric screening of biothiols. *Analyst*, 137(4), pp. 924–931.

Xu, L., Chopdat, R., Li, D. and Al-Jamal, K.T., 2020. Development of a simple, sensitive and selective colorimetric aptasensor for the detection of cancer-derived exosomes. *Biosensors and Bioelectronics*, 169, p. 112576.

Xu, L., Jiang, Z., Mu, Y., Zhang, Y., Zhan, Q., Cui, J., Cheng, W. and Ding, S., 2018. Colorimetric assay of rare disseminated tumor cells in real sample by aptamer-induced rolling circle amplification on cell surface. *Sensors and Actuators B: Chemical*, 259, pp. 596–603.

Xu, S., Jiang, L., Liu, Y., Liu, P., Wang, W. and Luo, X., 2019. A morphology-based ultrasensitive multicolor colorimetric assay for detection of blood glucose by enzymatic etching of plasmonic gold nanobipyramids. *Analytica Chimica Acta*, 1071, pp. 53–58.

Xu, S., Ouyang, W., Xie, P., Lin, Y., Qiu, B., Lin, Z., Chen, G. and Guo, L., 2017. Highly uniform gold nanobipyramids for ultrasensitive colorimetric detection of influenza virus. *Analytical Chemistry*, 89(3), pp. 1617–1623.

Yadav, S., Sadique, M.A., Ranjan, P., Kumar, N., Singhal, A., Srivastava, A.K. and Khan, R., 2021. SERS based lateral flow immunoassay for point-of-care detection of SARS-CoV-2 in clinical samples. *ACS Applied Bio Materials*, 4(4), pp. 2974–2995.

Yang, L., Fung, C.W., Cho, E.J. and Ellington, A.D., 2007. Real-time rolling circle amplification for protein detection. *Analytical Chemistry*, 79(9), pp. 3320–3329.

Yang, T., Wang, Z., Song, Y., Yang, X., Chen, S., Fu, S., Qin, X., Zhang, W., Man, C. and Jiang, Y., 2021. A novel smartphone-based colorimetric aptasensor for on-site detection of *Escherichia coli* O157: H7 in milk. *Journal of Dairy Science*, 104(8), pp. 8506–8516.

Yang, W., Bai, Z.Q., Shi, W.Q., Yuan, L.Y., Tian, T., Chai, Z.F., Wang, H. and Sun, Z.M., 2013. MOF-76: from a luminescent probe to highly efficient U VI sorption material. *Chemical Communications*, 49(88), pp. 10415–10417.

Yu, H., Alkhamis, O., Canoura, J., Liu, Y. and Xiao, Y., 2021. Advances and challenges in small-molecule DNA aptamer isolation, characterization, and sensor development. *Angewandte Chemie International Edition*, 60(31), pp. 16800–16823.

Yuan, F., Zhao, H., Wang, X. and Quan, X., 2017. Determination of oxytetracycline by a graphene—gold nanoparticle-based colorimetric aptamer sensor. *Analytical Letters*, 50(3), pp. 544–553.

Zhang, J., Qian, J., Mei, Q., Yang, L., He, L., Liu, S., Zhang, C. and Zhang, K., 2019. Imaging-based fluorescent sensing platform for quantitative monitoring and visualizing of fluoride ions with dual-emission quantum dots hybrid. *Biosensors and Bioelectronics*, 128, pp. 61–67.

Zhang, J., Wang, L., Pan, D., Song, S., Boey, F.Y., Zhang, H. and Fan, C., 2008. Visual cocaine detection with gold nanoparticles and rationally engineered aptamer structures. *Small*, 4(8), pp. 1196–1200.

Zhang, W., Wang, Y., Nan, M., Li, Y., Yun, J., Wang, Y. and Bi, Y., 2021. Novel colorimetric aptasensor based on unmodified gold nanoparticle and ssDNA for rapid and sensitive detection of T-2 toxin. *Food Chemistry*, 348, p. 129128.

Zhang, Z., Li, J., Gu, J., Amini, R., Stacey, H.D., Ang, J.C., White, D., Filipe, C.D., Mossman, K., Miller, M.S. and Salena, B.J., 2022. A universal DNA aptamer that recognizes spike proteins of diverse SARS-CoV-2 variants of concern. *Chemistry–A European Journal*, 28(15), p. e202200078.

Zhang, Z., Wang, Z., Wang, X. and Yang, X., 2010. Magnetic nanoparticle-linked colorimetric aptasensor for the detection of thrombin. *Sensors and Actuators B: Chemical*, 147(2), pp. 428–433.

Zhao, C., Hong, C.Y., Lin, Z.Z., Chen, X.M. and Huang, Z.Y., 2019. Detection of Malachite Green using a colorimetric aptasensor based on the inhibition of the peroxidase-like activity of gold nanoparticles by cetyltrimethylammonium ions. *Microchimica Acta*, 186(5), pp. 1–8.

Zhao, W., Chiuman, W., Brook, M.A. and Li, Y., 2007. Simple and rapid colorimetric biosensors based on DNA aptamer and noncrosslinking gold nanoparticle aggregation. *ChemBioChem*, 8(7), pp. 727–731.

Zhao, W., Chiuman, W., Lam, J.C., McManus, S.A., Chen, W., Cui, Y., Pelton, R., Brook, M.A. and Li, Y., 2008. DNA aptamer folding on gold nanoparticles: from colloid chemistry to biosensors. *Journal of the American Chemical Society*, 130(11), pp. 3610–3618.

Zhao, Y., Yavari, K. and Liu, J., 2022. Critical evaluation of aptamer binding for biosensor designs. *TrAC Trends in Analytical Chemistry*, 146, p. 116480.

Zhou, Q. and Tang, D., 2020. Recent advances in photoelectrochemical biosensors for analysis of mycotoxins in food. *TrAC Trends in Analytical Chemistry*, 124, p. 115814.

Zhou, W., Kong, W., Dou, X., Zhao, M., Ouyang, Z. and Yang, M., 2016. An aptamer based lateral flow strip for on-site rapid detection of ochratoxin A in Astragalus membranaceus. *Journal of Chromatography B*, 1022, pp. 102–108.

Zhou, X., Wang, L., Shen, G., Zhang, D., Xie, J., Mamut, A., Huang, W. and Zhou, S., 2018. Colorimetric determination of ofloxacin using unmodified aptamers and the aggregation of gold nanoparticles. *Microchimica Acta*, 185(7), pp. 1–9.

Zhou, Z., Du, Y. and Dong, S., 2011. DNA–Ag nanoclusters as fluorescence probe for turn-on aptamer sensor of small molecules. *Biosensors and Bioelectronics*, 28(1), pp. 33–37.

Zhu, D., Liu, B. and Wei, G., 2021a. Two-dimensional material-based colorimetric biosensors: A review. *Biosensors*, 11(8), p. 259.

Zhu, L., Feng, X., Yang, S., Wang, J., Pan, Y., Ding, J., Li, C., Yin, X. and Yu, Y., 2021b. Colorimetric detection of immunomagnetically captured rare number CTCs using mDNA-wrapped single-walled carbon nanotubes. *Biosensors and Bioelectronics*, 172, p. 112780.

Zhu, L., Li, C., Zhu, Z., Liu, D., Zou, Y., Wang, C., Fu, H. and Yang, C.J., 2012. In vitro selection of highly efficient G-quadruplex-based DNAzymes. *Analytical Chemistry*, 84(19), pp. 8383–8390.

Zhu, X., Zhuo, X., Li, Q., Yang, Z. and Wang, J., 2016. Gold nanobipyramid-supported silver nanostructures with narrow plasmon linewidths and improved chemical stability. *Advanced Functional Materials*, 26(3), pp. 341–352.

Zhuang, Y., Liu, L., Wu, X., Tian, Y., Zhou, X., Xu, S., Xie, Z. and Ma, Y., 2019. Size and shape effect of gold nanoparticles in "far-field" surface plasmon resonance. *Particle & Particle Systems Characterization*, 36(1), p. 1800077.

Zovoilis, A., Cifuentes-Rojas, C., Chu, H.P., Hernandez, A.J. and Lee, J.T., 2016. Destabilization of B2 RNA by EZH2 activates the stress response. *Cell*, 167(7), pp. 1788–1802.

Zuo, X., Song, S., Zhang, J., Pan, D., Wang, L. and Fan, C., 2007. A target-responsive electrochemical aptamer switch (TREAS) for reagentless detection of nanomolar ATP. *Journal of the American Chemical Society*, 129(5), pp. 1042–1043.

7 Aptamer beacon probes for the detection and visualization of miRNA

Jayavigneeswari Suresh Babu, Sailaja V. Eluchuri, and Janakiraman Narayanan

7.1 INTRODUCTION

The term "Aptamer" was invented by Andy Ellington and is derived from the Latin words "aptus" (to fit) and "meros" (part). Aptamers are single-stranded DNA/RNA molecules that have a high affinity and selectivity for a wide range of substrates including biomolecules, toxins, and cells. Peptide aptamers, which were discovered in 1996 and are similar to nucleotide aptamers, feature a peptide scaffold attached to a variable loop area. The protein scaffold gives flexibility and stability to the loop form by limiting improper binding. The variable loop segment recognizes and binds to sequences, while the protein scaffold adds flexibility and stability by avoiding inadvertent binding. Aptamers attach to their targets by changing conformation from single-stranded residues to tertiary structures, stems, hairpins, and other secondary structures by a combination of van der Waals, hydrogen bonding, hydrophobic, and electrostatic interactions. Aptamers add specificity to the identification of the target molecule. Initially, aptamers were assumed to primarily target certain surface proteins or cellular proteins. Surprisingly, when paired with molecular beacon probes, their applications are expanded, particularly in diagnostic sensor creation. The reason for this is that molecular beacon probes allow for better sensitivity detection of the target molecule by various detection modalities such as fluorescence, luminescence, electrochemical, and colorimetry. The combination of aptamer and molecular beacon enabled us to increase the sensitivity of biomolecular detection in cells and tissues both in situ and in vitro. A molecular beacon is a diagnostic tool that uses an aptamer molecule with a low detection limit, easy operation, rapid response, and repeatability. The fluorescence resonance energy transfer (FRET) phenomenon underpins the notion of guiding molecular beacon probes for biomolecule identification (Yongsheng Li, Zhou, and Ye 2008). It improves the sensitivity of biomolecule detection when paired with nanoparticle technology (Janakiraman et al. 2012). Hamaguchi, Ellington, and Stanton (2001) produced three molecular beacon probes using aptamers for thrombin detection, however only one was employed in the detection method. J. J. Li, Fang, and Tan (2002) went on to create MB with G-quadruplex to detect thrombin molecules. Finally, the thrombin detection sensitivity was increased up to 0.5 nM sensitivity (L. Hao and Zhao 2015).

Biomolecular detection sensitivity advancements have had a substantial influence on the molecular diagnosis of various disease disorders. Exosomes are nanovesicles generated by cells that range in size from 30 to 150 nm and contain a variety of biological compounds, including lipids, proteins, and nucleic acids, and are considered to be necessary for intercellular communication(Yáñez-Mó et al. 2015). Because of their unique features, such as intrinsic stability, minimal immunogenicity, and high tissue/cell penetration capability, exosomes are emerging as viable vehicles for targeted drug/gene delivery (D. Zhang et al. 2017). However, its actual applicability may be limited in some instances due to poor targeting abilities or ineffectiveness. Exosomes will reach their potential when it is tagged with the right ligand like aptamer for therapy or beacon probes for diagnostics (He et al. 2019).

This chapter will examine the many methods for choosing and characterizing aptamers (DNA/RNA/peptides). We will also discuss the design and testing of molecular beacon probes. We will also highlight significant developments in biological applications, such as exosome-based diagnostics and treatment, made possible by combining aptamer and molecular beacon probes. We will first introduce methods that are available for the synthesis of aptamers.

7.1.1 Aptamer and Beacon Probes

The term aptamer refers to a molecule that adheres well to the target molecule. Aptamers are typically composed of nucleotide or peptide sequences. Aptamers develop secondary structures that allow them to attach to the target molecule. The aptamer-like molecule's specificity and selectivity find increased applicability in biosensor devices. Tan's group first integrated cDNA into the loop sequence of the molecular beacon probe. Later, the loop was replaced by an aptamer to increase target protein detection. Replacing the cDNA sequence with an aptamer targeting a particular protein molecule was a watershed moment in the field, increasing both the detection limit and specificity. Biomolecule identification in patient serum is critical in molecular diagnosis. The current COVID-19 pandemic has further highlighted the necessity of fast identification in clinical laboratories.

The first group (Tan) found that adding aptamer in the molecular beacon probe enhanced sensitivity when compared to merely using cDNA. To increase detection, the researchers altered the cDNA in the loop region using an aptamer molecule. Surprisingly, it formed G- Quadruplex and was near the quencher. The first aptamer to be employed with molecular beacon probes was the thrombin aptamer. The sensitivity was further tested using denatured thrombin protein, and the fluorescence was unaffected. As a result, it was established that thrombin recognition was caused by the 3D structure generated by the thrombin molecule. Later, G15 nucleotides were utilized to detect thrombin, although this resulted in a number of variations. It was not satisfactory *in vivo*. In a complex matrix, recognition of the target molecule was compromised with non-specificity.

7.2 SYNTHESIS OF NUCLEIC ACID APTAMERS

Aptamers are generated utilizing the systematic evolution of ligands by exponential enrichment (SELEX) approach, which was established by Tuerk and Ellington in 1990 (Tuerk and Gold 1990). SELEX routinely screens and identifies aptamers for specific ligands from a chemically synthesized random DNA/RNA oligonucleotide library of diverse sequences (Figure 7.1). After the non-aptamers are washed away, the remaining aptamers are amplified using polymerase chain reaction (PCR) to establish a pool of sequences for the next round of selection. Further optimization is used to shorten, alter, and stabilize aptamers with high affinity. Six to twenty SELEX cycles are required to select target-specific aptamers.

SELEX procedures are commonly categorized as *in vitro* and *in vivo* (cell-based SELEX) based on the conditions utilized for obtaining the aptamer. Cell-based SELEX is identical to *in vitro* SELEX, except the aptamer selection target is expressed in living cells. The benefit of cell-based SELEX in this case is that it targets natural proteins expressed on cell surfaces, which retain their native conformation and function while being selected and are suited for generating aptamers to target cancer cells. There have been several variations in the SELEX technologies recently, which are reviewed below.

7.2.1 VARIANTS OF SELEX BASED ON TARGET TYPES

The SELEX technologies are categorized into four principal types based on the target and the conditions used for the aptamer synthesis. These are (1) immobilised target protein, (2) immobilised aptamer, (3) in solution, and (4) cell or tissues as the target for aptamer selection (Figures 7.2 and 7.3).

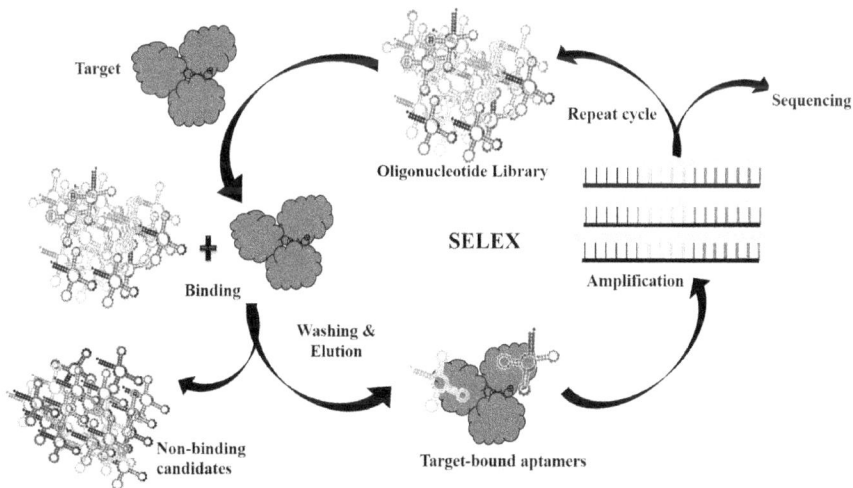

FIGURE 7.1 Schematic representation of the SELEX process with its steps in creating target-specific ligand preparation.

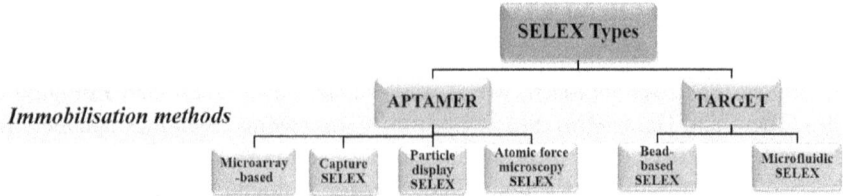

FIGURE 7.2 SELEX variants based on Immobilisation methods including ligand and target for SELEX process.

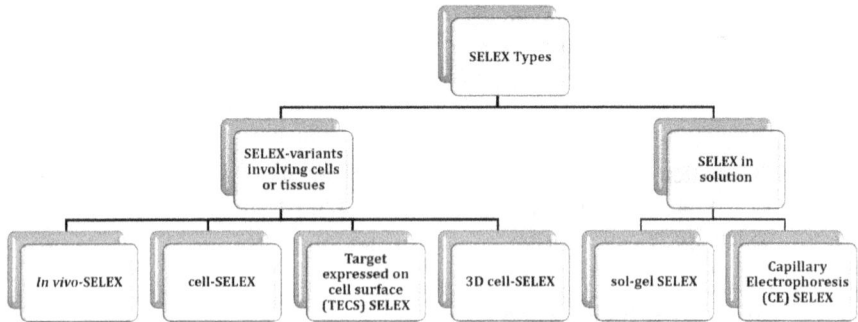

FIGURE 7.3 SELEX variants involving cells or tissues and SELEX in solution.

7.2.2 SELEX VARIANTS WITH IMMOBILIZED TARGETS

7.2.2.1 Microfluidic SELEX

Microfluidic SELEX, which enables automation even with picomolar concentrations of the target molecule. Here, aptamers are selected based on their binding characteristics after being incubated with target-coupled beads on a microchip (Oh et al. 2009).

7.2.2.2 Bead-based SELEX

Bead-based SELEX: In this method, the target molecules are attached to the magnetic beads, and aptamer sequences are allowed to interact with the target molecule. The best pairing aptamer sequence is selected based on the affinity between the sequence and the target molecule. In this method, magnetic beads are immobilized with the target molecules which improves the selection process significantly (Stoltenburg, Reinemann, and Strehlitz 2005).

7.2.3 SELEX VARIANTS INVOLVING CELLS OR TISSUES

7.2.3.1 Cell-SELEX

Foldable aptamers are incubated with whole cells as a target in Cell-SELEX to generate aptamers that detect certain cell types or conformations. Cell-SELEX may also be used to generate aptamers for specific proteins via a technique known as target expressed on the cell surface SELEX. In this case, eukaryotic cells are modified to express a specific protein on their surface, which is advantageous if a complicated protein cannot be generated in high enough quantity utilizing heterologous expression methods. Aptamers for the target protein in its natural configuration can be produced following the participation of the counter-selection process (Ohuchi, Ohtsu, and Nakamura 2006).

7.2.3.2   3D Cell-SELEX

In 3D Cell-SELEX, aptamers are developed for cells that are aligned in a three-dimensional grid. The cells are more actively in contact with the media and one another as if they were a tissue due to the spatial separation, which may result in the availability of new target epitopes (Souza et al. 2016).

7.2.3.3   In vivo SELEX

In in vivo SELEX, which involves injecting a library into an animal's bloodstream and then harvesting the desired organ along with the attached aptamers, can be used to produce aptamers. This method involves using xenografts in laboratory animals to produce oligonucleotides specific to human cancer cells (Mi et al. 2016).

7.2.4   **SELEX** VARIANTS WITH IMMOBILIZED APTAMERS

7.2.4.1   AFM-SELEX

AFM-SELEX is another SELEX technology that scans the surface of a small sample with a cantilever probe, detecting the weak force between the sample surface and the probe and producing pictures of the sample surface. The target molecules were immobilized on the gold chip, and avidin was used to immobilize the biotinylated random ssDNA on the cantilever. The cantilever and gold chip in the AFM were changed using DNA-probe and thrombin, respectively. The DNA aptamer that binds target molecules would bind the cantilever as it neared the target set on the gold chip. When the avidin-biotin connection is disrupted by the target's adhesion force, the leftover DNA is retrieved using heat elution and PCR, and the AFM-SELEX selection cycle is repeated three times (Miyachi et al. 2010).

Researchers recently employed Pheno SELEX to find an aptamer for an entire process. Rather than targeting a single protein, they intended to create an aptamer for the entire process. In comparison to a non-invasive cell line, they chose aptamer against an aggressive prostate cancer cell line. The aptamer has the potential to particularly target invasive cancer cell lines. The approach selected a metastatic phenotype (Shelley et al. 2021).

7.2.5   **SELEX** IN SOLUTION

7.2.5.1   Capillary electrophoresis (CE) SELEX

The target molecule and the oligonucleotide library are utilized in the solution in the capillary electrophoresis (CE) SELEX technique. This approach identifies target aptamer complexes using electrophoretic mobility patterns and manufactures high-affinity aptamers in a relatively short amount of time. In fact, aptamers may be discovered after just one selection in the highly specialized CE-based non-SELEX approach (Berezovski et al. 2006).

7.2.5.2 Sol–gel SELEX

Sol–gel SELEX is a high-tech technique that traps target molecules in a porous substance on a microchip. The aptamers are then added to the porous material in solution, travel through it at a steady flow rate, and bind to the native target molecules as they do so (S.M. Park et al. 2009). Additionally, several nanoparticles such as gold nanoparticles and graphene oxide silver nanoparticles have been employed to aid SELEX technology (Kim et al. 2021).

The SELEX system is time-consuming. Several *insilico* tools using deep learning methods have been developed to understand and predict protein aptamer interactions (Z. Chen et al. 2021). Recently a web-based protein aptamer interactions have been developed that use machine learning approaches. The interactions can be obtained at http://39.96.85.9/PPAI (Jianwei Li et al. 2020). A web-based tool available with more machine learning principles is AptaNet (https://github.com/nedaemami/AptaNet) (Emami and Ferdousi 2021). The prediction was based on using neural networks and random forest algorithms. They were able to get 91.38% accuracy in their testing set. The SELEX technologies can be used to synthesize DNA, RNA, and peptide aptamers (Figure 7.4). The synthesized aptamers must be characterized before they can be utilized for biological applications.

The process, systematic evolution of ligands by exponential enrichment (SELEX), can generate aptamers, single-stranded DNAs, or RNAs and peptides that bind targets with great specificity and affinity.

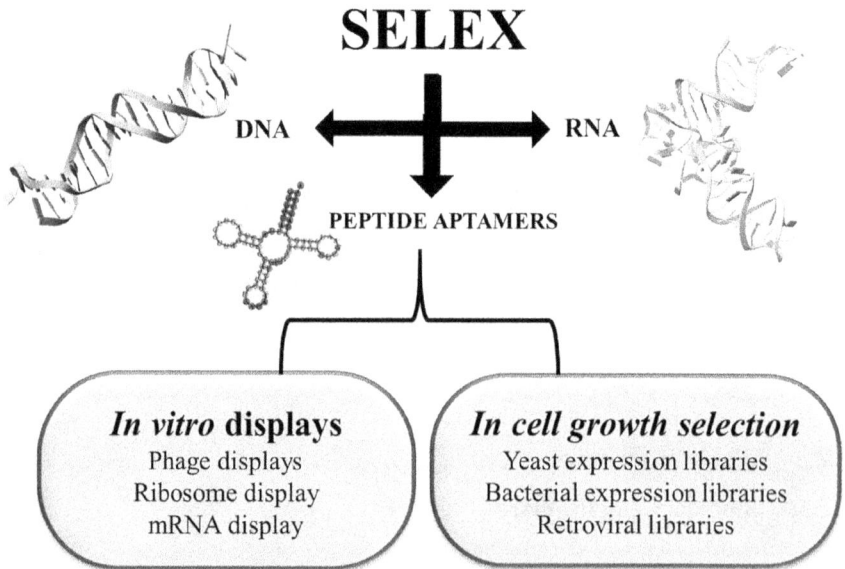

FIGURE 7.4 SELEX for DNA, RNA, and Peptide ligands explained with their methods.

7.3   CHARACTERIZATION OF APTAMERS

Aptamers are used in diagnostics and pharmaceuticals by determining binding properties such as affinity, kinetics, and thermodynamics. Surface plasmon resonance (SPR), isothermal titration calorimetry (ITC), fluorescence polarization/ anisotropy (FA/FP), and flow cytometry are current techniques that successfully evaluate aptamer-target interactions (Plach and Schubert 2020).

7.3.1   SURFACE PLASMON RESONANCE (SPR)

SPR technology is used to assess the affinity and kinetic characteristics of an aptamer and its target. The target or aptamer is initially immobilized on the surface of a sensor chip, after which different quantities of unbound analytes are allowed to flow through. The changes in refractive index caused by the development of the binding complex are measured in order to compute kinetic parameters (Kon and Koff) and steady-state affinity (KD; Chang, McKeague, and Smolke 2014).

7.3.2   FLUORESCENCE POLARIZATION OR FLUORESCENCE ANISOTROPY (FP OR FA)

Fluorescence anisotropy, also known as fluorescence polarization (FP), is a measurement of a molecule's shifting orientation in space as a function of time between absorption and emission events. If vertically polarized light is used to stimulate the fluorophore population, the emitted light will retain some of that polarization depending on how fast it rotates in solution. The more depolarized the emitted light is, the faster the orientation motion is. The affinity (KD) of the aptamer-target interaction is calculated using FP. During the experiment, a target or aptamer is monitored using an attached fluorescent dye and kept at a consistent concentration. The other binding element is titrated throughout a concentration range and assesses the rotational mobility of polarised light-excited fluorophores (Yapiao Li and Zhao 2019).

Efforts to improve FA assay efficiency by lowering assay volume and time from mixing to measurement may save time and costs by reducing reagent use. A recent work employed thrombin and two thrombin-binding aptamers as a model system to demonstrate the plate-based FA investigations with volumes as low as 2 μL per well in 20-minute incubations with no loss in assay accuracy. The downsizing of this test has ramifications for drug development and aptamer selection workflow efficiency since it allows for higher throughput aptamer analysis (Weaver and Whelan 2021). Aptamers that alter the fluorescence properties of a fluorophore connected to the aptamers (for non-competitive tests) or the analyte (for competitive assays) would be beneficial because of the smaller distance between the aptamer and analyte.

7.3.3   ISOTHERMAL TITRATION CALORIMETRY (ITC)

ITC is a label-free approach for determining thermodynamic characteristics including entropy, enthalpy, equilibrium-binding affinity (KD), and interaction stoichiometry of molecular interactions by measuring the heat generated during aptamer-target complex formation. This strategy delivers extra information without requiring any changes to the objectives. The adenosine DNA aptamer (also for AMP and ATP) is a highly conserved sequence found in a few samples. A typical biosensor model is an aptamer, and its nuclear magnetic resonance structure reveals that each aptamer binds two AMP molecules. In this study, each binding site was deleted independently using a rational sequence design, yet the remaining site kept a similar binding affinity and specificity as evaluated by ITC. The thermodynamic aspects of binding, as well as their biological ramifications, are explored. The number of binding sites in a single DNA sequence may also be expanded, with up to four sites added. Finally, utilizing the structure-switching signalling aptamer design, the different sequences are built into fluorescent biosensors. The one-site aptamer has a 3.8-fold better sensitivity at lower adenosine concentrations, with a detection limit of 9.1 μM adenosine, but a weaker fluorescence signal at higher adenosine concentrations (Zijie Zhang, Oni, and Liu 2017).

7.3.4 FLOW CYTOMETRY

Flow cytometry is a laser-based approach that involves incubating target cells with increasing quantities of fluorescently tagged aptamers. The fluorescence intensity shows the aptamer's affinity for the targeted cell. Flow cytometry has the benefit of characterizing the binding capacity of aptamers and targets in their native conformational state for the analysis of aptamer-cell interactions. The binding of aptamers to their associated proteins on cell surfaces has been detected using flow cytometry. A DNA aptamer designed to detect human neutrophil elastase (HNE) was modified to attach fluorescein at various sites distant from the target-binding site using different linkers and was used to stain HNE-coated beads for flow cytometry. Although every aptamer derivative examined bound the target-coated beads, the fluorescein attachment technique determined the signal intensity (Davis et al. 1996).

After being divided into two moieties, a few aptamers still bind to their targets. Split aptamers have demonstrated considerable promise in the construction of aptameric sensors. However, due to a lack of understanding about the binding structure of their parent aptamers, only a few split aptamers have been created. A new split aptamer as well as a flow cytometric bead sandwich assay that uses a split aptamer rather than two antibodies were developed to detect selectin (Shen et al. 2018). The target-binding moiety and the structure-stabilizing moiety of the l-selectin aptamer, Sgc-3b, were identified using DMS foot printing and mutation assays. The researchers developed a split-aptamer-based cytometric bead assay (SACBA) for the detection of soluble l-selectin after optimizing one part of the split-sequence to eliminate non-specific binding of the split-sequence pair. SACBA had strong l-selectin sensitivity and selectivity, and it was successfully used to detect spiked l-selectin in human serum. The procedures for generating split aptamers and constructing the split-aptamer-based sandwich test are straight forward and demonstrate good applicability in aptamer engineering.

7.4   APPLICATIONS OF APTAMERS

The characterized aptamers find a significant role in biotechnology, medicine, pharmacology, and cell biology. Within 15 years of their discovery, one aptamer as medication was pegaptanib (marketed as Macugen), became ready for public use to treat wet age-related macular degeneration. Aptamer-based biosensors and assays are being developed to replace traditional antibody-based technology because they have the potential to be a fantastic tool for rapid analytical instruments. Aptamers have the potential to be crucial in the development of biosensors and nanotechnology in the future. Aptamer chimaeras are being developed to transport therapeutic agents such as siRNAs, miRNAs, and chemotherapeutic drugs to cancer cells, such as aptamer-drug or aptamer-oligonucleotide connected with nano-vehicles.

A few applications of aptamers are discussed below.

7.4.1   APTASENSORS

Aptasensors have been used to identify biomarkers for cancer and other diagnostic purposes, leading to an increase in the manufacture of multi-analyte aptasensors using optical detecting devices. McCauley et al. created a fluorescence-based aptasensor-chip in 2003 for the detection of several analytes in complicated samples, including thrombin, inosine monophosphate dehydrogenase (IMPDH), vascular endothelial growth factor (VEGF), and basic fibroblast growth factor (bFGF). The major detection method for the Ap-analyte binding test in this study was based on the change in fluorescence polarisation caused by binding targets to the appropriate aptamers. This phenomenon happens due to a change in the rotation of aptamers during Ap-target complex formation, and hence the resulting fluorescence polarisation might be quantified as a direct indicator of the concentration of analyte in the samples (McCauley, Hamaguchi, and Stanton 2003). In a recent study by Maehashi et al, they used carbon nanotube field-effect transistors (CNTFETs) in a label-free sensor for the detection of immunoglobulin E (IgE) in the range 250 pm–160 nm (Maehashi and Matsumoto 2009). In another investigation, a hairpin sequence was utilized as the capture probe, with a restriction site added to the stem segment. The efficient and precise reaction mediated by EcoRI, the enzymatic cleavage reaction happens only on probes that preserve their stem-loop structure without catching the target, resulting in a decreased background signal. The biotin-streptavidin complexation binds to Au NPs that have been modified with a large number of Fc-signalling probes. Furthermore, following EcoRI therapy. Fc tags can be pulled in close proximity to the electrode surface by hybridization between the signalling probes and the capture probe residues, allowing for additional signal augmentation. This sensor has an extremely low detection limit in the zeptomole area (Qiu et al. 2013). Aptamer binding to their targets is typically dependent on certain conformations, such as G-quadruplex and hairpin. The conformational shift that occurs before and after the formation of aptamer-ligand complexes opens several possibilities for the development of aptamer-based biosensors. Using chimeric aptamers, multivalent nanoparticles such as dendrimers with a high potential for performing many tasks concurrently may be created. Aptamer chimaeras may thus prove valuable in the future for the diagnosis of a wide spectrum of disorders.

7.4.2 CHEMICAL TOXINS DETECTION

Bisphenol A (BPA) is a tiny carcinogenic chemical and an endocrine disruptor that mimics estrogen's action and poses a concern to the environment and human health. Jo et al. chose an ssDNA MRE specific for Bisphenol A, with a reported Kd of 8.3 nM and only little binding to structurally comparable chemical compounds such as 6F biophenol A, bisphenol B, and 4,4'-bisphenol. A cy-3 labelled MRE pair was mounted on a Sol–gel biochip, and a sandwich detection technique with nanomolar range sensitivity was devised (Jo et al. 2011). Aptamer-based biosensors and assays are now being developed to replace traditional antibody-based technology since they may be a great tool for quick analytical devices. Aptamers will play an essential role in the development of nanosensors in the next years. Aptamer chimaeras are being created to deliver therapeutic agents to cancer cells, such as siRNAs, miRNAs, and chemotherapeutic chemicals, such as aptamer-drug or aptamer-oligonucleotide associated with nano-vehicles.

7.4.3 PATHOGEN DETECTION

The aptamer's usage for the sensitive detection of pathogens has been another application in addition to toxin detection. The sensitive detection of pathogens has a prominent role in the environmental and medical applications. The disease-causing microbes could be bacteria, fungi, and viruses. Several microbes are resistant to medicinal treatments and sensitive detection, which is an important concern (Zhanhong Li et al. 2019). The aptasensors fabrication for microbial detections has been revived recently (Ziółkowski et al. 2021). There is an ongoing need to improve the detection limits of the microbes and use various aptamer probes and nanoparticles.

7.4.3.1 Bacterial detection

Abbaspour et al. developed an aptamer-based biosensor system that detects *S. aureus* by combining an aptamer-based sandwich immunosensor with electrochemical techniques (Abbaspour et al. 2015). It was done by employing two distinct aptamer sequences against the target bacteria, as well as magnetic beads to capture *S. aureus* in a liquid phase. When compared to traditional detection methods, the electrochemical detection approach has a few advantages, including simplicity, quick turnaround time, low cost, and ultra-low detection limits. Hua et al. created a photoelectrochemical aptasensor based on a three-dimensional graphene hydrogel filled with carbon quantum dots (3DGH) and a graphene-like carbon nitride sheet with a sensitive potentiometric resolved ratio metric (ratio of cathodic current to anodic current) (g-C3N4) (Hua et al. 2018). The differential bias voltages application results in the cathodic and anodic currents produced by C-dots/3DGH and g-C3N4, which could be detected and differentiated; the proposed dual signal system allowed not only to detect an analyte selectively but also to consider the possible influence of the environment on the sensor response. The detection limit of the aptasensor utilized for *E.*

coli detection is 2.9 CFU/ML. Joshi et al. (2009) used selective enrichment against outer membrane proteins to create a DNA-based aptamer for detecting *Salmonella enterica* serovar *Typhimurium* (OMPs). The conjugate of SMNPs–aptamer–ssDNA1 was generated by combining aptamer–magnetic separation with multifold AuNPs to complete the enrichment and signal transduction of *S. Typhimurium*. Among them, ssDNA1 was the aptamer's base pair, and it opened the aptamer's secondary structure. When *S. typhimurium* was present, the aptamer established a particular connection with the strain, releasing ssDNA1, which Joshi et al. designed to complement an outer membrane protein identified in *S. typhimurium* as a specific binding target. Using pure cultures of *S. typhimurium*, a dilution-to-extinction capture strategy was developed and aptamers were chosen with detection limits of 10–40 CFU. Further, another useful application is the sensitive detection of tuberculosis (TB) disease. MPT64 is a 24-kDa protein that is only released by *Mycobacterium tuberculosis* during the early and middle stages of bacterial development and is utilised as a diagnostic target for sensitive detection of diseases utilizing aptamers. Qin et al. developed and selected ssDNA aptamers against the MPT64 protein, which may be employed as a fast diagnostic tool for detecting active TB infection (Qin et al. 2009).

7.4.3.2 Virus detection

The viruses cause several diseases and some are fatal. Therefore, early and sensitive detection of the disease-causing viruses could help in finding therapy options for these diseases. The notable viruses that inflict disease burden at the human population level are HIV and Corona viruses. Sensitive detection of the HIV virus is achieved by Y.-T. Lai and DeStefano (2012). They created a 38-mer DNA aptamer that binds to HIV-1 reverse transcriptase and may be utilized for HIV-1 detection through radioactivity-based reverse transcriptase nucleotide incorporation assays with a detection limit of 100–300 virions. The aptamer utilized in this study is designed to resemble a primer-template, which is the natural substrate for RT[50]. Valero et al. (2021) created dimeric and trimeric RBD-PB6-Ta aptamers via scaffolding or poly (A) linkage to detect the SARS-Cov-2 virus. The presence of RBD-PB6 impeded the interaction of the SARS-CoV-2 spike protein with the host receptor ACE2 and hampered viral entry into cells, demonstrating that the binding sites on the spike for RBD-PB6 and ACE2 overlap. The multimerization of the aptamer to dimeric and trimeric forms led to a 10-fold and 100-fold increase in binding affinity, as shown by an increased inhibitory effect on SARS-CoV-2 infection, with IC_{50} values in the low nanomolar range.

7.4.3.3 Fungi detection

The sensitive detection of fungi has applications in the food and environmental industries. Identifying the aflatoxins generated by fungal species allows for sensitive detection of fungal contamination in food. C. Wang, Sun, and Zhao (2019) used the simple aptamer molecular beacon test to identify aflatoxin B1 (AFB1) injected in wine, methanol, and corn flour samples, and the assay showed promise for the quick detection of AFs in food. They describe a simple aptamer molecular beacon test for the rapid detection of AFB1 that uses an aptamer with a fluorescein (FAM) label at the 5′ end and a fluorescence quencher (black hole quencher 1, BHQ1) at the 3′ end. When AFB1 was present, the aptamer probe formed a hairpin shape, bringing FAM and BHQ1 together and inducing fluorescence quenching. This assay allowed for a detection limit of 3.9 nmol/L and a dynamic range from 3.9 nmol/L to 4 mmol/L. The aptamers are useful for the detection of other biomolecules in addition to microbial detections. The sensitive detection of these biomolecules could help in understanding disease progressions and metabolic changes in humans.

7.4.4 DETECTION OF BIOLOGICALLY RELEVANT MOLECULES

Dual aptamers, Adenosine aptamer, and Malachite green aptamers were used to detect adenosine without the need for a label (Stojanovic and Kolpashchikov 2004). In the presence of adenosine, W. Xu and Lu (2010) placed a bridging strand that may modulate the fluorescence of malachite green. The technique was considerably superior since this sensor detected adenosine specifically as an analyte even when guanosine and cytosine were present. This approach made use of DNA hybridization as a tool, opening the path for this technology to be used as a label-free solution for adenosine detection. Similarly, Wu et al. used this method to detect PDGF-BB homogeneously with a detection limit of 6.8 pM (picomolar concentration). The leftover circular DNA sequences were then used as templates to extend unbound aptamers using RCA. Using AuNP-enhanced silver staining to identify RCA products, they were able to detect as little as 10 fM human VEGF (W. Cheng et al. 2010). Similarly, Nishira et al. detected adenosine 5′-monophosphate (AMP) using a DNA aptamer (Nishihira et al. 2004). The detection of platelet-derived growth factor directly from blood serum using an aptamer-based electrosensor with a limit of pM concentration has been demonstrated (R. Y. Lai, Plaxco, and Heeger 2007).

7.4.5 DETECTION OF DIFFERENT CLASSES OF CELLS

Human tissues are comprised of different kinds of cells with different functions. Homeostasis of cells and tissue environment is based on the functions of every different cell in our human body. When the homeostasis is disturbed the cellular arrangements are altered. For example, blood tissue is considered, and the mixture of cells such as lymphocytes, red blood cells, monocytes, neutrophils, mast cells, eosinophils, basophils, and platelets contribute to its function. The presence of distinct cellular components in the blood indicates a diseased pathological state. Hence human cell type detection becomes a must when it comes to the identification of the disease progression of therapeutics (Toepfner et al. 2018).

7.4.5.1 Stem cell recognition

Ababneh et al. (2013) highlighted that only a few aptamers have been created to target stem cell indicators, including cancer stem cells (CSCs), which comprise cancer cell surface biomarkers such as epithelial cell adhesion molecule (EpCAM), CD133, CD117, and CD44. The fibroblast growth factor receptor (FGFR1)-binding aptamer SL38.2 was employed as a fibroblast growth factor mimic in four DNA aptamer assemblies, according to a recent study(Ueki et al. 2019). Because it is constructed completely of 76-mer single-stranded DNA, the most powerful aptamer assembly,

TD0, can sustain the self-renewal and pluripotency of induced pluripotent stem cells (iPSCs). This is the first time a DNA aptamer has been employed in iPSC cell maintenance. TA6NT-AKTin-DOX is an aptamer-conjugated DNA nanotrain designed by Z. Xu, Ni, and Chen (2019) for the simultaneous delivery of DOX and AKTin (an AKT inhibitor peptide). The effectiveness of TA6NT-AKTin-DOX was investigated on MCF-7 (Breast cancer stemcells) BCSCs and tumours produced by injecting BCSCs into nude mice. The results indicated that TA6NT-AKTin-DOX was more effective than free DOX and various DNA nanotrains in vitro and in vivo. AKTin, which can overcome drug resistance in Breast cancer stem cells (BCSCs) by inhibiting the AKT signalling pathway, could explain the synergistic effect of TA6NT-AKTin-DOX.

Stem cells carry an important property of pluripotency which can be tapped for patient care activity. Stem cells are unique in their expression of their surface proteins. Based on the cellular surface protein expression, the stem cells can be identified which holds true humanitarian value in therapy. Hence, the identification and sorting of stem cells are of paramount importance in clinical theragnostics (Wiraja et al. 2014).

7.4.5.2 Aptamers for identifying and characterizing circulating tumour cells

The discovery of circulating tumour cells (CTCs) in patient blood, as demonstrated by Wu et al., enables a non-invasive "liquid biopsy" for monitoring therapy effects, forecasting disease progression, and assessing survival. Modifications to nucleic acids also enhance aptamer stability, which may provide a solution to the limited stability of RNA-based aptamers. Biotin is utilized to mark peptide substrates for the construction of heterogeneous biosensors since it has a binding coefficient of 1015 M1 with avidin or its analogues neutravidin (NA) and streptavidin (SA). At the solid–liquid interface, such a contact enables the immobilization and identification of peptide substrate present in CTCs (Wu et al. 2021). Several aptamers are identified for stem cell markers, such as EpCAM (Macdonald et al. 2017), CD44 (Kim et al. 2019), and CD20 (Zeng et al. 2018) which are present on the surface of the CTCs. These aptamers could recognize CTCs as these usually contain stem cell-like properties to go to distant sites from the tissue of origin. Targeting these molecules helped not only in the diagnosis of the disease but also enhanced therapeutic potential when they could diagnose, target, and kill stem cells. The utility of CTCs in tumour diagnosis and utilizing aptamers to diagnose them using electrochemical sensors are reviewed recently by Mo et al. (2022) and Abd-Ellatief and Abd-Ellatief (2021).

7.4.5.3 Detection of immune cells

In recent years, catalytic hairpin assembly (CHA) has been proposed as a novel signal amplification strategy to address the constraints of enzymatic amplification, such as complicated procedures and specialized reaction conditions. CHA was a signal amplification method that depended on self-assembly and disassembly processes between nucleic acid hairpins, offering new avenues for on-site detection and bifunctional aptamers. The CHA response was initiated by a recognition domain that linked to particular cancer cells. In the presence of target cells, the bifunctional aptamer was freed from the inhibitor, resulting in a cascade reaction of hairpin formation and disassembly. Fluorescence signals were obtained by separating the fluorophores from the quenchers. The proposed method demonstrated good discrimination specificity of normal cells and leukocytes (J. Liu et al. 2018). Aptamers are widely used for detecting cells. However, they can be applied for the detection of nanovesicles secreted from cells.

7.4.6 Nanovescicles secreted from human tissues
and cells detection by aptamer

Exosomes are extra cellular vesicles secreted by human cells. These exosomes are tools for the communication between the cell types. Importance of exosomes in various diseases and why studying them is important? Recently, Esposito et al. (2021) developed an RNA aptamer targeting Breast cancer exosomes specifically which may be used for targeted tumour therapy. In the other example, Zhao et al. used the CRISPR-Cas system to identify the transmembrane protein, CD63, in an exosome (Zhao et al. 2020).

For the purpose of quantifying tumour-derived exosomal PD-L1, a dual-target-specific aptamer recognition induced in situ connection system on exosome membrane in conjunction with droplet digital PCR (ddPCR) (TRACER) was developed (Exo-PD-L1) by Lin et al. (2021). The level of tumour-derived Exo-PD-L1 measured by TRACER was for the first time found to be a more accurate tumour diagnostic marker than total Exo-PD-L1 due to its exceptional sensitivity, which allows it to discriminate cancer patients from healthy donors. Exosomes can be made into trustworthy clinical markers using the TRACER approach, and their biological roles can be investigated.

Ding et al. created a fluorescent assay for the sensitive, precise, and simultaneous quantification of exosome and cancer-related exosomal proteins [epidermal growth factor receptor (EGFR) and EpCAM] by using triple-coloured probes to recognize EGFR and EpCAM or naturally anchor to the lipid bilayer. A waxberry-like magnetic bead with a large surface area and strong affinity was produced in this study to pair with an aptamer for the collection and recovery of exosomes (Ding et al. 2021).

Exosomes are commonly used as a cancer biomarker in cancer detection. Wang et al. suggested a SERS (surface-enhanced Raman spectroscopy)-based technique for the simultaneous multiple detection of exosomes using magnetic substrates and SERS probes. The capturing substrates are aptamer-modified gold shell magnetic nanobeads, which can capture the majority of exosome types by recognizing the universal surface protein CD63. When the target exosome is present, the other non-specific SERS probes are suspended. Between the target exosomes, the substrate, and the suitable SERS probes, an apta-immunocomplex can form. Exosomes in real blood samples have also been effectively detected using this detection technique (Z. Wang et al. 2018). The utilization of aptamers has increased the detection, characterization, and functionalization of the exosomes, enabling these particles to be efficient biomarkers and drug delivery systems. However, aptamers alone can be drug delivery vehicles for targeted drug delivery.

7.4.7 Aptamers as drug delivery systems

Rabiee et al. (2020) described aptamers as targeting components for antibiotic delivery systems using nanocarriers. By increasing lipophilicity, the drug's metabolism and distribution improved, allowing the dose to be increased. The findings for the chemotherapeutic drug are encouraging, and the optimizations for the nanocomposite-to-drug ratio are relevant for preclinical testing.

Aptamers are frequently digested by nucleases, limiting their use in many biomedical applications. A xeno-nucleic acid system has been developed that is totally resistant to nuclease digestion and is based on a-l-threofuranosyl nucleic acid (TNA). The use of an engineered TNA polymerase allowed the isolation of functional TNA aptamers with KDs of 0.4–4.0 nM that bind to HIV reverse transcriptase (HIV RT). The aptamers were discovered utilizing a display technique that allows for a strong genotype–phenotype correlation. TNA aptamers are significantly more thermally stable than monoclonal antibodies and remain active in the presence of nuclease. TNA aptamers (Dunn et al. 2020) are a strong system to produce diagnostic and therapeutic medicines because of their biological stability, high binding affinity, and thermal stability.

The nucleotide bases are changed to prevent enzymatic or chemical cleavage of single-stranded oligonucleotides. The modification of the phosphodiester backbone, which is commonly done by utilizing athio-substituted deoxynucleotide triphosphates, has been found to be more effective with DNA aptamers than with RNA aptamers. To be more specific, insilico molecular dynamics can be utilized to determine whether aptamer and therapeutic medication have any influence on each other prior to in vitro studies (Athyala et al. 2016).

Thus, nucleic aptamers are a section of aptamers with wide biological applications. Further, there is another class of aptamers termed peptide aptamers that found applications in biomedical fields. These are similar to antibodies as they selectively recognize target proteins.

7.5 PEPTIDE APTAMERS

Peptide aptamers are typically 5–20 amino acids long and have a secondary structure that allows them to attach to target proteins. Aptamers and antibodies have comparable qualities, except that aptamers are more versatile and can be cost-effectively manufactured in large quantities with a long shelf life. They can be readily chemically changed using signalling molecules like probes, nanoparticles, and fluorophores. They are non-toxic, less immunogenic because they can't initiate MHC- Class I & II signalling, smaller in size, and heat resistant.

7.5.1 Selection of peptide aptamers

The pioneering of generating small peptide aptamers was performed by Cohen, Colas, and Brent (1998). They have developed peptide aptamers that could specifically target Cyclin-dependent kinase2. The first scaffold introduced by them that is widely used is *Escherichia coli* thioredoxin (trxA) (Colas et al. 1996). Thioredoxin is a non-toxic, highly soluble, tiny, and structurally rigid 12 kDa oxidoreductase enzyme important in maintaining the *E. coli* cytosolic thiol/disulfide equilibrium. Thioredoxin contains an active site made up of a Cys-Gly-Pro-Cys stretch that can accommodate lengthy peptide insertions but at the expense of enzymatic activity. The peptides are placed into the loop within the biologically active centre of the molecule, disrupting its catalytic activity, because the scaffold should be biologically inert (LaVallie et al. 1993). Thioredoxin is a single-domain protein that is well-folded, with four -helices flanking a core five-stranded -sheet and an active site disulphide group projecting from the protein surface. Thioredoxin has been shown in research to be more stable than other scaffolds.

The approach is similar to that of nucleotide aptamers in that 5–20 residue peptide loops are inserted on a scaffold that provides a rich and diverse environment for choosing high affibodies to a target protein from combinatorial libraries (Borghouts, Kunz, and Groner 2008).

The combinatorial libraries of peptide aptamers are used as random "mutagens" that interfere with biological processes via the mechanisms outlined below.

1. Incorporating combinatorial expression libraries of peptide aptamers into cells,
2. Screens and selects cells that carry peptide aptamers that cause the desired function, and
3. Identifies the targets of the peptide aptamers by screening the aptamers for interactions against groups of proteins or of cDNA libraries using the two-hybrid system.

Peptide aptamers are synthesized and chosen through yeast expression libraries (Bickle et al. 2006), bacterial expression libraries (Ahmadvand, Rahbarizadeh, and Moghimi 2011), and retroviral libraries (Figure 7.3). Phage-, ribosome-, and mRNA-displays are employed to isolate the necessary aptamer for *in vitro* synthesis. A phage display means, on one phage one peptide will be displayed. Then ligands will be screened to get peptide aptamers with high binding affinity. The diversity of the library can be limited to $<10^9$. However, to increase the diversity polypeptides are linked to the mRNA to form mRNA-ribosome -nascent peptide complex. The complexes will be purified, and peptide ligands will be isolated thus increasing the aptamer generation efficiency (Sussman, Nix, and Wilson 2000). Recently, retroviral plasmids were used for peptide aptamer generation. Aptamers were specifically generated for five protein interaction pairs. For example, P53 and MDM2 were well known for their interaction where aptamer was employed to understand the protein-protein interactions.

Peptide aptamer libraries differ depending on the scaffold used, the length of the peptide, and the selection process. The following characteristics should be included in an ideal aptamer scaffold:

1. The scaffold should have good solubility properties to prevent aggregation of aptamers with hydrophobic variable regions;
2. The scaffold should be small, stable, and non-toxic; and
3. The scaffold should have high adaptability to modifications such as localization sequences, epitope tags, purification tags, and other protein moieties.

Peptide aptamer against viral UL84 open reading frame of cytomegalovirus was a potential antiviral compound (Kaiser et al. 2009). The secondary structure of peptide aptamers is determined by the peptide sequence. Ligands such as peptide aptamers were created in such a way that they attach to the surface of target proteins with high affinity. When cyclic peptides interact with another linear peptide sequence, they achieve their full potential. New, Bui, and Bogus (2020) demonstrated that the impact of cyclic peptide sequence and their interaction with linear peptides were considerably more efficient than the same linear sequence alone. Another way to identify ligands that target a specific protein surface is phage display. When phage display is used in peptide aptamer selection, the effectiveness of the peptide aptamer is increased manyfold. To create an aptamer against calmodulin protein binding, Manandhar et al. (2017) used phage display in conjunction with nonfluorogenic compounds such as amino acid and 7-nitro-2,1,3-benzoxadiazole. Interestingly, Kashima and Kawahara (2021) created a platform for monitoring peptide–protein interactions inside the cellular environment by combining interleukin 3 dependent murine cells chimeric protein including receptor tyrosine kinase c-kit to detect and choose the protein binders (KIPPIS). Using the kit, the scientists discovered six peptide aptamers that detect cell growth. Aptamer design, whether peptide or oligonucleotide-based, necessitates both design and validation. In some cases, the induced fit theory may be used for aptamer-based beacon probes. Even online tools like as PATCHDOCK and YASARA may not accurately reflect the induced fit hypothesis between aptamers and their targets (Bruno and Phillips 2019). Peptide-based aptamers are being studied not just in fundamental research but also in translational research. Corda et al. (2018) have created a peptide-based aptamer to target prion protein-promoting cleavage of the PrPc domain for neurodegenerative disorders. Not only in neurological illnesses but also in the present pandemic COVID-19 detection, an in silico investigation for developing peptide-based aptamers targeting spike protein of the SARS CoV2 variant was investigated (Devi and Chaitanya 2022). Not just in insilico viral detection, but also in the creation of a diagnostic approach for Zika virus detection using a peptide aptamer targeting the Virus epitope (Bao et al. 2017) was done by researchers. Peptide-based medicinal compounds have also been investigated for their ability to affect cellular signalling, particularly the interaction of the proteins p53 and MDM2. Stapled peptides also exhibit significant cellular internalization against protease activity (Thean et al. 2017).

7.5.2 CHARACTERIZATION OF PEPTIDE APTAMERS

Peptide aptamers are characterized by two different methods like structural and functional characterisation. Structural validation of the peptide aptamer is done through circular dichroism spectroscopy, SPR, and thermogravimetry assay. Functional validation of peptide aptamer is done through yeast two-hybrid system, flow cytometry (d'Orlyé et al. 2021).

7.5.3 APPLICATIONS OF PEPTIDE APTAMERS

Recently a label-free detection system was developed using peptide aptamer for experimental troponin protein. The fluorescence from detector proteins that were preferentially coupled to the aptamer was transformed into a longer wavelength that could be detected by a CCD camera in a microfluidic device system containing Zinc Sulphide compounds as luminophores in this reported work (Sitkov et al. 2021). Recently, parts of antibodies (monobodies) have been engineered instead of using whole antibodies for undruggable targets (Gupta et al. 2018).

Many proteins have been fused to GFP to highlight their subcellular distribution, dynamics, and activities. GFP has also been utilized as a scaffold to increase the production of peptide aptamers. The luminous features give the added benefit of allowing the placed aptamers to be traced. Furthermore, this scaffold has been demonstrated to stabilize linear peptides, increase target binding, and inhibit neighbouring binding sites. Another significant advantage is the ability to monitor the intracellular expression level of the peptide aptamers simply and quantitatively. Peptide aptamers can be attached to GFP's C- or N-terminus. In addition, two loops have been identified that accommodate peptide insertions of different sizes without seriously disturbing GFP protein function (Abedi, Caponigro, and Kamb 1998). Aptamer molecules bring the specificity for targeting the biological molecules, while the molecular beacon probes that are designed for specific target molecule brings sensitivity to the detection methods. When combining aptamer with a molecular beacon probe increases the sensitivity and specificity in detecting the biomolecules in complex biological fluids such as serum (Goulko, Li, and Le 2009).

7.6   MOLECULAR APTAMER BEACON PROBES

Molecular aptamer beacon (MAB) probes detect specific biomolecular targets by combining a fluorophore and a quencher. Because of the inherent practicality of molecular engineering in beacon probes, new avenues for molecular diagnostics in sensing, imaging, and treatments are opened. The advantage of MAB probes in detecting chemicals is their strong fluorescence and specificity. The length of the aptamer sequence and the quencher molecule both have an impact on the probe's performance. The probe is composed of two components: a stem and a loop structure. The stem is always built using the AT/GC pairing rule, and the loop is supposed to be complementary to the target sequence.

The MAB produces a stem-loop structure under a particular situation or in the absence of a target analyte. When the target molecule is present in the environment, the loop structure opens and attaches to it because of the complementary sequence. Due to the obvious opening of the loop structure, the two ends of the beacon probes become separated, and the fluorophore attached begins to produce fluorescence without the presence of a quencher molecule nearby.

7.6.1   BASIC PRINCIPLE OF MOLECULAR BEACON PROBES

The beacon probe operates using the concept of fluorescence energy transfer (FRET) (Figure 7.5). The fluorophore and quencher are positioned in the sequence so that the FRET distance is maintained (1–10 nm). The FRET distance is crucial in FRET-based probes. Because the excitation-emission peak coincides with the absorption maximum of the quencher molecule, the energy released is transferred to the quencher molecule when the fluorophore is excited with the right wavelength. As a result, when the target is not there, the fluorophore and quencher are adjacent, and hence fluorescence is not visible. In the presence of the target molecule, the fluorophore and the quencher are well separated, and fluorescence is emitted.

MiRNAs are short oligonucleotides with important physiological and biological functions such as tissue-specific expression and regulation. MiRNAs are generated and circulated inside the human body to perform a variety of important cellular tasks. It not only has cellular activities, but it also exhibits disease phenotypes in many pathological conditions. The identification and quantification of miRNAs produced by the cellular/tissue compartment would indicate early alterations in the clinical state (Backes, Meese, and Keller 2016). As a result, it has the potential to be a biomarker for the early detection of disease patterns. MiRNAs have proven to be useful as biomarkers not just in diagnostics but also in prognostics and therapeutics. When combined with an aptamer, molecular beacon probes have previously demonstrated increased sensitivity and specificity in the detection of miRNAs directly from human clinical samples (Ferapontova, Olsen, and Gothelf 2008).

7.6.2 BEACON PROBES WITH APTAMER ENGINEERING FOR BIOMOLECULE DETECTION

Adenosine molecules can be detected by various techniques. However, selective action of Adenosine triphosphate and Adenosine diphosphate could not be achieved before. Therefore, aptamers to differentiate these moieties were obtained by SELEX technology and utilized for sensitive detection of ATP in the serum samples. An aptamer chimaera was constructed using a novel aptamer, a restriction site, and a primer binding region and this molecule was adsorbed onto the Graphene Oxide (GO) nanoparticles. The ATP when binds to the aptamer, is released from the GO for amplification reactions. This is followed by using molecular beacon probes 5'FAM and 3'dabcyl for the detection of ATP. The recovery of FAM fluorescence after hybridization is proportional (Xin Chen et al. 2022) to the ATP concentration.

The aptamer is split into two parts by definition in order to self-assemble with the target sequence. If an aptamer sequence is designed to target Molecule A, it is divided into two parts. The target is then allowed to bind to the first half of the aptamer. FRET probes between the fluorescent label and quencher are used to quantify the complex formed between the target and split aptamer. Without any enzyme-substrate reaction, the bisphenol molecule is identified using split aptamers at a sensitivity of 0.89 ng/mL (W. Wang et al. 2022). Gerasimova, Nedorezova, and Kolpashchikov (2022) developed recently split light-up aptamer sequences to detect DNA at ambient temperature without fluorophore conjugation. Quencher-free molecular beacon probes were also made to detect biomolecules like DNA. Even single base pair match was identified directly and the discrimination factor was found to be 14.7 using the method developed by Hwang, Seo, and Kim (2004).

7.6.3 APTAMER-BASED BEACON PROBES FOR PATHOGEN DETECTIONS

Bacterial detection by aptamer and its role in Fungi detection: Different methods have been employed by various groups. Whole cells are used as target molecules to select the aptamers. There are a few groups that tried different biomolecules in the target pathogen. Whole pathogens such as *Bacillus anthracis* (Ziółkowski et al. 2018), *Trypanosoma cruzi* (Ulrich et al. 2002), *Mycobacterium tuberculosis* (Kumar et al. 2009), *Staphylococcus aureus* (Sinsimer et al. 2005), *Pseudomonas aeruginosa* (Zhong et al. 2018), *Campylobacter jejuni* (Dwivedi, Smiley, and Jaykus 2010) etc were used as target whole cell and aptamers have been developed against the pathogens. These aptamers will find a potential role in molecular diagnostics as well as in rapid detection kits. Different viral Pathogens causing human disease are impacting human life significantly. The advances are happening holistically such as diagnosis, prognosis, and therapeutics. Infectious diseases are also impacting the country's economy severely which needs regular monitoring. The molecular diagnostics of viral detection have improved with the development of molecular ligands like aptamer. Rous sarcoma virus detection was developed by Percze et al. (2017). Similarly, various viral pathogen-detecting aptamers were developed by different groups such as Human Influenza A virus particles (R. Wang et al. 2013), Vaccinia virus particles (Nitsche et al. 2007), g Hepatitis C E2 envelope glycoprotein (J. H. Park et al. 2013). SARS Covid RNA virus detection using a DNA aptamer and green fluorescent protein. The detection of RNA in biological cells is critical for diagnostics and therapies. The COVID SARS CoV2 viral RNA was recently isolated and detected using a DNA aptamer (Yang et al. 2021).

7.6.4 DETECTION OF RNA IN LIVING CELLS USING MOLECULAR BEACON PROBES

To monitor the RNA state inside cells, fluorescent RNAs that bind to specific RNA have been produced. These probes are exceedingly stable and may be able to bind to RNA with minimal disruption to transcription. These pepper probes were created by Xianjun Chen et al. (2019).

Luo et al. recently published an article on an antibody aptamer dual probe for the detection of target molecules that provides both specificity and selectivity. The detection limit of Interleukin 06 was determined to be 0.5pg/ml, while control studies revealed no absorption, implying selective detection. The IL for the arthritic disease was identified using a dual-probed ELISA (Luo et al. 2022).

Detection of tumour-derived extracellular vehicles-miRNA with better selectivity and specificity utilizing an aptamer and molecular beacon technique is explained. To recapitulate, exosomes derived from tumour cells are crucial biomarkers for disease staging. As a result, detecting miRNA in extracellular carriers is critical without sacrificing selectivity and specificity. When a Molecular beacon aptamer is engineered in such a way that it may fuse with extracellular vehicles generated by tumour cells and be identified, it is said to be a beacon aptamer.

7.6.5 MIRNA DETECTION METHODS

MicroRNAs (miRNAs) are non-coding RNA molecules that control mRNA degradation and alter protein levels (J. Wang, Chen, and Sen 2016). In recent years, significant progress has been made in understanding the genesis and particular activities of miRNA, with an emphasis on their potential value in both research and

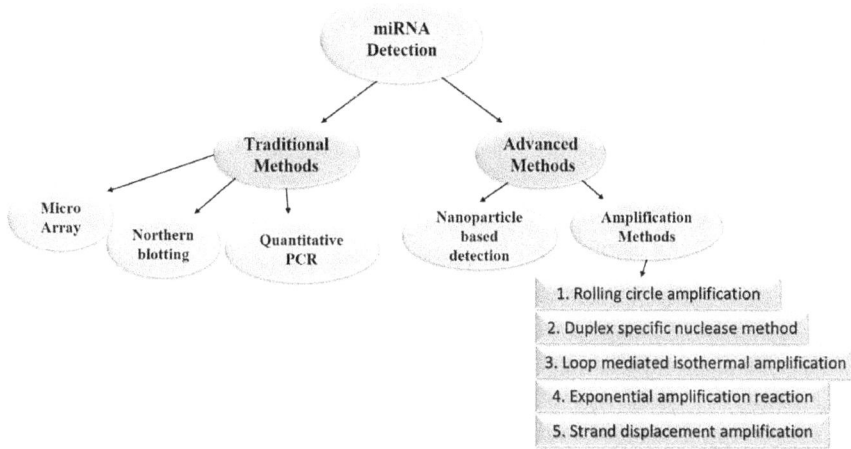

FIGURE 7.5   Classification of sensitive detection of miRNA by traditional and advanced methods.

therapeutic situations. MiRNA's principal role in the human body is gene regulation (Kai, Dittmar, and Sen 2018), which it accomplishes by affecting mRNA degradation as well as controlling transcription and translation through both conventional and non-canonical ways. MiRNA also plays an important role in intercellular signalling. Even though the majority of miRNAs are found within cells, a significant fraction migrates outside of them and can be found in bodily fluids (Weber et al. 2010). The early and incredibly sensitive detection of miRNA in physiological fluids is essential for high-end molecular diagnostics, prognostics, and therapeutic benefits (Figure 7.5). Northern blotting, microarray, and quantitative PCR make up the standard method of miRNA detection. The traditional approaches are insensitive and time-consuming. Through the development of nanotechnology, several improvements were made to the sensitivity of detection. Recent developments include nucleic acid amplification techniques and nanoparticle-based miRNA detection. The development of the amplification technique also includes the Rolling circle amplification method, Duplex specific nuclease approach, Loop-mediated isothermal amplification, Exponential amplification response, and Strand displacement amplification.

7.6.6 HYBRIDIZATION OF THE MATURE BEACON TO THE MATURE MIRNA TARGET

In the absence of a complementary target, a mature beacon molecular beacon forms a stem-loop structure, bringing the quencher close to the fluorophore and thereby quenching the fluorescence emission. When the beacon attaches to its miRNA target, the hairpin is opened, disrupting the stem and physically detaching the fluorophore from the quencher, permitting fluorescence emission upon stimulation (Figure 7.6).

Hairpin allosteric molecular beacon probes are being developed for detection by strand displacement and cascade amplification. The detection limit reached picomolar concentrations. MiRNA 21 was detected in serum using this approach, and the sensitivity was determined to be 0.7 pM in both serum and NSCLC A549 samples, as reported by Zheng et al. (2022).

As previously mentioned, the combination of aptamer and molecular beacon probes strengthens the sensitivity and specificity of miRNA detection in tissues and cells.

7.6.7 APTAMERS BEACON PROBES FOR THE DETECTION OF MIRNAS IN DIFFERENT DISEASES

7.6.7.1 Detection of miRNA

Recently, molecular beacon probes mediated sensitive detection of Let7a was achieved using electrochemical detection. They used the technique of molecular beacon-mediated isothermal circular strand displacement (ICSDPR). The technique involves recycling the target MiRNA and opening the hairpin capture probe immobilized on a gold electrode. The primers enable the synthesis of further Let7a strand molecules enabling the sensitive detection of this miRNA (Zhang Zhang et al. 2021). Beta et al (2015) published a direct assessment of the miRNA copy number for Retinoblastoma tumour from human serum utilizing a locked nucleic acid (LNA) modified beacon probe in a single step employing fluorescence spectroscopy and microscopy. They sensitively detected the levels of mir18-a. The method proved to be clinically important as detection of the miRNA was achieved in 0.1 mL of patient serum samples (Beta et al. 2015). Recently, multiplexed detection of several miRNAs in the serum and cancer cells has been developed. A fluorophore is attached to RNA aptamer, Fluorogenic RNA aptamer (FRA) that can bind to specific miRNA used here. Usually, it is an antisense sequence of the stem-loop region of the miRNA and consists of a stem-loop primer. This would be reverse transcribed to single-strand DNA and the target miRNA is now degraded. The cDNA with fluorescence signal is now made into a double strand and then amplified for detection. Several miRNAs could be detected by varying the initial RNA aptamers that target-specific miRNAs and the colour of the fluorophores used (Y. Park et al. 2022).

Another nanoparticle system that was employed for miRNA detection is metal-organic frameworks. They are biocompatible, easy to make, and have been used as drug delivery systems as reviewed by Wang et al. 2017 (Y. Liu, Jiang, and Liu 2022). Many of them possess fluorescence quenching properties enabling the use of these particles for sensitive detection of miRNAs. Zeolitic imidazolate framework-8 (ZIF-8) has excellent biocompatibility properties. However, it has low fluorescence quenching properties. To improve this property, Lanthanide ions were doped on these structures. A well-studied miR-21 with a significant role in various cancers regulating apoptosis and proliferation was detected using these nanostructures. The mir-21 aptamers conjugated to FAM and TAMRA fluorophores were adsorbed onto the La-doped nanostructures. The fluorescence intensity of FAM decreased with an increase in TAMRA fluorescence when MIR-21 was present enabling sensitive detection of this miRNA (Y.-B. Hao et al. 2019). Recent advances in imaging nanostructures enabled the characterization of Iodine absorption at the single particle level on the Zeolite imidazole frameworks (ZIF) (Lei et al. 2021). This is meaningful as this property of ZIF has been utilized for cheaper calorimetric detection of miRNA. The

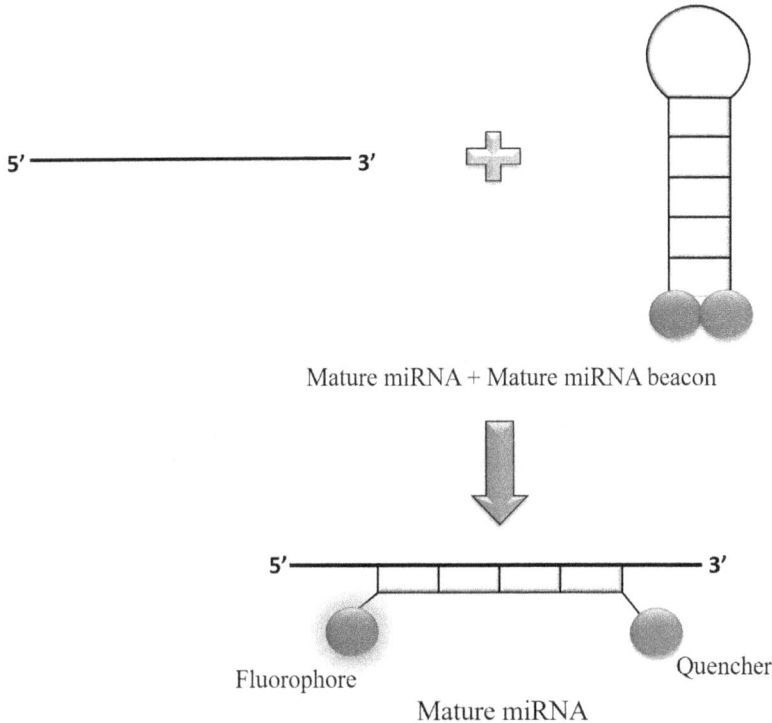

5′ ─────────────────── 3′   +

Mature miRNA + Mature miRNA beacon

5′ ─────────────────────── 3′

Fluorophore   Quencher

Mature miRNA

FIGURE 7.6   Schematic illustration of molecular beacon - miRNA hybridization assays.

ZIFs were encapsulated with different starch moieties and tannic acids. The visual colour of adding I_2/KI or $FeCl_3$ was used to detect miRNA. Specific aptamers were used that can bind miRNA efficiently and can be adsorbed onto the ZIF-based nanomaterial. This was fine-tuned to increase the detection limits of miRNA (J. Zhang et al. 2020).

7.6.7.2   Visualising miRNA abundance using live cell imaging

The miRNAs are low-abundant RNA making them difficult to visualize in living cells. Several methods have been employed recently for the sensitive detection of miRNAs in living cells. Interestingly, the use of self-powered FRET flares (SPF) has become popular for visualizing the expression of low-abundant miRNA. In this method, aptamer was specifically used to target cancer cells. AS411 aptamer that specifically targets Nucleolin protein which is overexpressed in cancer cells is used for targeted detection. In addition, it employed AS1411 aptamer to target-specific cancer cells and then SPFs to amplify and detect miRNA-21 and image its expression in live cancer cells. The SPF flares self-assembly inside a live cell form a DNA nanostructure, when cellular miRNA-21 is present, and they do not need additional signal amplification (Jing Li et al. 2021). Another recent study used a method of rolling circle amplification of the target miRNA for imaging low-copy number miRNAs specifically in cancer cells. They sensitively visualized Let7 family of miRNAs (a, b, c, d, f, I, g) in live cancer cells. They first created a padlock probe containing a miRNA recognition region, T7 promoter binding region, malachite green (MG) aptamer template, and a spacer. The miRNA recognition region is complementary to the specific miRNA that is being visualized. The padlock probe in the presence of specific endogenous miRNA in the cancer cells amplified the miRNA using a rolling circle process of amplification. Now there are several copies of the MG aptamer and when Malachite green is added bright fluorescence is observed and could reflect the expression of that miRNA. The single-cell visualization enables documentation of the differential expression of the miRNAs in the cell types (D. Li et al. 2020). A Nucleolin aptamer tethered DNA Nanowire was made with probe sets and then targeted to cancer cells such as MCF-7 cells. There are donor and acceptor fluorescence probes. When this structure is taken by the cancer cell specifically, the target, mir-21T could hybridize to the recognition probe and can displace fluorescence flares. The hairpin structure comes back again and brings donor and accepter fluorophores close to each other. The intensity of fluorescence increases due to the phenomenon of FRET enabling the visualization of the miRNA inside the cancer cell. The gold nanoparticles possess the property of fluorescence quenching (A. Wang et al. 2020). DNA nanostructures are fabricated containing tetrahedron shapes. If these two are in close proximity the fluorescence is quenched by Gold nanoparticles and minimal signal is present. When mir-21 (target) was present the fluorescence intensity was greatly enhanced enabling visualization of miRNA (Bai et al. 2018).

7.7 THERAPEUTIC ADVANCES

Aptamers, molecular beacons, miRNA, and exosomes or extracellular vesicles are some of the components that are helping to advance therapeutic outcomes with more accuracy and robustness. Aptamers and molecular beacon probes, which are generated *in vitro* and target-specific biomolecules, are considerably enhancing treatments. Similarly, identifying extracellular molecules released by human cells, such as micro RNAs and exosomes, plays a crucial role in increasing therapeutic outcomes.

7.7.1 SMALL RNA AS THERAPY MOLECULES

There are several small RNA molecules that are explored for disease regulation. These are siRNA, miRNA, Antisense nucleotides (ASO), short activating RNAs (saRNAs), and RNA guides for engineered nucleases (gRNAs) are therapy molecules. These non-coding RNAs have several functions. The miRNA emerged as important regulatory molecules when overexpressed/underexpressed causing changes in the molecular reprogram of the cell. They have been identified as biomarkers and potential therapy targets in several diseases including cancer. Therefore, estimating the abundance of miRNA and its expression in live cells has been an intense area of research recently. Several miRNAs are diagnostic markers and tools are developed for early detection as they can help therapy processes with early detection. Additionally, they could predict chemotherapy response. Let7 miRNA (Chin et al. 2008) could be a prediction marker in lung cancer. This miRNA could be dysregulating Rsf-1 protein that could mediate radiation response. The

Ras/mapkinase signalling system was altered interfering with the response of the tumour to radiation (F. Liu, Tai, and Ma 2018).

The antigomirs targeted against miRNA (Mattes, Yang, and Foster 2007) have several functions. Systemic therapy of tumour-bearing mice with miR-10b antagomirs a family of chemically modified anti-miRNA oligonucleotides reduces breast cancer metastasis, according to Ma et al. MiR-10b silencing with antagomirs both *in vitro* and *in vivo* significantly reduces miR-10b levels while increasing levels of a functionally important miR-10b target, Hoxd10. The administration of miR-10b antagomirs to animals containing highly metastatic cells does not diminish primary mammary tumour development but significantly reduces lung metastasis formation. This anti-metastasis action is sequence-specific. The miR-10b antagomir looks to be a potential contender and a starting point for the creation of novel anti-metastasis treatments, as it is well tolerated by normal animals (Ma et al. 2010). When some microRNAs, known as oncomiRs, are overexpressed, they have a causal role in the initiation and maintenance of cancer. Cheng et al. report a unique antimiR delivery platform that targets the acidic tumour microenvironment, bypasses liver clearance, and permits cells to enter via a non-endocytic channel. Attaching peptide nucleic acid antimiRs to a peptide with a low pH-induced transmembrane structure (pHLIP) results in a novel construct that can target the tumour microenvironment, transport antimiRs across plasma membranes under acidic conditions (pH around 6), and effectively inhibit the miR-155 oncomiR in a mouse model of lymphoma. This study proposes a fresh approach to using antimiRs as anti-cancer drugs, which has the potential to have far-reaching implications in the field of targeted drug delivery (C. J. Cheng et al. 2015).

7.7.2 CHEMICAL MODIFICATIONS OF MIRNA-BASED THERAPEUTICS

MicroRNA (miRNA)-based treatments are divided into two categories: miRNA mimics and miRNA inhibitors (also known as antimiRs). MiRNA mimics are synthetic double-stranded ds short RNA molecules that have the same sequence as the relevant miRNA and hence attempt to restore lost miRNA expression in illnesses. AntimiRs, on the other hand, are single-stranded and based on first-generation antisense oligonucleotides (ASOs) intended to target mRNAs or modified with LNAs. AntagomiRs are antimiRs with a 2-O-methoxyethyl alteration. These synthesized short RNA molecules contain a complementary sequence to the miRNA to be suppressed and firmly attached to it to impede its activity. Chemical changes to the nucleotide backbone have resulted in significant increases in the binding affinity, stability, and target modulation effects of miRNA mimics and antimiRs throughout the years.

7.7.3 COMBINATION OF MIRNA AND APTAMERS FOR THERAPY

As previously stated, miRNAs secreted by cells play important biological roles in cellular functioning. Aptamer is a synthetic molecule that may be programmed to target certain molecules. Combining the aptamer with miRNAs for therapeutic reasons considerably improves the specificity of the treatment. Esposito and colleagues were the first to use nucleic acid aptamers as carriers for delivering let-7g, a tumour suppressor miRNA, to cells. They explain the production of aptamer-miRNA conjugates as multifunctional drugs that use an aptamer that binds to and antagonizes the oncogenic receptor tyrosine kinase Axl to inhibit the development of Axl-expressing tumours (GL21.T). Let-7g miRNA conjugation to GL21.T demonstrated preferential transport to target cells, RNA interference processing, and silencing of let-7g target genes. In addition, the multifunctional combination inhibited tumour development in a lung adenocarcinoma xenograft model. As a result, aptamer-miRNA conjugates (Esposito et al. 2014) are now recognized as a unique technique for the targeted delivery of miRNAs with therapeutic potential. RNA nanotechnology is applied to regulate mir-21 in animal models of breast cancer (Iaboni et al. 2016). This technology consists of using RNA particles as core complexes/scaffolds on which therapeutic RNA molecules are engineered and the use of RNA aptamers to specifically target cancer cells. Shu et al. (2015) used bacteriophage phi29 packing RNA 50 as a scaffold. Then they attached an anti-mRNA sequence for mir-21. An RNA aptamer that specifically binds to EGFR was attached to the scaffold to enable targeted delivery to the tumour in a preclinical orthotopic triple-negative breast cancer model. They used fluorophore 647 to visualize the uptake and see the off-target effects of the aptamer. They could demonstrate successful therapy in this type of tumour which usually harbours drug-resistant phenotype (Guo et al. 2020). Another recent study used AS1411 aptamer for targeted therapy to breast cancer cells. They used gold nanoparticles functionalized with miR-155 antagomir and AS1411 aptamer that targets nucleolin (Kardani et al. 2020). According to the literature, combining an aptamer with a miRNA molecule dramatically improves therapeutic options.

7.7.4 APTAMER-MODIFIED EXOSOMES AS THERAPY

Exosomes are used as drug delivery vehicles to specifically deliver therapeutic molecules such as siRNA to knock down genes involved in tumour progression. The siRNA is unstable in body fluids and delivery vehicles are needed for the successful delivery of siRNA to knockdown genes in tumours. Exosomes have been employed recently to knock down genes in tumour samples. They are better delivery vehicles compared to liposomes. These nanostructures can be used to deliver siRNA to regulate targets for which small molecule inhibitors are not present. For example, mutated KRAS Oncogene drives prostate cancer progression. There are not many efficient small molecules to inhibit the mutated protein. Exosome-mediated delivery of siRNA to the mutated KRAS protein enabled the death of prostate cancer cells in the orthotopic mouse models of Prostate cancer. Exosomes are more efficient than liposomes that are used in the delivery of siRNA. The exosomes had cell surface marker CD 47 that could enable the body's immune system to not recognize the delivery system by the macrophages and the circulation time of the drug molecule was increased enabling the reduction in tumour burden (Kamerkar et al. 2017). Exosomes are in clinical trials by MD Anderson for prostate cancer and they are recruiting patients.

Initially, peptides such as RGD were used to modify exosomes for targeted delivery to the tumour sites. However, peptides interferes with Exosome stability and biogenesis. Therefore, aptamers are used for targeted delivery. The Prostate-specific membrane antigen (PSMA) RNA aptamer was used to modify Exosomes containing siRNA to regulate Survivin levels. This nanocomplex was tested in prostate cancer

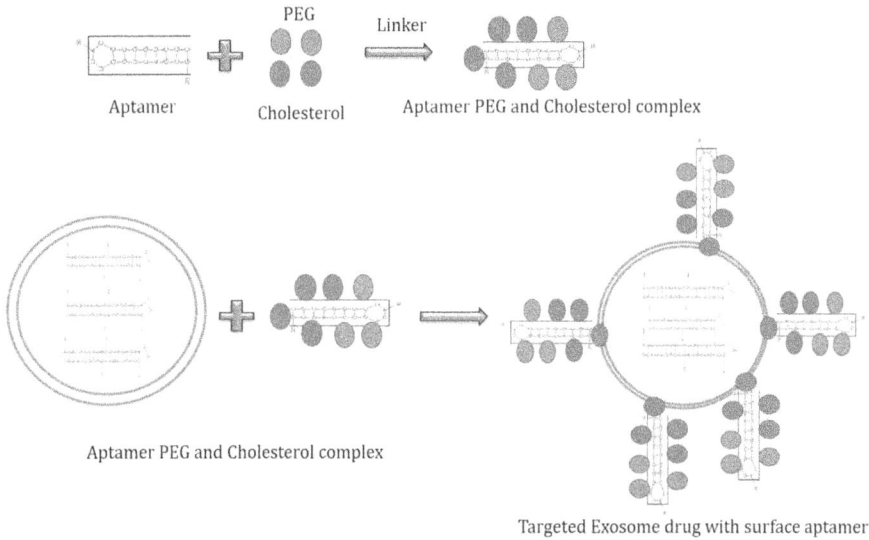

Aptamer   Cholesterol   Aptamer PEG and Cholesterol complex

Aptamer PEG and Cholesterol complex   Targeted Exosome drug with surface aptamer

FIGURE 7.7   Schematic illustration of the procedure for the targeted aptamer-modified siRNA-loaded exosomes.

TABLE 7.1
Cell surface protein aptamers and their applications

Aptamer	Target	Application
TTA140,41/ GBI1042 (DNA)	Tenascin-C (TN-C)	Blocks TN-C-involved pathways Potential therapeutic drug for tumours with TN-C overexpression like GBM (Daniels et al. 2003)
tJBA8.1 (DNA)	Transferrin receptor (TfR)	Binds to transferrin receptor 1 (TFR1) a receptor upregulated by cancer cells and depletion of cancer cells by tJBA8.1.(E. L. Cheng et al. 2022)
A30 (RNA)	Human epidermal growth factor 3 (HER3)	Inhibits tyrosine phosphorylation and reduces heregulin-specific growth stimulation, and may be useful as an HER-3 inhibitor in malignancies with high HER-3 expression as PAC (C.-H. B. Chen et al. 2003)
A9g (RNA)	PSMA	Bind to PSMA and prostate cancer cells expressing PSMA on the surface, Inhibits PC *in vitro* and *in vivo* metastasis (Dassie et al. 2014)
E0727/CL428/ KD1130/ TuTu2231 (RNA)	Epidermal growth factor receptor variant (EGFR)	Bind to newly synthesized EGFRvIII in aptamer-transfected cancer cells and block its glycosylation, Induces *in vitro* cell apoptosis, and inhibits *in vivo* LC growth (Esposito et al. 2011)

cells and mouse xenograft models (Pi et al. 2018). Similarly, EGFR aptamer was used to target Survivin by siRNA-loaded Exosomes in EGFR-expressing Cancer cells. Further, exosomes functionalized with aptamers for target-specific delivery have increased the effectiveness of the Exosome loaded drugs as they selectively target tumours (Zhefeng Li et al. 2021). A thiolated E3 aptamer was utilized, followed by a linker maleimide to connect PEG and Cholesterol (Figure 7.7). The E3 aptamer has been shown to particularly target prostate cancer cells. This aptamer is subsequently coupled to Exosomes containing siRNA in order to target an oncogene that is overexpressed in tumours. In mice models of prostate cancer, the aforesaid technique was used to silence Sirtuin 6 (SIRT6), and a decrease in tumour burden and metastasis was reported (Han et al. 2021). The aptamers were able to guide the siRNA-loaded Exosomes to the tumour site thus reducing the off-target effect of the drugs. In the future, such drugs could help in personalized medicine.

7.8   FUTURE PROSPECTIVE

Because peptide aptamers may play critical functions in cancer cells with high specificity and affinity, they should be ideally suited to influence target activities in transformed cells. Aptamers can be used to evaluate a target's biological significance as well as druggability, guiding the creation of small compounds for therapeutic applications. Peptide aptamers can enhance RNA interference techniques that eliminate all protein interactions with the target protein because they can bind to

TABLE 7.2
Commercially available aptamers

Aptamer	Target	Condition	References
Macugen (Pegaptanib)	VEGF	Age-related macular degeneration	Ng et al. (2006)
NOX-A12	Stromal cell-derived factor-1 (SDF-1)	Multiple myeloma (MM) and non-Hodgkin's lymphoma (NHL)	Suarez-Carmona et al. (2021)

TABLE 7.3
Aptamers withdrawn from clinical trials

Aptamer	Target	Condition	References
AS1411	Nucleolin	Acute myeloid leukaemia	Carvalho et al. (2019)
ARC1779	A1 domain of von Willebrand factor (vWF)	von Willebrand disease	Halawa et al. (2021)
E10030	Platelet-derived growth factor-B (PDGF-B)	Age-related macular degeneration	Sadiq et al. (2016)

distinct domains of the target protein and disrupt particular functions. Additionally, peptide aptamers have the potential to be turned into medications.

Several nucleic acid aptamers have been authorized by the FDA or are under clinical studies for potential approval (Table 7.1). Macugen (Pegaptanib) and Nox-A12 are authorized aptamers for a variety of medical problems. However, due to unsuccessful clinical studies, numerous aptamers are not in clinical use (Table 7.2). There is continuing research and clinical trials on new aptamers as medications. Kaur et al. (2018) analyzed the list of aptamers in clinical trials as well as potential aptamers in the preclinical setting. Several aptamers that are in clinical trials were recalled or terminated. The recalled aptamers were reviewed by Kumar Kulabhusan, Hussain, and Yüce (2020). Several variables influence aptamer performance, including stability and toxicity buildup in non-targeted tissues. Continuous research is being conducted to enhance these parameters and conduct clinical studies in order to bring them to market. Clinicaltrials.gov provides access to ongoing clinical studies. Complement factor 5 aptamer studies for AMD and idiopathic polypoidal choroidal vasculopathy are two significant trials now underway. A Fovista® (aptamer medication I) clinical study for AMD has been completed or ended. The results are still awaiting. The latter was a clinical experiment in its second phase. The study is finished, but the findings have not yet been revealed. Several point-of-care devices, however, are under clinical trials for the detection of HIV, COVID-19, the pregnancy hormone Oxytocin, and bladder cancer (Table 7.3). Table 7.4 summarises the present status of aptamer therapies in clinical studies. Aptamer medicines and sensors are expected to be available for general therapeutic usage after studies are completed. All the new developments should pave the path for future personalized medicine.

TABLE 7.4

Current status of the aptamer therapeutics undergoing clinical trails

Clinical trial number	Device/diagnosis and key aptamer constituents used	Disease	Status
NCT04974203	COVID-19 virus By DNA aptamer for virus detection	Flu cold and respiratory disease caused by COVID-19	Recruiting patients for rapid tests using Saliva to help patients in countries with low resources
NCT04870671	An aptasensor to detect AIDS drug Tenofovir sensitively in blood plasma to monitor drug efficacy	AIDS	Completed
NCT02957370	Calorimetric aptasensor for biomarkers	Bladder cancer	Recruiting by UC Irvine
NCT03140709	Aptamer-based electrochemical assay is a point-of-care device for Oxytocin detection in body fluids	Pregnant women	Recruiting by Stanford University

REFERENCES

Ababneh, Nidaa, Walhan Alshaer, Omar Allozi, Azmi Mahafzah, Mohammed El-Khateeb, Hervé Hillaireau, Magali Noiray, Elias Fattal, and Said Ismail. 2013. "In Vitro Selection of Modified RNA Aptamers against CD44 Cancer Stem Cell Marker." *Nucleic Acid Therapeutics* 23 (6): 401–407. https://doi.org/10.1089/nat.2013.0423.

Abbaspour, Abdolkarim, Fatemeh Norouz-Sarvestani, Abolhassan Noori, and Noushin Soltani. 2015. "Aptamer-Conjugated Silver Nanoparticles for Electrochemical Dual-Aptamer-Based Sandwich Detection of Staphylococcus Aureus." *Biosensors & Bioelectronics* 68 (June): 149–155. https://doi.org/10.1016/j.bios.2014.12.040.

Abd-Ellatief, Ragaa, and Maha Ragaa Abd-Ellatief. 2021. "Electrochemical Aptasensors: Current Status and Future Perspectives." *Diagnostics (Basel, Switzerland)* 11 (1). https://doi.org/10.3390/diagnostics11010104.

Abedi, Majid R, Giordano Caponigro, and Alexander Kamb. 1998. "Green Fluorescent Protein as a Scaffold for Intracellular Presentation of Peptides." *Nucleic Acids Research* 26 (2): 623–630. https://doi.org/10.1093/nar/26.2.623.

Ahmadvand, Davoud, Fatemeh Rahbarizadeh, and Seyed Moein Moghimi. 2011. "Biological Targeting and Innovative Therapeutic Interventions with Phage-Displayed Peptides and Structured Nucleic Acids (Aptamers)." *Current Opinion in Biotechnology* 22 (6): 832–838. https://doi.org/10.1016/j.copbio.2011.02.012.

Athyala, Prasanna Kumar, Jagat Rakesh Kanwar, Mohamed Alameen, Rupinder Kaur Kanwar, Subramanian Krishnakumar, Jon Watson, Umashankar Vetrivel, and Janakiraman Narayanan. 2016. "Probing the Biophysical Interaction between Neocarzinostatin Toxin and EpCAM RNA Aptamer." *Biochemical and Biophysical Research Communications* 469 (2): 257–262. https://doi.org/10.1016/j.bbrc.2015.11.109.

Backes, Christina, Eckart Meese, and Andreas Keller. 2016. "Specific MiRNA Disease Biomarkers in Blood, Serum and Plasma: Challenges and Prospects." *Molecular Diagnosis & Therapy* 20 (6): 509–518. https://doi.org/10.1007/s40291-016-0221-4.

Bai, Shulian, Bangtian Xu, Yongcan Guo, Juhui Qiu, Wen Yu, and Guoming Xie. 2018. "High-Discrimination Factor Nanosensor Based on Tetrahedral DNA Nanostructures and Gold Nanoparticles for Detection of MiRNA-21 in Live Cells." *Theranostics* 8 (9): 2424–2434. https://doi.org/10.7150/thno.23852.

Bao, Duong Tuan, Do Thi Hoang Kim, Hyun Park, Bui Thi Cuc, Nguyen Minh Ngoc, Nguyen Thi Phuong Linh, Nguyen Chien Huu, et al. 2017. "Rapid Detection of Avian Influenza Virus by Fluorescent Diagnostic Assay Using an Epitope-Derived Peptide." *Theranostics* 7 (7): 1835–1846. https://doi.org/10.7150/thno.18857.

Berezovski, Maxim, Michael Musheev, Andrei Drabovich, and Sergey N Krylov. 2006. "Non-SELEX Selection of Aptamers." *Journal of the American Chemical Society* 128 (5): 1410–1411. https://doi.org/10.1021/ja056943j.

Beta, Madhu, Subramanian Krishnakumar, Sailaja V Elchuri, Bindu Salim, and Janakiraman Narayanan. 2015. "A Comparative Fluorescent Beacon-Based Method for Serum MicroRNA Quantification." *Analytical Sciences : The International Journal of the Japan Society for Analytical Chemistry* 31 (3): 231–235. https://doi.org/10.2116/analsci.31.231.

Bickle, Marc B T, Eric Dusserre, Olivier Moncorgé, Hélène Bottin, and Pierre Colas. 2006. "Selection and Characterization of Large Collections of Peptide Aptamers through Optimized Yeast Two-Hybrid Procedures." *Nature Protocols* 1 (3): 1066–1091. https://doi.org/10.1038/nprot.2006.32.

Borghouts, Corina, Christian Kunz, and Bernd Groner. 2008. "Peptide Aptamer Libraries." *Combinatorial Chemistry & High Throughput Screening* 11 (2): 135–145. https://doi.org/10.2174/138620708783744462.

Bruno, John G, and Taylor Phillips. 2019. "Beacons Contribute Valuable Empirical Information to Theoretical 3-D Aptamer-Peptide Binding." *Journal of Fluorescence* 29 (3): 711–717. https://doi.org/10.1007/s10895-019-02380-6.

Carvalho, Josué, Artur Paiva, Maria Paula Cabral Campello, António Paulo, Jean-Louis Mergny, Gilmar F Salgado, João A Queiroz, and Carla Cruz. 2019. "Aptamer-Based Targeted Delivery of a G-Quadruplex Ligand in Cervical Cancer Cells." *Scientific Reports* 9 (1): 7945. https://doi.org/10.1038/s41598-019-44388-9.

Chang, Andrew L, Maureen McKeague, and Christina D Smolke. 2014. "Facile Characterization of Aptamer Kinetic and Equilibrium Binding Properties Using Surface Plasmon Resonance." *Methods in Enzymology* 549: 451–466. https://doi.org/10.1016/B978-0-12-801122-5.00019-2.

Chen, Chi-Hong B, George A Chernis, Van Q Hoang, and Ralf Landgraf. 2003. "Inhibition of Heregulin Signaling by an Aptamer That Preferentially Binds to the Oligomeric Form of Human Epidermal Growth Factor Receptor-3." *Proceedings of the National Academy of Sciences of the United States of America* 100 (16): 9226–9231. https://doi.org/10.1073/pnas.1332660100.

Chen, Xianjun, Dasheng Zhang, Ni Su, Bingkun Bao, Xin Xie, Fangting Zuo, Lipeng Yang, et al. 2019. "Visualizing RNA Dynamics in Live Cells with Bright and Stable Fluorescent RNAs." *Nature Biotechnology* 37 (11): 1287–1293. https://doi.org/10.1038/s41587-019-0249-1.

Chen, Xin, Yangkun Feng, Haohan Chen, Yuting Zhang, Xiaoli Wang, and Nandi Zhou. 2022. "Fluorescent Aptasensor for Highly Specific Detection of ATP Using a Newly Screened Aptamer." *Sensors (Basel, Switzerland)* 22 (7). https://doi.org/10.3390/s22072425.

Chen, Zihao, Long Hu, Bao-Ting Zhang, Aiping Lu, Yaofeng Wang, Yuanyuan Yu, and Ge Zhang. 2021. "Artificial Intelligence in Aptamer-Target Binding Prediction." *International Journal of Molecular Sciences* 22 (7). https://doi.org/10.3390/ijms22073605.

Cheng, Christopher J, Raman Bahal, Imran A Babar, Zachary Pincus, Francisco Barrera, Connie Liu, Alexander Svoronos, et al. 2015. "MicroRNA Silencing for Cancer Therapy Targeted to the Tumour Microenvironment." *Nature* 518 (7537): 107–110. https://doi.org/10.1038/nature13905.

Cheng, Emmeline L, Ian I Cardle, Nataly Kacherovsky, Harsh Bansia, Tong Wang, Yunshi Zhou, Jai Raman, et al. 2022. "Discovery of a Transferrin Receptor 1-Binding Aptamer and Its Application in Cancer Cell Depletion for Adoptive T-Cell Therapy Manufacturing." *Journal of the American Chemical Society* 144 (30): 13851–13864. https://doi.org/10.1021/jacs.2c05349.

Cheng, Wei, Lin Ding, Yunlong Chen, Feng Yan, Huangxian Ju, and Yibing Yin. 2010. "A Facile Scanometric Strategy for Ultrasensitive Detection of Protein Using Aptamer-Initiated Rolling Circle Amplification." *Chemical Communications* 46 (36): 6720–6722. https://doi.org/10.1039/C002078H.

Chin, Lena J, Elena Ratner, Shuguang Leng, Rihong Zhai, Sunitha Nallur, Imran Babar, Roman-Ulrich Muller, et al. 2008. "A SNP in a Let-7 MicroRNA Complementary Site in the KRAS 3' Untranslated Region Increases Non-Small Cell Lung Cancer Risk." *Cancer Research* 68 (20): 8535–8540. https://doi.org/10.1158/0008-5472.CAN-08-2129.

Cohen, Barak A, Pierre Colas, and Roger Brent. 1998. "An Artificial Cell-Cycle Inhibitor Isolated from a Combinatorial Library." *Proceedings of the National Academy of Sciences of the United States of America* 95 (24): 14272–14277. https://doi.org/10.1073/pnas.95.24.14272.

Colas, Pierre, Barak Cohen, Timm Jessen, Irina Grishina, John McCoy, and Roger Brent. 1996. "Genetic Selection of Peptide Aptamers That Recognize and Inhibit Cyclin-Dependent Kinase 2." *Nature* 380 (6574): 548–550. https://doi.org/10.1038/380548a0.

Corda, Erica, Xiaotang Du, Su Yeon Shim, Antonia N Klein, Jessica Siltberg-Liberles, and Sabine Gilch. 2018. "Interaction of Peptide Aptamers with Prion Protein Central Domain Promotes α-Cleavage of PrP(C)." *Molecular Neurobiology* 55 (10): 7758–7774. https://doi.org/10.1007/s12035-018-0944-9.

Daniels, Dion A, Hang Chen, Brian J Hicke, Kristine M Swiderek, and Larry Gold. 2003. "A Tenascin-C Aptamer Identified by Tumor Cell-SELEX: Systematic Evolution of Ligands by Exponential Enrichment." *Proceedings of the National Academy of Sciences of the United States of America* 100 (26): 15416–15421. https://doi.org/10.1073/pnas.2136683100.

Dassie, Justin P, Luiza I Hernandez, Gregory S Thomas, Matthew E Long, William M Rockey, Craig A Howell, Yani Chen, et al. 2014. "Targeted Inhibition of Prostate Cancer Metastases with an RNA Aptamer to Prostate-Specific Membrane Antigen." *Molecular Therapy : The Journal of the American Society of Gene Therapy* 22 (11): 1910–1922. https://doi.org/10.1038/mt.2014.117.

Davis, Kenneth A, Barnaby Abrams, Yun Lin, and Sumedha D Jayasena. 1996. "Use of a High Affinity DNA Ligand in Flow Cytometry." *Nucleic Acids Research* 24 (4): 702–706. https://doi.org/10.1093/nar/24.4.702.

Devi, Arpita, and Nyshadham S N Chaitanya. 2022. "Designing of Peptide Aptamer Targeting the Receptor-Binding Domain of Spike Protein of SARS-CoV-2: An in Silico Study." *Molecular Diversity* 26 (1): 157–169. https://doi.org/10.1007/s11030-020-10171-6.

Ding, Lihua, Li-E Liu, Leiliang He, Clement Yaw Effah, Ruiying Yang, Dongxun Ouyang, Ningge Jian, Xia Liu, Yongjun Wu, and Lingbo Qu. 2021. "Magnetic-Nanowaxberry-Based Simultaneous Detection of Exosome and Exosomal Proteins for the Intelligent Diagnosis of Cancer." *Analytical Chemistry* 93 (45): 15200–15208. https://doi.org/10.1021/acs.analchem.1c03957.

d'Orlyé, Fanny, Laura Trapiella-Alfonso, Camille Lescot, Marie Pinvidic, Bich-Thuy Doan, and Anne Varenne. 2021. "Synthesis, Characterization and Evaluation of Peptide Nanostructures for Biomedical Applications." *Molecules (Basel, Switzerland)* 26 (15). https://doi.org/10.3390/molecules26154587.

Dunn, Matthew R, Cailen M McCloskey, Patricia Buckley, Katherine Rhea, and John C Chaput. 2020. "Generating Biologically Stable TNA Aptamers That Function with High Affinity and Thermal Stability." *Journal of the American Chemical Society* 142 (17): 7721–7724. https://doi.org/10.1021/jacs.0c00641.

Dwivedi, Hari P, R Derike Smiley, and Lee-Ann Jaykus. 2010. "Selection and Characterization of DNA Aptamers with Binding Selectivity to Campylobacter Jejuni Using Whole-Cell SELEX." *Applied Microbiology and Biotechnology* 87 (6): 2323–2334. https://doi.org/10.1007/s00253-010-2728-7.

Emami, Neda, and Reza Ferdousi. 2021. "AptaNet as a Deep Learning Approach for Aptamer-Protein Interaction Prediction." *Scientific Reports* 11 (1): 6074. https://doi.org/10.1038/s41598-021-85629-0.

Esposito, Carla L, Laura Cerchia, Silvia Catuogno, Gennaro De Vita, Justin P Dassie, Gianluca Santamaria, Piotr Swiderski, Gerolama Condorelli, Paloma H Giangrande, and Vittorio de Franciscis. 2014. "Multifunctional Aptamer-MiRNA Conjugates for Targeted Cancer Therapy." *Molecular Therapy: The Journal of the American Society of Gene Therapy* 22 (6): 1151–1163. https://doi.org/10.1038/mt.2014.5.

Esposito, Carla Lucia, Diana Passaro, Immacolata Longobardo, Gerolama Condorelli, Pina Marotta, Andrea Affuso, Vittorio de Franciscis, and Laura Cerchia. 2011. "A Neutralizing RNA Aptamer against EGFR Causes Selective Apoptotic Cell Death." *PLoS One* 6 (9): e24071. https://doi.org/10.1371/journal.pone.0024071.

Esposito, Carla Lucia, Cristina Quintavalle, Francesco Ingenito, Deborah Rotoli, Giuseppina Roscigno, Silvia Nuzzo, Renato Thomas, Silvia Catuogno, Vittorio de Franciscis, and

Gerolama Condorelli. 2021. "Identification of a Novel RNA Aptamer That Selectively Targets Breast Cancer Exosomes." *Molecular Therapy Nucleic Acids* 23 (March): 982–994. https://doi.org/10.1016/j.omtn.2021.01.012.

Ferapontova, Elena E, Eva M Olsen, and Kurt V Gothelf. 2008. "An RNA Aptamer-Based Electrochemical Biosensor for Detection of Theophylline in Serum." *Journal of the American Chemical Society* 130 (13): 4256–4258. https://doi.org/10.1021/ja711326b.

Gerasimova, Yulia V, Daria D Nedorezova, and Dmitry M Kolpashchikov. 2022. "Split Light up Aptamers as a Probing Tool for Nucleic Acids." *Methods (San Diego, Calif.)* 197 (January): 82–88. https://doi.org/10.1016/j.ymeth.2021.05.008.

Goulko, Alevtina A, Feng Li, and X Chris Le. 2009. "Bioanalytical Applications of Aptamer and Molecular-Beacon Probes in Fluorescence-Affinity Assays." *TrAC Trends in Analytical Chemistry* 28 (7): 878–892. https://doi.org/https://doi.org/10.1016/j.trac.2009.03.014.

Guo, Sijin, Mario Vieweger, Kaiming Zhang, Hongran Yin, Hongzhi Wang, Xin Li, Shanshan Li, et al. 2020. "Ultra-Thermostable RNA Nanoparticles for Solubilizing and High-Yield Loading of Paclitaxel for Breast Cancer Therapy." *Nature Communications* 11 (1): 972. https://doi.org/10.1038/s41467-020-14780-5.

Gupta, Ankit, Jing Xu, Shirley Lee, Steven T Tsai, Bo Zhou, Kohei Kurosawa, Michael S Werner, et al. 2018. "Facile Target Validation in an Animal Model with Intracellularly Expressed Monobodies." *Nature Chemical Biology* 14 (9): 895–900. https://doi.org/10.1038/s41589-018-0099-z.

Halawa, Omar A, Jonathan B Lin, Joan W Miller, and Demetrios G Vavvas. 2021. "A Review of Completed and Ongoing Complement Inhibitor Trials for Geographic Atrophy Secondary to Age-Related Macular Degeneration." *Journal of Clinical Medicine* 10 (12). https://doi.org/10.3390/jcm10122580.

Hamaguchi, Nobuko, Andrew Ellington, and Martin Stanton. 2001. "Aptamer Beacons for the Direct Detection of Proteins." *Analytical Biochemistry* 294 (2): 126–131. https://doi.org/10.1006/abio.2001.5169.

Han, Qing, Qian Rueben Xie, Fan Li, Yirui Cheng, Tingyu Wu, Yanshuang Zhang, Xin Lu, Alice S T Wong, Jianjun Sha, and Weiliang Xia. 2021. "Targeted Inhibition of SIRT6 via Engineered Exosomes Impairs Tumorigenesis and Metastasis in Prostate Cancer." *Theranostics* 11 (13): 6526–6541. https://doi.org/10.7150/thno.53886.

Hao, Lihua, and Qiang Zhao. 2015. "A Fluorescein Labeled Aptamer Switch for Thrombin with Fluorescence Decrease Response." *Analytical Methods* 7 (9): 3888–3892. https://doi.org/10.1039/C5AY00464K.

Hao, Ya-Bo, Zhen-Shu Shao, Chen Cheng, Xiao-Yu Xie, Jie Zhang, Wen-Jun Song, and Huai-Song Wang. 2019. "Regulating Fluorescent Aptamer-Sensing Behavior of Zeolitic Imidazolate Framework (ZIF-8) Platform via Lanthanide Ion Doping." *ACS Applied Materials & Interfaces* 11 (35): 31755–62. https://doi.org/10.1021/acsami.9b12253.

He, Dinggeng, Huizhen Wang, See-Lok Ho, Hei-Nga Chan, Luo Hai, Xiaoxiao He, Kemin Wang, and Hung-Wing Li. 2019. "Total Internal Reflection-Based Single-Vesicle in Situ Quantitative and Stoichiometric Analysis of Tumor-Derived Exosomal MicroRNAs for Diagnosis and Treatment Monitoring." *Theranostics* 9 (15): 4494–4507. https://doi.org/10.7150/thno.33683.

Hua, Rong, Nan Hao, Jinwen Lu, Jing Qian, Qian Liu, Henan Li, and Kun Wang. 2018. "A Sensitive Potentiometric Resolved Ratiometric Photoelectrochemical Aptasensor for Escherichia Coli Detection Fabricated with Non-Metallic Nanomaterials." *Biosensors & Bioelectronics* 106 (May): 57–63. https://doi.org/10.1016/j.bios.2018.01.053.

Hwang, Gil Tae, Young Jun Seo, and Byeang Hyean Kim. 2004. "A Highly Discriminating Quencher-Free Molecular Beacon for Probing DNA." *Journal of the American Chemical Society* 126 (21): 6528–6529. https://doi.org/10.1021/ja049795q.

Iaboni, Margherita, Valentina Russo, Raffaela Fontanella, Giuseppina Roscigno, Danilo Fiore, Elvira Donnarumma, Carla Lucia Esposito, et al. 2016. "Aptamer-MiRNA-212 Conjugate Sensitizes NSCLC Cells to TRAIL." *Molecular Therapy. Nucleic Acids* 5 (3): e289. https://doi.org/10.1038/mtna.2016.5.

Janakiraman, Narayanan, Abhilash Mohan, Ashwin Kannan, and Gautam Pennathur. 2012. "Resonance Energy Transfer between Protein and Rhamnolipid Capped ZnS Quantum Dots: Application in in-Gel Staining of Proteins." *Spectrochimica Acta. Part A, Molecular and Biomolecular Spectroscopy* 95 (April): 478–482. https://doi.org/10.1016/j. saa.2012.04.025.

Jo, Minjoung, Ji-Young Ahn, Joohyung Lee, Seram Lee, Sun Woo Hong, Jae-Wook Yoo, Jeehye Kang, et al. 2011. "Development of Single-Stranded DNA Aptamers for Specific Bisphenol a Detection." *Oligonucleotides* 21 (2): 85–91. https://doi.org/10.1089/ oli.2010.0267.

Joshi, Raghavendra, Harish Janagama, Hari P Dwivedi, T M A Senthil Kumar, Lee-Ann Jaykus, Jeremy Schefers, and Srinand Sreevatsan. 2009. "Selection, Characterization, and Application of DNA Aptamers for the Capture and Detection of Salmonella Enterica Serovars." *Molecular and Cellular Probes* 23 (1): 20–28. https://doi.org/10.1016/j. mcp.2008.10.006.

Kai, Kazuharu, Rachel L Dittmar, and Subrata Sen. 2018. "Secretory MicroRNAs as Biomarkers of Cancer." *Seminars in Cell & Developmental Biology* 78 (June): 22–36. https://doi.org/10.1016/j.semcdb.2017.12.011.

Kaiser, Nina, Peter Lischka, Nadine Wagenknecht, and Thomas Stamminger. 2009. "Inhibition of Human Cytomegalovirus Replication via Peptide Aptamers Directed against the Nonconventional Nuclear Localization Signal of the Essential Viral Replication Factor PUL84." *Journal of Virology* 83 (22): 11902–11913. https://doi.org/10.1128/ JVI.01378-09.

Kamerkar, Sushrut, Valerie S LeBleu, Hikaru Sugimoto, Sujuan Yang, Carolina F Ruivo, Sonia A Melo, J Jack Lee, and Raghu Kalluri. 2017. "Exosomes Facilitate Therapeutic Targeting of Oncogenic KRAS in Pancreatic Cancer." *Nature* 546 (7659): 498–503. https://doi.org/10.1038/nature22341.

Kardani, Arefeh, Hajar Yaghoobi, Abbas Alibakhshi, and Mehrdad Khatami. 2020. "Inhibition of MiR-155 in MCF-7 Breast Cancer Cell Line by Gold Nanoparticles Functionalized with Antagomir and AS1411 Aptamer." *Journal of Cellular Physiology* 235 (10): 6887–6895. https://doi.org/10.1002/jcp.29584.

Kashima, Daiki, and Masahiro Kawahara. 2021. "Evolution of KIPPIS as a Versatile Platform for Evaluating Intracellularly Functional Peptide Aptamers." *Scientific Reports* 11 (1): 11758. https://doi.org/10.1038/s41598-021-91287-z.

Kaur, Harleen, John G Bruno, Amit Kumar, and Tarun Kumar Sharma. 2018. "Aptamers in the Therapeutics and Diagnostics Pipelines." *Theranostics* 8 (15): 4016–4032. https://doi. org/10.7150/thno.25958.

Kim, Dong-Min, Myeong-June Go, Jingyu Lee, Dokyun Na, and Seung-Min Yoo. 2021. "Recent Advances in Micro/Nanomaterial-Based Aptamer Selection Strategies." *Molecules (Basel, Switzerland)* 26 (17). https://doi.org/10.3390/molecules26175187.

Kim, Dong-Min, Minhee Kim, Hee-Bin Park, Keun-Sik Kim, and Dong-Eun Kim. 2019. "Anti-MUC1/CD44 Dual-Aptamer-Conjugated Liposomes for Cotargeting Breast Cancer Cells and Cancer Stem Cells." *ACS Applied Bio Materials* 2 (10): 4622–4633. https://doi.org/10.1021/acsabm.9b00705.

Kumar, Parameet, Kapili Nath, Bimba Rath, Manas K Sen, Potharaju Vishalakshi, Devender S Chauhan, Vishwa M Katoch, et al. 2009. "Visual Format for Detection of Mycobacterium Tuberculosis and M. Bovis in Clinical Samples Using Molecular Beacons." *The Journal of Molecular Diagnostics: JMD* 11 (5): 430–438. https://doi.org/10.2353/ jmoldx.2009.080135.

Kumar Kulabhusan, Prabir, Babar Hussain, and Meral Yüce. 2020. "Current Perspectives on Aptamers as Diagnostic Tools and Therapeutic Agents." *Pharmaceutics* 12 (7). https://doi.org/10.3390/pharmaceutics12070646.

Lai, Rebecca Y, Kevin W Plaxco, and Alan J Heeger. 2007. "Aptamer-Based Electrochemical Detection of Picomolar Platelet-Derived Growth Factor Directly in Blood Serum." *Analytical Chemistry* 79 (1): 229–233. https://doi.org/10.1021/ac061592s.

Lai, Yi-Tak, and Jeffrey J DeStefano. 2012. "DNA Aptamers to Human Immunodeficiency Virus Reverse Transcriptase Selected by a Primer-Free SELEX Method: Characterization and Comparison with Other Aptamers." *Nucleic Acid Therapeutics* 22 (3): 162–176. https://doi.org/10.1089/nat.2011.0327.

LaVallie, Edward R, Elizabeth A DiBlasio, Sharlotte Kovacic, Kathleen L Grant, Paul F Schendel, and John M McCoy. 1993. "A Thioredoxin Gene Fusion Expression System That Circumvents Inclusion Body Formation in the *E. coli* Cytoplasm." *Bio/Technology (Nature Publishing Company)* 11 (2): 187–193. https://doi.org/10.1038/nbt0293-187.

Lei, Yuting, Guihua Zhang, Qinglan Zhang, Ling Yu, Hua Li, Haili Yu, and Yi He. 2021. "Visualization of Gaseous Iodine Adsorption on Single Zeolitic Imidazolate Framework-90 Particles." *Nature Communications* 12 (1): 4483. https://doi.org/10.1038/s41467-021-24830-1.

Li, Daxiu, Fang Yang, Ruo Yuan, and Yun Xiang. 2020. "Lighting-up RNA Aptamer Transcription Synchronization Amplification for Ultrasensitive and Label-Free Imaging of MicroRNA in Single Cells." *Analytica Chimica Acta* 1102 (March): 84–90. https://doi.org/10.1016/j.aca.2019.12.040.

Li, Jianwei J, Xiaohong Fang, and Weihong Tan. 2002. "Molecular Aptamer Beacons for Real-Time Protein Recognition." *Biochemical and Biophysical Research Communications* 292 (1): 31–40. https://doi.org/10.1006/bbrc.2002.6581.

Li, Jianwei, Xiaoyu Ma, Xichuan Li, and Junhua Gu. 2020. "PPAI: A Web Server for Predicting Protein-Aptamer Interactions." *BMC Bioinformatics* 21 (1): 236. https://doi.org/10.1186/s12859-020-03574-7.

Li, Jing, Anmin Wang, Xiaohai Yang, Kemin Wang, and Jin Huang. 2021. "Orderly Assembled, Self-Powered FRET Flares for MicroRNA Imaging in Live Cells." *Analytical Chemistry* 93 (15): 6270–6277. https://doi.org/10.1021/acs.analchem.1c00873.

Li, Yapiao, and Qiang Zhao. 2019. "Aptamer Structure Switch Fluorescence Anisotropy Assay for Small Molecules Using Streptavidin as an Effective Signal Amplifier Based on Proximity Effect." *Analytical Chemistry* 91 (11): 7379–7384. https://doi.org/10.1021/acs.analchem.9b01253.

Li, Yongsheng, Xiaoyan Zhou, and Duyun Ye. 2008. "Molecular Beacons: An Optimal Multifunctional Biological Probe." *Biochemical and Biophysical Research Communications* 373 (4): 457–461. https://doi.org/https://doi.org/10.1016/j.bbrc.2008.05.038.

Li, Zhanhong, Mona A Mohamed, A M Vinu Mohan, Zhigang Zhu, Vinay Sharma, Geetesh K Mishra, and Rupesh K Mishra. 2019. "Application of Electrochemical Aptasensors toward Clinical Diagnostics, Food, and Environmental Monitoring: Review." *Sensors (Basel, Switzerland)* 19 (24). https://doi.org/10.3390/s19245435.

Li, Zhefeng, Linlin Yang, Hongzhi Wang, Daniel W Binzel, Terence M Williams, and Peixuan Guo. 2021. "Non-Small-Cell Lung Cancer Regression by SiRNA Delivered Through Exosomes That Display EGFR RNA Aptamer." *Nucleic Acid Therapeutics* 31 (5): 364–374. https://doi.org/10.1089/nat.2021.0002.

Lin, Bingqian, Tian Tian, Yinzhu Lu, Dan Liu, Mengjiao Huang, Lin Zhu, Zhi Zhu, Yanling Song, and Chaoyong Yang. 2021. "Tracing Tumor-Derived Exosomal PD-L1 by Dual-Aptamer Activated Proximity-Induced Droplet Digital PCR." *Angewandte Chemie (International Ed. in English)* 60 (14): 7582–7586. https://doi.org/10.1002/anie.202015628.

Liu, Fei, Yong Tai, and Jiqing Ma. 2018. "LncRNA NEAT1/Let-7a-5p Axis Regulates the Cisplatin Resistance in Nasopharyngeal Carcinoma by Targeting Rsf-1 and Modulating the Ras-MAPK Pathway." *Cancer Biology & Therapy* 19 (6): 534–542. https://doi.org/1 0.1080/15384047.2018.1450119.

Liu, Jumei, Ye Zhang, Qianwen Zhao, Bo Situ, Jiamin Zhao, Shihua Luo, Bo Li, et al. 2018. "Bifunctional Aptamer-Mediated Catalytic Hairpin Assembly for the Sensitive and Homogenous Detection of Rare Cancer Cells." *Analytica Chimica Acta* 1029 (October): 58–64. https://doi.org/10.1016/j.aca.2018.04.068.

Liu, Yanfei, Ting Jiang, and Zhenbao Liu. 2022. "Metal-Organic Frameworks for Bioimaging: Strategies and Challenges." *Nanotheranostics* 6 (2): 143–160. https://doi.org/10.7150/ntno.63458.

Luo, Jian, Subash C B Gopinath, Sreeramanan Subramaniam, and Zaifeng Wu. 2022. "Arthritis Biosensing: Aptamer-Antibody-Mediated Identification of Biomarkers by ELISA." *Process Biochemistry* 121: 396–402. https://doi.org/https://doi.org/10.1016/j.procbio.2022.07.022.

Ma, Li, Ferenc Reinhardt, Elizabeth Pan, Jürgen Soutschek, Balkrishen Bhat, Eric G Marcusson, Julie Teruya-Feldstein, George W Bell, and Robert A Weinberg. 2010. "Therapeutic Silencing of MiR-10b Inhibits Metastasis in a Mouse Mammary Tumor Model." *Nature Biotechnology* 28 (4): 341–347. https://doi.org/10.1038/nbt.1618.

Macdonald, Joanna, Justin Henri, Lynda Goodman, Dongxi Xiang, Wei Duan, and Sarah Shigdar. 2017. "Development of a Bifunctional Aptamer Targeting the Transferrin Receptor and EpCAM for the Treatment of Brain Cancer Metastases." *ACS Chemical Neuroscience* 8 (4): 777–784. https://doi.org/10.1021/acschemneuro.6b00369.

Maehashi, Kenzo, and Kazuhiko Matsumoto. 2009. "Label-Free Electrical Detection Using Carbon Nanotube-Based Biosensors." *Sensors (Basel, Switzerland)* 9 (7): 5368–5378. https://doi.org/10.3390/s90705368.

Manandhar, Yasodha, Wei Wang, Jin Inoue, Nobuhiro Hayashi, Takanori Uzawa, Yutaka Ito, Toshiro Aigaki, and Yoshihiro Ito. 2017. "Interactions of in Vitro Selected Fluorogenic Peptide Aptamers with Calmodulin." *Biotechnology Letters* 39 (3): 375–382. https://doi.org/10.1007/s10529-016-2257-2.

Mattes, Joerg, Ming Yang, and Paul S Foster. 2007. "Regulation of MicroRNA by Antagomirs: A New Class of Pharmacological Antagonists for the Specific Regulation of Gene Function?" *American Journal of Respiratory Cell and Molecular Biology* 36 (1): 8–12. https://doi.org/10.1165/rcmb.2006-0227TR.

McCauley, Thomas G, Nobuko Hamaguchi, and Martin Stanton. 2003. "Aptamer-Based Biosensor Arrays for Detection and Quantification of Biological Macromolecules." *Analytical Biochemistry* 319 (2): 244–250. https://doi.org/10.1016/s0003-2697(03)00297-5.

Mi, Jing, Partha Ray, Jenny Liu, Chien-Tsun Kuan, Jennifer Xu, David Hsu, Bruce A Sullenger, Rebekah R White, and Bryan M Clary. 2016. "In Vivo Selection Against Human Colorectal Cancer Xenografts Identifies an Aptamer That Targets RNA Helicase Protein DHX9." *Molecular Therapy. Nucleic Acids* 5 (4): e315. https://doi.org/10.1038/mtna.2016.27.

Miyachi, Yusuke, Nobuaki Shimizu, Chiaki Ogino, and Akihiko Kondo. 2010. "Selection of DNA Aptamers Using Atomic Force Microscopy." *Nucleic Acids Research* 38 (4): e21. https://doi.org/10.1093/nar/gkp1101.

Mo, Tong, Xiyu Liu, Yiqun Luo, Liping Zhong, Zhikun Zhang, Tong Li, Lu Gan, et al. 2022. "Aptamer-Based Biosensors and Application in Tumor Theranostics." *Cancer Science* 113 (1): 7–16. https://doi.org/10.1111/cas.15194.

New, Roger R C, Tam T T Bui, and Michal Bogus. 2020. "Binding Interactions of Peptide Aptamers." *Molecules* 25 (24). https://doi.org/10.3390/molecules25246055.

Ng, Eugene W M, David T Shima, Perry Calias, Emmett T Jr Cunningham, David R Guyer, and Anthony P Adamis. 2006. "Pegaptanib, a Targeted Anti-VEGF Aptamer for Ocular Vascular Disease." *Nature Reviews. Drug Discovery* 5 (2): 123–132. https://doi.org/10.1038/nrd1955.

Nishihira, Akifumi, Hiroaki Ozaki, Masayuki Wakabayashi, Masayasu Kuwahara, and Hiroaki Sawai. 2004. "Detection of Biomolecule by Aptamer Beacon." *Nucleic Acids Symposium Series (2004)* (48): 135–136. https://doi.org/10.1093/nass/48.1.135.

Nitsche, Andreas, Andreas Kurth, Anna Dunkhorst, Oliver Pänke, Hendrik Sielaff, Wolfgang Junge, Doreen Muth, et al. 2007. "One-Step Selection of Vaccinia Virus-Binding DNA Aptamers by MonoLEX." *BMC Biotechnology* 7 (1): 48. https://doi.org/10.1186/1472-6750-7-48.

Oh, Seung Soo, Jiangrong Qian, Xinhui Lou, Yanting Zhang, Yi Xiao, and H Tom Soh. 2009. "Generation of Highly Specific Aptamers via Micromagnetic Selection." *Analytical Chemistry* 81 (13): 5490–5495. https://doi.org/10.1021/ac900759k.

Ohuchi, Shoji P, Takashi Ohtsu, and Yoshikazu Nakamura. 2006. "Selection of RNA Aptamers against Recombinant Transforming Growth Factor-Beta Type III Receptor Displayed on Cell Surface." *Biochimie* 88 (7): 897–904. https://doi.org/10.1016/j.biochi.2006.02.004.

Park, Ji Hoon, Min Hyeok Jee, Oh Sung Kwon, Sun Ju Keum, and Sung Key Jang. 2013. "Infectivity of Hepatitis C Virus Correlates with the Amount of Envelope Protein E2: Development of a New Aptamer-Based Assay System Suitable for Measuring the Infectious Titer of HCV." *Virology* 439 (1): 13–22. https://doi.org/10.1016/j.virol.2013.01.014.

Park, Seung-Min, Ji-Young Ahn, Minjoung Jo, Dong-Ki Lee, John T Lis, Harold G Craighead, and Soyoun Kim. 2009. "Selection and Elution of Aptamers Using Nanoporous Sol-Gel Arrays with Integrated Microheaters." *Lab on a Chip* 9 (9): 1206–1212. https://doi.org/10.1039/b814993c.

Park, Yeonkyung, Junhyeok Yoon, Jinhwan Lee, Seoyoung Lee, and Hyun Gyu Park. 2022. "Multiplexed MiRNA Detection Based on Target-Triggered Transcription of Multicolor Fluorogenic RNA Aptamers." *Biosensors & Bioelectronics* 204 (May): 114071. https://doi.org/10.1016/j.bios.2022.114071.

Percze, Krisztina, Zoltán Szakács, Éva Scholz, Judit András, Zsuzsanna Szeitner, Corné H van den Kieboom, Gerben Ferwerda, Marien I de Jonge, Róbert E Gyurcsányi, and Tamás Mészáros. 2017. "Aptamers for Respiratory Syncytial Virus Detection." *Scientific Reports* 7 (February): 42794. https://doi.org/10.1038/srep42794.

Pi, Fengmei, Daniel W Binzel, Tae Jin Lee, Zhefeng Li, Meiyan Sun, Piotr Rychahou, Hui Li, et al. 2018. "Nanoparticle Orientation to Control RNA Loading and Ligand Display on Extracellular Vesicles for Cancer Regression." *Nature Nanotechnology* 13 (1): 82–89. https://doi.org/10.1038/s41565-017-0012-z.

Plach, Maximilian, and Thomas Schubert. 2020. "Biophysical Characterization of Aptamer-Target Interactions." *Advances in Biochemical Engineering/Biotechnology* 174: 1–15. https://doi.org/10.1007/10_2019_103.

Qin, Lianhua, Ruijuan Zheng, Zhanzhong Ma, Yonghong Feng, Zhonghua Liu, Hua Yang, Jie Wang, et al. 2009. "The Selection and Application of SsDNA Aptamers against MPT64 Protein in Mycobacterium Tuberculosis." *Clinical Chemistry and Laboratory Medicine* 47 (4): 405–411. https://doi.org/10.1515/CCLM.2009.097.

Qiu, Liping, Li Qiu, Zai-Sheng Wu, Guoli Shen, and Ru-Qin Yu. 2013. "Cooperative Amplification-Based Electrochemical Sensor for the Zeptomole Detection of Nucleic Acids." *Analytical Chemistry* 85 (17): 8225–8231. https://doi.org/10.1021/ac401300a.

Rabiee, Navid, Sepideh Ahmadi, Zeynab Arab, Mojtaba Bagherzadeh, Moein Safarkhani, Behzad Nasseri, Mohammad Rabiee, Mohammadreza Tahriri, Thomas J Webster, and Lobat Tayebi. 2020. "Aptamer Hybrid Nanocomplexes as Targeting Components for Antibiotic/Gene Delivery Systems and Diagnostics: A Review." *International Journal of Nanomedicine* 15: 4237–4256. https://doi.org/10.2147/IJN.S248736.

Sadiq, Mohammad Ali, Mostafa Hanout, Salman Sarwar, Muhammad Hassan, Aniruddha Agarwal, Yasir Jamal Sepah, Diana V Do, and Quan Dong Nguyen. 2016. "Platelet-Derived Growth Factor Inhibitors: A Potential Therapeutic Approach for Ocular Neovascularization." *Developments in Ophthalmology* 55: 310–316. https://doi.org/10.1159/000438953.

Shelley, Greg, Jinlu Dai, Jill M Keller, and Evan T Keller. 2021. "Pheno-SELEX: Engineering Anti-Metastatic Aptamers through Targeting the Invasive Phenotype Using Systemic Evolution of Ligands by Exponential Enrichment." *Bioengineering (Basel, Switzerland)* 8 (12). https://doi.org/10.3390/bioengineering8120212.

Shen, Luyao, Tao Bing, Xiangjun Liu, Junyan Wang, Linlin Wang, Nan Zhang, and Dihua Shangguan. 2018. "Flow Cytometric Bead Sandwich Assay Based on a Split Aptamer." *ACS Applied Materials & Interfaces* 10 (3): 2312–2318. https://doi.org/10.1021/acsami.7b16192.

Shu, Dan, Hui Li, Yi Shu, Gaofeng Xiong, William E 3rd Carson, Farzin Haque, Ren Xu, and Peixuan Guo. 2015. "Systemic Delivery of Anti-MiRNA for Suppression of Triple Negative Breast Cancer Utilizing RNA Nanotechnology." *ACS Nano* 9 (10): 9731–9740. https://doi.org/10.1021/acsnano.5b02471.

Sinsimer, Daniel, Surbhi Leekha, Steven Park, Salvatore A E Marras, Larry Koreen, Barbara Willey, Steve Naidich, Kimberlee A Musser, and Barry N Kreiswirth. 2005. "Use of a Multiplex Molecular Beacon Platform for Rapid Detection of Methicillin and Vancomycin Resistance in Staphylococcus Aureus." *Journal of Clinical Microbiology* 43 (9): 4585–4591. https://doi.org/10.1128/JCM.43.9.4585-4591.2005.

Sitkov, Nikita, Tatiana Zimina, Alexander Kolobov, Vladimir Karasev, Alexander Romanov, Viktor Luchinin, and Dmitry Kaplun. 2021. "Toward Development of a Label-Free Detection Technique for Microfluidic Fluorometric Peptide-Based Biosensor Systems." *Micromachines* 12 (6). https://doi.org/10.3390/mi12060691.

Souza, Aline G, Karina Marangoni, Patrícia T Fujimura, Patrícia T Alves, Márcio J Silva, Victor Alexandre F Bastos, Luiz R Goulart, and Vivian A Goulart. 2016. "3D Cell-SELEX: Development of RNA Aptamers as Molecular Probes for PC-3 Tumor Cell Line." *Experimental Cell Research* 341 (2): 147–156. https://doi.org/10.1016/j.yexcr.2016.01.015.

Stojanovic, Milan N, and Dmitry M Kolpashchikov. 2004. "Modular Aptameric Sensors." *Journal of the American Chemical Society* 126 (30): 9266–9270. https://doi.org/10.1021/ja032013t.

Stoltenburg, R, C Reinemann, and B Strehlitz. 2005. "FluMag-SELEX as an Advantageous Method for DNA Aptamer Selection." *Analytical and Bioanalytical Chemistry* 383 (1): 83–91. https://doi.org/10.1007/s00216-005-3388-9.

Suarez-Carmona, Meggy, Anja Williams, Jutta Schreiber, Nicolas Hohmann, Ulrike Pruefer, Jürgen Krauss, Dirk Jäger, et al. 2021. "Combined Inhibition of CXCL12 and PD-1 in MSS Colorectal and Pancreatic Cancer: Modulation of the Microenvironment and Clinical Effects." *Journal for Immunotherapy of Cancer* 9 (10). https://doi.org/10.1136/jitc-2021-002505.

Sussman, Django, Jay C Nix, and Charles Wilson. 2000. "The Structural Basis for Molecular Recognition by the Vitamin B 12 RNA Aptamer." *Nature Structural Biology* 7 (1): 53–57. https://doi.org/10.1038/71253.

Thean, D, J S Ebo, T Luxton, Xue'Er Cheryl Lee, T Y Yuen, F J Ferrer, C W Johannes, D P Lane, and C J Brown. 2017. "Enhancing Specific Disruption of Intracellular Protein Complexes by Hydrocarbon Stapled Peptides Using Lipid Based Delivery." *Scientific Reports* 7 (1): 1763. https://doi.org/10.1038/s41598-017-01712-5.

Toepfner, Nicole, Christoph Herold, Oliver Otto, Philipp Rosendahl, Angela Jacobi, Martin Kräter, Julia Stächele, et al. 2018. "Detection of Human Disease Conditions by Single-Cell Morpho-Rheological Phenotyping of Blood." *ELife* 7 (January). https://doi.org/10.7554/eLife.29213.

Tuerk, Craig, and Larry Gold. 1990. "Systematic Evolution of Ligands by Exponential Enrichment: RNA Ligands to Bacteriophage T4 DNA Polymerase." *Science (New York, N.Y.)* 249 (4968): 505–510. https://doi.org/10.1126/science.2200121.

Ueki, Ryosuke, Saki Atsuta, Ayaka Ueki, Junya Hoshiyama, Jingyue Li, Yohei Hayashi, and Shinsuke Sando. 2019. "DNA Aptamer Assemblies as Fibroblast Growth Factor Mimics and Their Application in Stem Cell Culture." *Chemical Communications (Cambridge, England)* 55 (18): 2672–2675. https://doi.org/10.1039/c8cc08080a.

Ulrich, Henning, Margaret H Magdesian, Maria Julia M Alves, and Walter Colli. 2002. "In Vitro Selection of RNA Aptamers That Bind to Cell Adhesion Receptors of Trypanosoma Cruzi and Inhibit Cell Invasion." *The Journal of Biological Chemistry* 277 (23): 20756–20762. https://doi.org/10.1074/jbc.M111859200.

Valero, Julián, Laia Civit, Daniel M Dupont, Denis Selnihhin, Line S Reinert, Manja Idorn, Brett A Israels, et al. 2021. "A Serum-Stable RNA Aptamer Specific for SARS-CoV-2 Neutralizes Viral Entry." *Proceedings of the National Academy of Sciences of the United States of America* 118 (50). https://doi.org/10.1073/pnas.2112942118.

Wang, Anmin, Qing Lin, Shiyuan Liu, Jing Li, Jiaoli Wang, Ke Quan, Xiaohai Yang, Jin Huang, and Kemin Wang. 2020. "Aptamer-Tethered Self-Assembled FRET-Flares for MicroRNA Imaging in Living Cancer Cells." *Chemical Communications* 56 (16): 2463–2466. https://doi.org/10.1039/C9CC09919K.

Wang, Chao, Linlin Sun, and Qiang Zhao. 2019. "A Simple Aptamer Molecular Beacon Assay for Rapid Detection of Aflatoxin B1." *Chinese Chemical Letters* 30 (5): 1017–1020. https://doi.org/https://doi.org/10.1016/j.cclet.2019.01.029.

Wang, Jin, Jinyun Chen, and Subrata Sen. 2016. "MicroRNA as Biomarkers and Diagnostics." *Journal of Cellular Physiology* 231 (1): 25–30. https://doi.org/10.1002/jcp.25056.

Wang, Ronghui, Jingjing Zhao, Tieshan Jiang, Young M Kwon, Huaguang Lu, Peirong Jiao, Ming Liao, and Yanbin Li. 2013. "Selection and Characterization of DNA Aptamers for Use in Detection of Avian Influenza Virus H5N1." *Journal of Virological Methods* 189 (2): 362–369. https://doi.org/10.1016/j.jviromet.2013.03.006.

Wang, Wenjing, Fei Zhai, Fupei Xu, and Min Jia. 2022. "Enzyme-Free Amplified and One-Step Rapid Detection of Bisphenol A Using Dual-Terminal Labeled Split Aptamer Probes." *Microchemical Journal* 183: 107977. https://doi.org/https://doi.org/10.1016/j.microc.2022.107977.

Wang, Zhile, Shenfei Zong, Yujie Wang, Na Li, Lang Li, Ju Lu, Zhuyuan Wang, Baoan Chen, and Yiping Cui. 2018. "Screening and Multiple Detection of Cancer Exosomes Using an SERS-Based Method." *Nanoscale* 10 (19): 9053–9062. https://doi.org/10.1039/C7NR09162A.

Weaver, Simon D, and Rebecca J Whelan. 2021. "Characterization of DNA Aptamer-Protein Binding Using Fluorescence Anisotropy Assays in Low-Volume, High-Efficiency Plates." *Analytical Methods : Advancing Methods and Applications* 13 (10): 1302–1307. https://doi.org/10.1039/d0ay02256j.

Weber, Jessica A, David H Baxter, Shile Zhang, David Y Huang, Kuo How Huang, Ming Jen Lee, David J Galas, and Kai Wang. 2010. "The MicroRNA Spectrum in 12 Body Fluids." *Clinical Chemistry* 56 (11): 1733–1741. https://doi.org/10.1373/clinchem.2010.147405.

Wiraja, Christian, David Yeo, Daniel Lio, Louai Labanieh, Mengrou Lu, Weian Zhao, and Chenjie Xu. 2014. "Aptamer Technology for Tracking Cells' Status & Function." *Molecular and Cellular Therapies* 2: 33. https://doi.org/10.1186/2052-8426-2-33.

Wu, Lingling, Yidi Wang, Xing Xu, Yilong Liu, Bingqian Lin, Mingxia Zhang, Jialu Zhang, Shuang Wan, Chaoyong Yang, and Weihong Tan. 2021. "Aptamer-Based Detection of Circulating Targets for Precision Medicine." *Chemical Reviews* 121 (19): 12035–12105. https://doi.org/10.1021/acs.chemrev.0c01140.

Xu, Weichen, and Yi Lu. 2010. "Label-Free Fluorescent Aptamer Sensor Based on Regulation of Malachite Green Fluorescence." *Analytical Chemistry* 82 (2): 574–578. https://doi.org/10.1021/ac9018473.

Xu, Zhiyuan, Ronghua Ni, and Yun Chen. 2019. "Targeting Breast Cancer Stem Cells by a Self-Assembled, Aptamer-Conjugated DNA Nanotrain with Preloading Doxorubicin." *International Journal of Nanomedicine* 14: 6831–6842. https://doi.org/10.2147/IJN.S200482.

Yáñez-Mó, María, Pia R-M Siljander, Zoraida Andreu, Apolonija Bedina Zavec, Francesc E Borràs, Edit I Buzas, Krisztina Buzas, et al. 2015. "Biological Properties of Extracellular Vesicles and Their Physiological Functions." *Journal of Extracellular Vesicles* 4: 27066. https://doi.org/10.3402/jev.v4.27066.

Yang, Ge, Ziyue Li, Irfan Mohammed, Liping Zhao, Wei Wei, Haihua Xiao, Weisheng Guo, Yongxiang Zhao, Feng Qu, and Yuanyu Huang. 2021. "Identification of SARS-CoV-2-against Aptamer with High Neutralization Activity by Blocking the RBD Domain of Spike Protein 1." *Signal Transduction and Targeted Therapy* 6, Article number 227. https://doi.org/10.1038/s41392-021-00649-6.

Zeng, Yi-Bin, Zuo-Chong Yu, Yan-Ni He, Tong Zhang, Ling-Bo Du, Yin-Mei Dong, Huai-Wen Chen, Ying-Ying Zhang, and Wu-Qing Wang. 2018. "Salinomycin-Loaded Lipid-Polymer Nanoparticles with Anti-CD20 Aptamers Selectively Suppress Human CD20+ Melanoma Stem Cells." *Acta Pharmacologica Sinica* 39 (2): 261–274. https://doi.org/10.1038/aps.2017.166.

Zhang, Duo, Heedoo Lee, Ziwen Zhu, Jasleen K Minhas, and Yang Jin. 2017. "Enrichment of Selective MiRNAs in Exosomes and Delivery of Exosomal MiRNAs in Vitro and in Vivo." *American Journal of Physiology. Lung Cellular and Molecular Physiology* 312 (1): L110–L121. https://doi.org/10.1152/ajplung.00423.2016.

Zhang, Jie, Xing Yu Wang, Yi Hui Wang, Dan Dan Wang, Zhen Song, Chang Dong Zhang, and Huai Song Wang. 2020. "Colorable Zeolitic Imidazolate Frameworks for Colorimetric Detection of Biomolecules." *Analytical Chemistry* 92 (18): 12670–12677. https://doi.org/10.1021/acs.analchem.0c02895.

Zhang, Zhang, Li Zhang, Youqiang Wang, Juan Yao, Ting Wang, Zhi Weng, Liu Yang, and Guoming Xie. 2021. "Ultrasensitive Electrochemical Biosensor for Attomolar Level Detection of Let 7a Based on Toehold Mediated Strand Displacement Reaction Circuits and Molecular Beacon Mediated Circular Strand Displacement Polymerization." *Analytica Chimica Acta* 1147 (February): 108–115. https://doi.org/10.1016/j.aca.2020.12.057.

Zhang, Zijie, Olatunji Oni, and Juewen Liu. 2017. "New Insights into a Classic Aptamer: Binding Sites, Cooperativity and More Sensitive Adenosine Detection." *Nucleic Acids Research* 45 (13): 7593–7601. https://doi.org/10.1093/nar/gkx517.

Zhao, Xianxian, Wenqing Zhang, Xiaopei Qiu, Qiang Mei, Yang Luo, and Weiling Fu. 2020. "Rapid and Sensitive Exosome Detection with CRISPR/Cas12a." *Analytical and Bioanalytical Chemistry* 412 (3): 601–609. https://doi.org/10.1007/s00216-019-02211-4.

Zheng, Cheng, Xuemei Hu, Shujuan Sun, Lingye Zhu, Ning Wang, Jing Zhang, Guoqiao Huang, et al. 2022. "Hairpin Allosteric Molecular Beacons-Based Cascaded Amplification for Effective Detection of Lung Cancer-Associated MicroRNA." *Talanta* 244 (July): 123412. https://doi.org/10.1016/j.talanta.2022.123412.

Zhong, Zitao, Xiaomei Gao, Ran Gao, and Li Jia. 2018. "Selective Capture and Sensitive Fluorometric Determination of Pseudomonas Aeruginosa by Using Aptamer Modified Magnetic Nanoparticles." *Microchimica Acta* 185 (8): 377. https://doi.org/10.1007/s00604-018-2914-3.

Ziółkowski, Robert, Marta Jarczewska, Łukasz Górski, and Elżbieta Malinowska. 2021. "From Small Molecules Toward Whole Cells Detection: Application of Electrochemical Aptasensors in Modern Medical Diagnostics." *Sensors (Basel, Switzerland)* 21 (3). https://doi.org/10.3390/s21030724.

Ziółkowski, Robert, Sławomir Oszwałdowski, Katarzyna Zacharczuk, Aleksandra Zasada, and Elżbieta Malinowska. 2018. "Electrochemical Detection of Bacillus Anthracis Protective Antigen Gene Using DNA Biosensor Based on Stem–Loop Probe." *Journal of The Electrochemical Society* 165 (January): B187–B195. https://doi.org/10.1149/2.0551805jes.

8 Microfluidics-enabled aptamer-based sensing devices – the aptafluidics microdevices

Vishal K. Sahu, Amit Ranjan, A.S.M. Shailaja, Jyotirmoi Aich, and Soumya Basu

8.1 INTRODUCTION

Aptasensors coupled with microfluidics (Aptafluidics) utilize the micro behaviour of fluids for qualitative, quantitative, and semi-quantitative analysis using aptamers as a recognition element that interacts with the transducer elements such as molecules or metals present in the media and environmental factors.

Microfluidics is a study to control the behaviour of fluids at a very minute scale, millilitre to femtoliter, where surface forces like surface tension, energy dissipation, and fluid resistance, dominate over volumetric forces responsible for physical behaviour in macrofluidics (Menz & Guber, 1994). It is widespread and has attracted interdisciplinary domains pertaining to basic sciences (physics, chemistry, and biology) to advanced applied sciences (nanotechnology, biotechnology, engineering, and information technology).

Microfluidics was developed in the 1980s and has been used for a diverse range of purposes, from inkjet print heads to manufacturing DNA chips, LOC, organs-on-chip, micro propulsion, and microthermal technologies. In the field of Life Sciences, microfluidics has revolutionized diagnostics devices in terms of precision, size, and time consumption. The study deals with fluids at a very small scale and in small quantities to manufacture small-sized flexible devices for personalized solutions, and medical, and industrial usage (Cai et al., 2022). Microfluidic systems, in general, use multiplexing to transport and process data across media.

Microfluidics-enabled aptasensors (MeAS or Aptafluidics microdevices) can be developed with or without an energy requirement for fluid transport. Microfluidics with no energy requirement or passive microfluidics is based on the phenomena of capillary actions which depend on cohesion and adhesion properties of the fluid. Further velocity of fluid due to capillary flow is controlled with design modification of capillary tubes. Active microfluidics requires micropumps, to displace the fluid and microvalves to control the flow. Often these processes are miniaturized

DOI: 10.1201/9781003304227-8

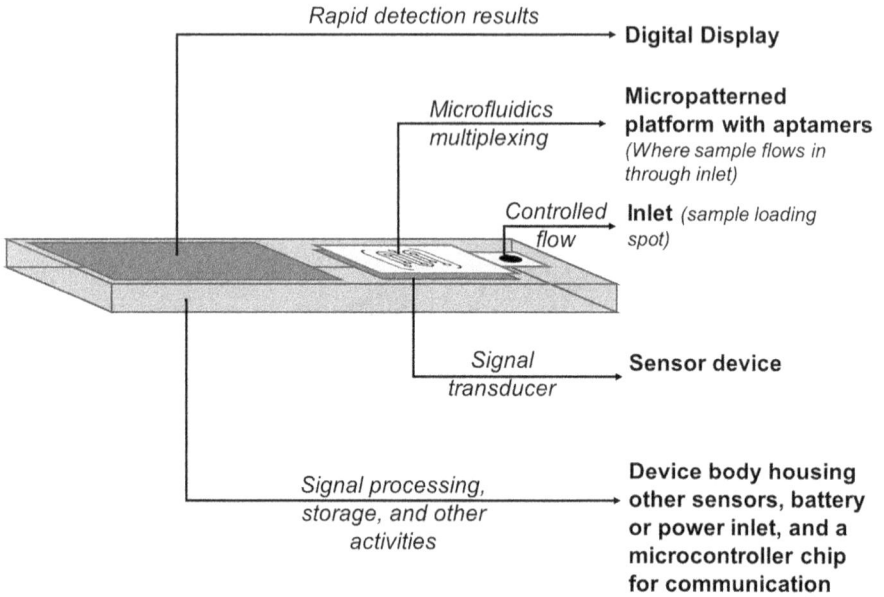

FIGURE 8.1 General diagram depicting components of miniaturized microfluidic aptasensor; it has a platform or stage where aptamers as a probe are fixed and the sample is loaded for detection through inlet, a sensor device screening for the signal by either moving the stage automatically or moving the sensor head, the signals are sent to microcontroller equipped in the device which further processes and analyses the signal, further the results can be stored or uploaded to the cloud through internet.

(Figure 8.1) on a single chip, allowing for greater efficiency and mobility while using less sample and reagent volume.

The MeAS are built on micropatterned platforms using lithography, printing, and etching techniques, and then functionalized with electronic chips on paper or glass platforms. Further, these patterns are post-processed for additional mechanical and chemical stability of the platforms.

8.2 MICROFLUIDIC PLATFORMS PATTERNING METHODS

Microdevices containing microfluidic patterns on platforms are the most important part as they provide guidance and a platform for microfluidic flow and analysis. The manufacturing methods for different microdevices vary from simple and inexpensive to complex and expensive. Inexpensive methods result in lower and usually lower resolution of patterning while costlier methods provide higher resolution of the patterns.

8.2.1 WAX PRINTING

Wax printing is the process of manufacturing paper-based MeAS where wax is printed on paper through a wax dispensing printer in the desired pattern designed using 3D paper-based microfluidic devices (µPADs) designing software. Later channels are created by melting the wax on a hotplate at around 150°C (Carrilho et al., 2009). Wax-printed design achieves fine design patterns and can be used for different assays.

8.2.2 INKJET PRINTING

To manufacture paper platforms with inkjet printing, paper is first coated with a hydrophobic layer and then subjected to chemicals in the form of ink for etching to get microfluidic patterns (Yamada et al., 2015). The basic concept of inkjet printing comes from the general inkjet printers used in offices and homes for normal printing which have multiple cartridges for different inks. Further, etching methods can be classified as dry etching or wet etching based on the principle involved by the fabricating equipment.

8.2.3 DIGITAL LIGHT PROCESSING (DLP) PRINTING

Digital Light Processing printing uses photo-curable polymers to form patterns on the platform. The DLP printing method can be used for printing the platform on both sides and the problem of evaporation can be overcome by printing additional layers. Extra polymer or resin used for fabrication can be removed using ethanol. The method is less expensive and requires readily available materials for its manufacturing (Park et al., 2018).

8.2.4 PLASMA PRINTING

The micropatterns using plasma printing can be generated using different monomers and stabilizers which can be non-toxic preferably and can readily polymerize and possess functional groups in their structures. For the plasma process, a gas (like argon or fluorocarbon) can be used with a spark discharge method known as hairline plasma to flow on the substrate from a jet nozzle controlled by a three-axis movement software. The process usually involves three steps, substrate activation through plasma, deposition of the monomer on the substrate, and plasma-based polymerization of the monomer (Barillas et al., 2020; Kao & Hsu, 2014).

8.2.5 LITHOGRAPHY

The microlithography technique is widely used for framing microdevices and microprocessors. Microfluidic chips can be manufactured using the microlithography technique (Thompson, 1983) to create a small protective pattern on a thin film on a substrate to protect the selected areas during the etching or deposition process. Various types of processes are involved in microlithography *viz.*, photolithography, electron beam lithography, nanoimprinting, interference lithography, magneto lithography, scanning probe, surface charge or diffraction lithography.

Photolithography is a modified version of the lithography technique where photo-resistant polymers are etched to obtain microfluidic patterns. The polymers on the platform are covered with a photomask and then exposed to light (Ultraviolet light) for patterning (Asano & Shiraishi, 2015). This technique achieves higher resolution but accounts for the cost of manufacturing.

8.3   DETECTION AND ANALYTICAL METHODS

Microfluidic aptasensor devices utilize the physical behaviour of fluids at a very small scale and utilize various physicochemical methods, like electrochemical, transistor, optics, and mass to build optimized biosensors.

8.3.1   Electrochemical method

Electrochemical-based techniques use electrophoretic movement of ions, biomolecules, and cells captured in the inlet and sequentially flow to the electrode for detection using a single electrochemical sensor (Hiramoto et al., 2019). In electrochemical-based detection, the occurring chemical reaction can be directly converted to an electrical signal. It involves the detection of specific variations in voltage (voltammetric detection), current (amperometry detection), or using phenomena of electrochemical impedance spectroscopy (EIS) (Khan & Song, 2020; Mahmoudpour et al., 2022). Further chains of reactions are implemented to process the sample within the device for amplification of the sample type to get an amplified signal through various techniques, hybridization chain reaction (HCR) amplification being one of them (Zhang et al., 2021a).

8.3.2   Transistor-based method

A field effect transistor (FET)-based aptafluidics device houses semiconducting channels between the source and the drain electrodes. The phenomena of adsorption of the analyte cause a change in the voltage or current applied on the medium in the channel read by the electrochemical sensor. The specific characteristics of variation by specified molecule or analyte can be characterized by the determined signal (Lu et al., 2009; Ohno et al., 2010).

8.3.3   Optical method

Optical detection methods result in visualization of the detected analyte through unaided eyes or through optical analysis devices like cameras, diodes, microscopes, or digital devices (Yildirim et al., 2012). LOC aptafluidics microdevices developed for optical detection are more efficient and quicker in detection. Optical detection involves measurements of fluorescence intensity (He et al., 2010), absorbance, luminescence, colorimetry (Zhang et al., 2016), or surface plasmon resonance (Chang, 2021; Lafleur et al., 2016). Among other optical methods, microdevices housing surface-enhanced Raman spectroscopy (SERS) (Lee et al., 2021) are miniaturized, highly sensitive for the level of trace amount, and provide very reliable solutions.

8.3.4 GRAVIMETRIC METHOD

Aptafluidics devices based on mass or gravitational forces work on the basic principle of change in the mass at the sensing surface because of the binding of an analyte to the aptamer, relying on piezoelectric quartz crystals. These crystal structures can be used as resonators or as surface acoustic waves. These sensors can be used for rapid detection of the analyte (Fu et al., 2019; Neethirajan et al., 2018; Ozalp et al., 2015).

8.4 THE DIVERSE MICROFLUIDICS PLATFORMS

Based on the platforms, microfluidics-based biosensors show a huge diversity in manufacturing, efficiency, target, and size scale that makes them suitable for their application in the development of microdevices.

8.4.1 PAPER MICROCHIPS

The paper-based MeAS contains filter papers, hydrophilic cellulose or nitrocellulose fibres, or chromatography papers that transport media through capillary action, i.e., follow phenomena of passive microfluidics or controlled flow by modifying interface wettability or tuning the geometry of the porous media (Liu et al., 2019; Ming et al., 2020; Yamada et al., 2015). With lateral flow it has been reported to detect cocaine (Wang et al., 2017), and glucose (Martinez et al., 2007). Paper-based microfluidic devices came into existence in the early twenty-first century to provide portable inexpensive medical diagnostic microdevices.

In paper-based MeAS samples are dispensed through an inlet made up of cellulose or nitrocellulose fibres which are further transported to the device through hydrophilic channels with pores with a range of millimetres. The transport is controlled for the steady state velocity of the fluid flow using the design of the device called flow amplifiers or flow resistors. The fluid is prevented from leaving the channel through hydrophobic regions known as barriers. Thus, controlled fluid is subjected to the outlet chamber where the chemical reactions take place, and the sensor scans for the signal (Xue et al., 2020).

Manufacturing of paper-based MeAS can be done through direct patterning; wax printing, inkjet printing, DLP printing, and plasma processing or indirect patterning; photolithography, etching, spraying, screen printing, or dipping (Yamada et al., 2015).

Furthermore, the platform can be integrated with electronic chips to provide micro total analysis systems (μTAS) through which automation of sample preparation to analysis is achieved.

8.4.2 GLASS OR PLASTIC-BASED MICROCHIPS

Apart from paper, micropatterns for microfluidic movement are fabricated on glass or thermoplastic platforms. Glass and plastic-based platforms are mostly fabricated on a polymeric substrate such as polydimethylsiloxane (PDMS), poly-methylmethacrylate (PMMA), polyester, polycarbonate (PC), polyethylene (PE), polystyrene

(PS) or cyclic olefin copolymer (COC) (Coltro et al., 2014). On these substrates, probes are trapped which in turn undergo conformational changes or participate in specific reactions to provide signals to the sensors (Khan & Song, 2020; Liu et al., 2022; Perréard et al., 2017).

8.5   ADVANTAGES

Aptasensors serve diverse purposes being smaller in size, showing high specificity and selectivity, and providing results promptly. The same is comparable with microarray-based cytogenetic analysis detecting thousands of probes simultaneously. In comparison to aptasensors the technique is time-consuming, costly, and requires professionals to prepare, process, and analyze the samples.

8.5.1   Rapid detection

In microfluidics fluids used are with high specificity of chemical and physical properties (i.e., pH, temperature, and shear force) which ensure a more uniform condition and higher grade aptasensors in single and multi-step (Abatemarco et al., 2017; Ozalp et al., 2015).

8.5.2   High sensitivity and selectivity

MeAS devices show excellent Limit of Detection (LoD) for small analytes like potassium to cells or organelles. A microdevice has been developed which can detect 2.5×10^3 to 1×10^7 exosomes (60–100 nm diameter extracellular vesicles) per millilitre of sample with LoD of 5×10^2 exosomes/mL (Zhang et al., 2021). Another aptafluidics device can detect *Vibrio parahaemolyticus* pathogen in the range of 10^6 CFU m/L with a LoD of 5.74 CFU m/L (Jiang et al., 2021). High sensitivity, efficiency and greater LoD are attributed to the small sample size which provides a higher surface-to-volume ratio (Khan & Song, 2020). To detect 18–22 nucleotide long microRNAs (miRNAs), Chu et al. (2021) have achieved an ultrasensitive level of detection in the attomolar (10^{-18} moles per litre) range. Their nanomaterial locally assembled microfluidic biochip can detect miRNAs in the given sample in the 1.0 aM to 10 nM range with a 0.146 aM LoD value.

8.5.3   Multiplexing of multiple signals

Microfluidics-based aptasensors may involve more than one type of fluids and they do not necessarily mix due to differences in their nature, differences in viscosity or density, thus suitable for multiplexing, a term used to indicate the process of mixing and separation of data transfer.

8.5.4   Miniaturized devices – LOC

Miniaturized design of the microfluidics has made LOC possible. These small devices are revolutionizing the field of healthcare and self-care. Aptamer-functionalized microdevices for bioanalysis (Xue et al., 2020). The prototype of the devices can be prepared on a three-dimensional (3D) modelling software printed with a 3D printer for rapid testing (Belmonte & White, 2022).

The microfluidics-based aptasensors fulfil the purpose of bringing technology within the reach of the common world as they are manufactured with probes to detect a set of specific analytes and can be operated and analyzed without the intervention of professionals or technical skills. It is cheaper than existing similar techniques like DNA Chip. By comparing different processes and steps involved (Figure 8.2) by existing medical laboratory diagnostic setups and sample analysis methods, the methods prove to be more costly though reliable than new technologies. MeAS will additionally provide benefits when a single analysis is required to be repeated. However, development costs involved in the research and development of such devices would vary to analyze the same number (1 to ~10^4) of probes or analytes. Sensor devices and other parts at low cost can be manufactured in small laboratories to develop a new kind of sensor detecting different analytes while keeping the operating procedure the same (Strong et al., 2019).

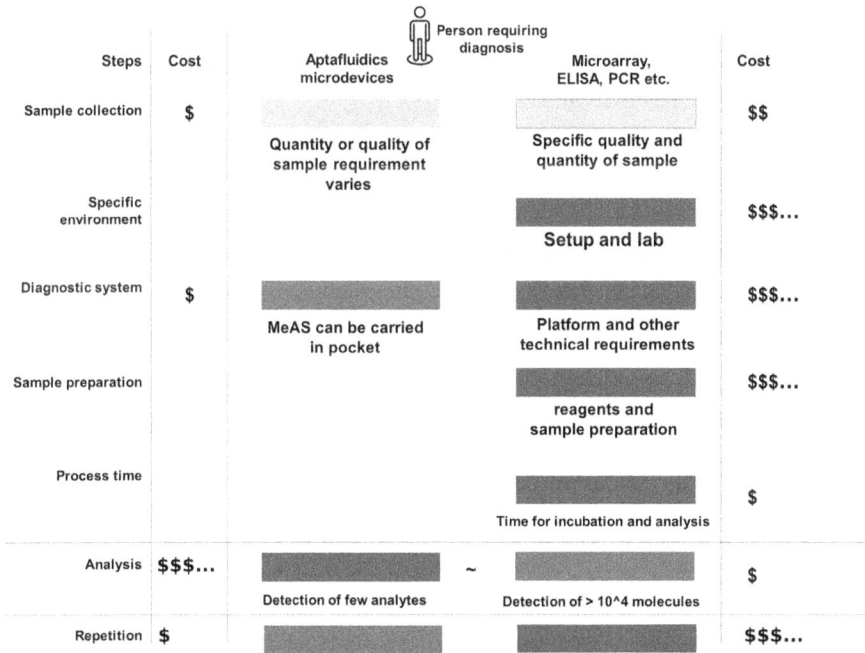

FIGURE 8.2 Comparison between aptafluidics microdevices and existing medical laboratory diagnostic techniques such as DNA microarray, ELISA, PCR, and cell culturing. The comparison is based on cost, sample analysis, and steps involved during the various techniques. Green bars and red bars compare the lower and higher costs respectively.

8.5.5 QUANTITATIVE AND QUALITATIVE DETECTION

With a very low LoD value quantitative and qualitative detection of analytes is feasible using MeAS. Detection involves label-free and labelled detection which can be visualized without aided eyes. Ochratoxin A, a type of mycotoxin can be detected and visualized on microfluidic chip platforms (Liu et al., 2015). A label-free and universal platform based on microchip electrophoresis has been developed to detect antibiotics using deploying aptamers (Zhou et al., 2017).

8.5.6 MULTIPLE ANALYTE DETECTION

MeAS can be developed with the ability to detect multiple analytes with a single probe or multiple probes housed on the chip extending the capability of the microdevices to cover a broad range of analytes. Microfluidic beads array aptasensor based on multienzyme-linked nanoparticles with quantum dot labels have been reported to detect multiple analytes simultaneously (Zhang et al., 2014). A single universal aptamer has also been developed to detect multiple strains of influenza viruses ruling out multiple tests for diagnosis (Wang et al., 2016).

8.5.7 REUSABILITY AND DISPOSABILITY

The microdevices, on completing their life-cycle can be easily disposed of and partially reused by separating their parts as electronic chips and the platforms fabricated on a glass or a plastic material. Most of the parts of these microdevices are not harmful or polluting to the environment.

8.6 APPLICATIONS OF APTAFLUIDICS MICRODEVICES (MEAS)

Microfluidics-enabled chips, well known as LOC, are widely used devices and are well explored in the field of biology, *viz.,* molecular biology, evolutionary biology, cell behaviour, cellular biophysics, optics, chromatographic techniques, fuel cells, astrobiology, and food technology. Aptasensors with microfluidics decoy the targets to achieve high precision, specificity, and real-time results. MeAS can detect or isolate viral particles, bacterial cells, tumour cells, and extracellular vesicles (exosomes) along with many biomolecular analytes with a low LoD and higher precision. Applications of aptafluidics microdevices include the detection and separation of cells, molecules, and cellular vesicles to the development and selection of new agents for biosensors.

8.6.1 WHOLE-CELL DETECTION AND SEPARATION

Influenza H1N1 virus has been detected using a sandwich-based aptamer assay in an integrated microfluidic system (Tseng et al., 2016). Bacterial cells and pathogens like *Acinetobacter baumannii* and *Vibrio parahaemolyticus* have been reported to be detected on different electrochemical-based microfluidic platforms (Jiang et al., 2021; Su et al., 2020; Yu et al., 2021). Rapid and continuous detection of microorganisms using aptamer functionalized on fluorescent nanoparticles fixed on an optofluidic platform has been achieved by Chung et al. (2015).

8.6.2 DETECTION AND EXTRACTION OF MOLECULES

8.6.2.1 Detection of biomarkers and metabolites

MeAS have been developed to detect biomolecules and metabolites that act as a biomarker for characterizing a metabolic dysregulation or disease. Aptafluidics microdevices are suitable to process and analyze biomarkers, hormones, and other biomolecules in the analyzed samples to provide rapid results and can be further subjected to artificial intelligence (AI) based analysis using the attached device to capture and analyze signals (Figure 8.3) (Son et al., 2017).

8.6.2.2 Growth factors, hormones, and other biomolecules

MeAS can detect and quantify growth factors, hormones, lysozymes, and other biomolecules (Li et al., 2010; Tseng et al., 2022). A new probe G-quadruplex-selective luminescent iridium (III) complex was used for rapid label-free quantitative determination of vascular epithelial growth factor (VEGF) (Crulhas et al., 2017; Lin et al., 2016). Vasopressin, a pituitary hormone related to renal function, was targeted, and detected without a label at very low abundance at picomolar concentration (Yang et al., 2016). In other research, cell-secreted Interferon-gamma (IFN-γ) (Qiu et al., 2017) and tumour necrosis factor-alpha (TNF-α) (Kwa et al., 2014) were detected on different platforms. Further immobilization-free electrochemical detection of cortisol, which plays a diverse regulatory role in physiological functions and stress conditions, was developed (Sanghavi et al., 2016). The advancements have the potential to

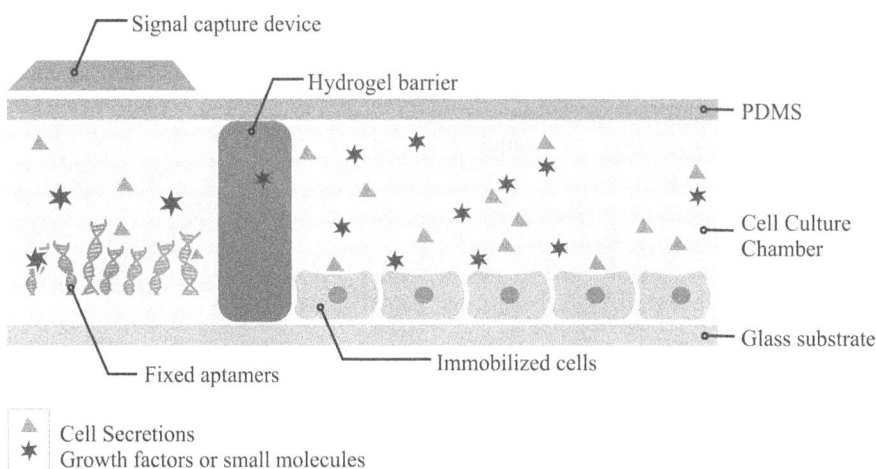

FIGURE 8.3 Design of microfluidic device for detection of cell-secreted growth factors or metabolites. The device body is separated for cell culture and fixed aptamers allowing diffusion of cell-secreted molecules through a hydrogel barrier. The molecules upon binding generate signals that can be detected by a signal capture device for further analysis.

be used for the study of intramolecular and intercellular communication and interactions to dive deep into the concept of cellular communication.

8.6.2.3 Toxins and other molecules

The real-time detection and quantification ability of the microdevices helped in developing biosensors for the detection of pesticides (Mahmoudpour et al., 2022), colorimetric determination of cocaine (Wang et al., 2017), mercury (II) ions (Liu et al., 2018), food allergens (Weng & Neethirajan, 2016), gentamicin in milk (Ramalingam et al., 2021), and mycotoxin (Liu et al., 2015). These devices have ensured the quality management of food products and lowered the cost of costly devices and procedures limited to specific laboratories. MeAS can be used for the detection and separation of biomolecules as aptasensors show precise and higher affinity towards their target. Acoustofluidic separation of proteins has been achieved using aptamer-attached microparticles (Afzal et al., 2021).

8.6.3 APTAFLUIDICS MICRODEVICES FOR CANCER

The MeAS-based diagnostics solutions for cancer have reduced the cost and detection time. The LOC has a great potential for designing novel approaches for diagnosis and monitoring treatment and follow-up of the disease. This will change the traditional experiments viz., *in vivo, ex vivo,* and *in vitro* methods for diagnosis, monitoring, and drug discovery and development (Huang et al., 2011; Silva et al., 2020).

8.6.3.1 Detection and separation of cancer cells

Symptoms of tumour generation remain dormant and are detected in critical stages after metastasis. Therefore, early diagnosis of tumour cells and biomarkers remains a challenge to defeating cancer (Crosby et al., 2022). Devices specific to cancer cell detection have been developed and are showing remarkable success (Figure 8.4) in providing early diagnosis and personalized treatment (Santiago et al., 2019). The devices can detect circulating tumour cells (Sheng et al., 2013; Zamay et al., 2017; Zhang et al., 2021, 2020;) or capture them (Song et al., 2019; Zhao et al., 2012) for monitoring of cancer progression or drug testing in Lung Carcinoma Cells. Nguyen et al. (2018) have successfully demonstrated real-time detection of migration of MDA-MB-231 cells in an electrochemical microfluidic platform. Other cell capturing and release methods have shown 83% release efficiency and 91% cell viability (Zhang et al., 2020) which have the potential for drug discovery and testing (Pulikkathodi et al., 2018; Zhang et al., 2018).

8.6.3.2 Cancer biomarkers

Diagnostic focuses on detecting a set of specific molecules or targets like miRNAs to characterize diseases or altered metabolism. Cancer is of high priority to preferably find biomarkers to characterize it for personalized treatment inexpensively. Cancer biomarkers can be detected using the MeAS (Jolly et al., 2016) along with confirmatory molecules differentially regulated in cancer (Wang et al., 2022). Epidermal growth factor receptor 2 (EGFR2) proteins quantify breast cancer biomarkers and

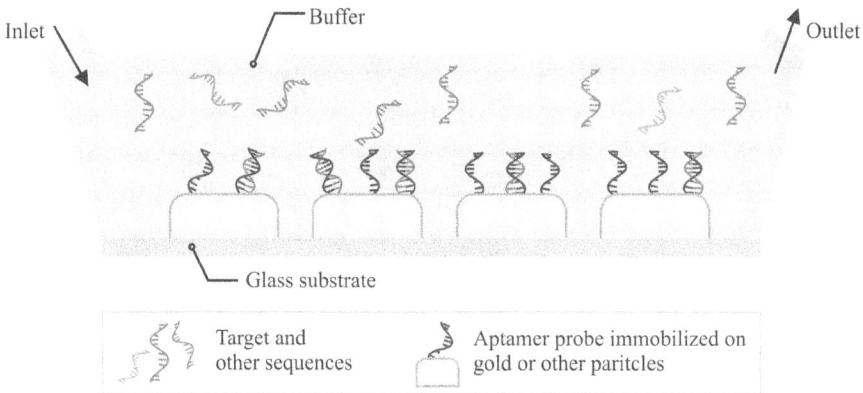

FIGURE 8.4 Circulating tumour cell detects MeAS having aptamers immobilized on a glass platform mounted with an optical detection system for real-time analysis. The captured cells can be later released by altering binding conditions.

have been successfully detected on microfluidics aptasensors in a range of 1.0 fM to 0.1 μM (Ali et al., 2016).

Differentially expressed miRNAs playing a vital role in cancer control and metastasis have gained significant focus in cancer studies. They enable the characterization of cancer types or other diseases as their expression level is studied using microarray chips, which provide accurate estimation of gene expression, however, the method is very expensive (He et al., 2013). Microfluidics-based platforms have shown significant advancement in detecting miRNAs (miR-125, miR-126, miR-191, miR-155, and miR-21) in breast cancer at attomolar concentration that promise the least expensive and highly efficient solutions in coming future (Figure 8.5) (Chu et al., 2021).

8.6.3.3 Exosomes

The role of exosomes has been well discovered (Tai et al., 2018) requiring new methods for detection and separation of exosomes in each sample for diagnostics is a need of the day. MeAS provides methods for rapid detection and isolation of exosomes to expedite research outcomes. Aptamers conjugated microfluidic biosensors have been successfully tested for improved targeting (Han et al., 2020) and detection (Chen et al., 2022; Zhang et al., 2021b).

8.6.4 DETECTION AND CHARACTERIZATION OF OTHER DISEASES

Microfluidics-enabled aptasensors (MeAS) have been proved to be a suitable candidate to provide minimally invasive solutions to diagnose a disease using least invasive or non-invasive body fluid samples. A microdevice was prototyped to detect Minimal Residual Disease (MRD) using peripheral blood of T-cell acute lymphoblastic leukemia patients (Liu et al., 2020). Additionally, antibodies formed during infectious diseases can also be detected with the MeAS (Zhou et al., 2017).

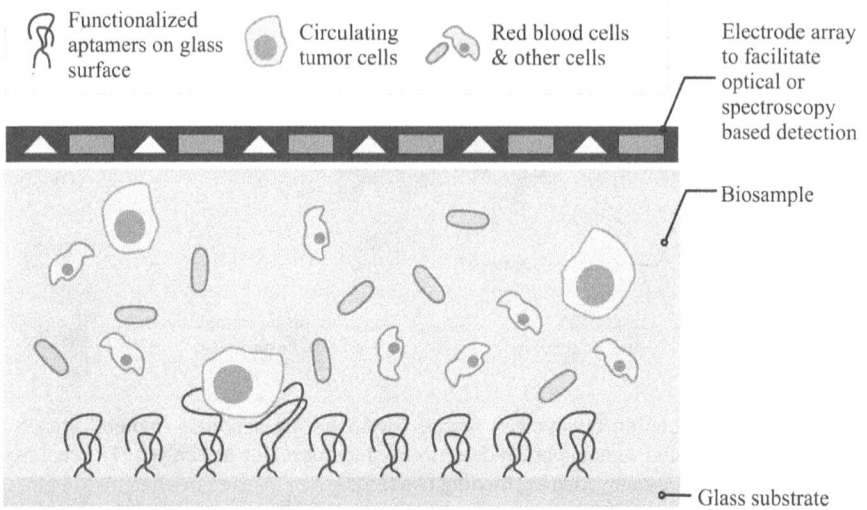

FIGURE 8.5 Aptamers immobilized on gold or other nano-particle combination fixed on a glass substrate. The device design allows the inflow of a preprocessed sample. Complementary oligomers like microRNAs as a biomarker bind specifically to aptamer probes which is further detected for their binding.

8.6.5 SCREENING AND DISCOVERY OF NEW POTENTIAL AGENTS FOR DIAGNOSTICS AND TREATMENT

Apart from detection, microfluidics technology has been deployed for aptamer selection (Liu et al., 2021). The efficient and small-sized MeAS have additional applications for discovering new potential agents for diagnostics and treatment. Aptamers are basically selected using the systematic evolution of ligands by exponential enrichment (SELEX) method (Ellington & Szostak, 1990) where these microdevices play an important role in reducing the cost and time to discover new agents (Xue et al., 2020). Single-stranded DNA (ssDNA) aptamer (Park et al., 2016), selection of DNA aptamers (Cho et al., 2010), aptamer selection optimization (Lin et al., 2021), and isolation (Kim et al., 2016) are a few exemplary achievements.

Additional applications involve cell separation or force measurements of adherent cells (Qi et al., 2022; Pawell et al., 2013; Pelletier et al., 2012), controlled study of chemical reactions (deMello, 2006), automated microfluidic parts verification (Pawell et al., 2014), and real time and continuous sampling of air, water, or other entities to detect toxins or other hazardous molecules (Jing et al., 2007).

8.7 CHALLENGES IN THE FABRICATION OF MEAS DEVICES AND PROSPECTS

Aptasensors fabricated on microfluidics platforms are highly sensitive, optimized, and show greater precision when compared to traditional and well-established devices for the same purpose. Their ability to work with very minimal sample requirements and favourable results is bundled with challenges with prospective to be improved in the near future.

1. Miniaturization comes at the cost and effectiveness of the originally devised method. With the miniaturization of circuits, electronic chips, and sensors have been decoupled or miniaturized to a significant level. By decoupling, MeAS needs to connect with the analyzing component which may be connected through the internet posing a possible threat of hacking or slightly delayed results.
2. Advancements in these microdevices increase their cost, limiting the possibilities of further development as higher cost and alternative solutions decline the demand resulting in the device remaining a proof of concept. Apart from such challenges SERS-based MeAS has been successfully employed to detect microRNAs in biological samples opening doors for cancer-specific detection devices.
3. Continuous use of the MeAS as compared to traditional methods poses fear of misguiding the diagnosis and treatment process. Traditional devices are equipped with partial self-maintenance, automated or manual calibration, and can be repaired by replacing original parts. However, microdevices may lack these functionalities in favour of cost, miniaturization, or quick diagnosis (Gowers et al., 2019).
4. Mass production and cost-effectiveness might result in higher usage of these microdevices in research and general purpose requiring further research in recycling, reusability, and safe discard of the devices as the fabricated devices contain electronics along with other chemicals.
5. The diversity of users handling the MeAS may result in biased results. As processing and handling of analytes differ among individual scholars and common users. Standard operating protocol may not be effective in such cases deviating from the purpose of MeAS. Hence, the utilization of the collection of data for machine learning studies might not be suitable for important projects.

Microfluidics-based devices enable quick development of prototypes for any variation of the analyte. These devices having prospective futures are rapidly enhanced for their ability to provide full-fledged and complete solutions in the field of diagnostics and pathology.

8.8 MEAS PATENTS

As the second decade of the twenty-first century has witnessed tremendous growth in MeAS devices, the rise in MeAS patents is also rising. Patents have been obtained for the different detection systems.

Lin et al. patented (Patent ID WO2016112079A1, year 2016) FETs-based microfluidic aptasensor including aptamer-functionalized graphene nanosensor. It additionally allows selective elution of analyte. Neethiranjan and Weng hold a patent (Patent ID US20170341077A1, year 2017) for the microdevice quantifying allergen or toxin that uses a probe with a fluorescent label applying the principle of fluorescence spectroscopy. However, the patent held by Hansang Cho (Patent ID US20100136551A1, year 2010) involves an aptamer-based detection system involving Raman active molecules. Non-invasive sample-based aptasensors have also been patented and a patent obtained by Heinkenfeld (Patent ID US20190231236A1, year 2018) uses sweat analytes involving enzymatic activity. The list is exhaustive based on detection methods, type of samples, analytes, and diseases.

8.9 CONCLUSION

Aptasensors, a highly developed category of biosensors aided with microfluidics technology, enhance the flexibility, selectivity, and precision of these microdevices. The Profound LOC concept has revolutionized diagnosis practices and enabled people with less technical knowledge to self-diagnose with the provided kit.

The role of microdevices to provide precise, efficient, and reliable solutions having excellent detection range in the droplets of samples to diagnose and characterize a disease, especially those having metabolic dysregulation, can be seen as a promising healthcare solution for all. This will ensure early diagnostics to control the diseases in their early stages.

These POC microdevices are mostly equipped with electronic chips and are connected to the internet to access the power of AI to enhance diagnostics. Being the least expensive these devices may not replace the expensive lab equipment but surely going to reduce the cost of diagnosis and the burden on the labs.

CONFLICT OF INTEREST

The authors have declared no conflict of interest.

ACKNOWLEDGEMENT

The authors are thankful to Dr. D. Y. Patil Biotechnology and Bioinformatics Institute, Dr. D. Y. Patil Vidyapeeth, Tathawade, Pune 411033, Maharashtra, India for providing research facilities. Vishal Kumar Sahu acknowledges the Council of Scientific and Industrial Research (CSIR) for Junior Research Fellowship [File No: 09/1340(11487)/2021-EMR-I].

LIST OF ABBREVATIONS

AI	Artificial intelligence
Aptafluidics	Aptasensors coupled with microfluidics
COC	Cyclic olefin copolymer
DLP	Digital light processing
DNA	Deoxyribonucleic Acid
EGFR2	Epidermal growth factor receptor 2
EIS	Electrochemical impedance spectroscopy
ELISA	Enzyme-linked immunosorbent assay

FETs	Field effect transistor
HCR	Hybridization chain reaction
IFN-γ	Interferon-gamma
LOC	Lab-on-a-chip
LoD	Limit of Detection
MeAS	Microfluidics-enabled aptasensors/Aptafluidics microdevices
MRD	Minimal Residual Disease
PC	Polycarbonate
PCR	Polymerase Chain Reaction
PDMS	Polydimethylsiloxane
PE	Polyethylene
PMMA	Poly-methyl-methacrylate
PS	Polystyrene
SELEX	Systematic evolution of ligands by exponential enrichment
SERS	Surface-enhanced Raman spectroscopy
ssDNA	Single-stranded DNA
TNF-α	Tumour necrosis factor-alpha
VEGF	Vascular epithelial growth factor
μM	Micromolar
μPADs	Microfluidic devices
μTAS	Micro total analysis systems

REFERENCES

Abatemarco, J., Sarhan, MF., Wagner, JM., Lin, JL., Liu, L., Hassouneh, W., Yuan, SF., Alper, HS., & Abate, AR. (2017). RNA-aptamers-in-droplets (RAPID) high-throughput screening for secretory phenotypes. *Nature Communications*, *8* (1). https://doi.org/10.1038/s41467-017-00425-7

Afzal, M., Park, J., Jeon, JS., Akmal, M., Yoon, TS., & Sung, HJ. (2021). Acoustofluidic separation of proteins using aptamer-functionalized microparticles. *Analytical Chemistry*, *93* (23), 8309–8317. https://doi.org/10.1021/acs.analchem.1c01198

Ali, MA., Mondal, K., Jiao, Y., Oren, S., Xu, Z., Sharma, A., & Dong, L. (2016). Microfluidic immuno-biochip for detection of breast cancer biomarkers using hierarchical composite of porous graphene and titanium dioxide nanofibers. *ACS Applied Materials & Interfaces*, *8* (32), 20570–20582. https://doi.org/10.1021/acsami.6b05648

Asano, H. & Shiraishi, Y. (2015). Development of paper-based microfluidic analytical device for iron assay using photomask printed with 3D printer for fabrication of hydrophilic and hydrophobic zones on paper by photolithography. *Analytica Chimica Acta*, *883*, 55–60. https://doi.org/10.1016/j.aca.2015.04.014

Barillas, L., Makhneva, E., Weltmann, KD., Seitz, H., & Fricke, K. (2020). Plasma printing – direct local patterning with functional polymer coatings for biosensing and microfluidics applications. *Microelectronic Engineering*, *233*, 111431. https://doi.org/10.1016/j.mee.2020.111431

Belmonte, I. & White, RJ. (2022). 3-D printed microfluidics for rapid prototyping and testing of electrochemical, aptamer-based sensor devices under flow conditions. *Analytica Chimica Acta*, *1192*, 339377. https://doi.org/10.1016/j.aca.2021.339377

Cai, T., Fang, Y., Fang, Y., Li, R., Yu, Y., & Huang, M. (2022). Electrostatic pull-in application in flexible devices: A review. *Beilstein Journal of Nanotechnology*, *13*, 390–403. https://doi.org/10.3762/bjnano.13.32

Carrilho, E., Martinez, AW., & Whitesides, GM. (2009). Understanding wax printing: A simple micropatterning process for paper-based microfluidics. *Analytical Chemistry*, *81* (16), 7091–7095. https://doi.org/10.1021/ac901071p

Chang, CC. (2021). Recent advancements in aptamer-based surface plasmon resonance biosensing strategies. *Biosensors*, *11* (7), 233. https://doi.org/10.3390/bios11070233

Chen, H., Bian, F., Guo, J., & Zhao, Y. (2022). Aptamer-functionalized barcodes in herringbone microfluidics for multiple detection of exosomes. *Small Methods*, *6* (6), 2200236. https://doi.org/10.1002/smtd.202200236

Cho, M., Xiao, Y., Nie, J., Stewart, R., Csordas, AT., Oh, SS., Thomson, JA., & Soh, HT. (2010). Quantitative selection of DNA aptamers through microfluidic selection and high-throughput sequencing. *Proceedings of the National Academy of Sciences*, *107* (35), 15373–15378. https://doi.org/10.1073/pnas.1009331107

Chu, Y., Gao, Y., Tang, W., Qiang, L., Han, Y., Gao, J., Zhang, Y., Liu, H., & Han, L. (2021). Attomolar-level ultrasensitive and multiplex microRNA detection enabled by a nanomaterial locally assembled microfluidic biochip for cancer diagnosis. *Analytical Chemistry*, *93* (12), 5129–5136. https://doi.org/10.1021/acs.analchem.0c04896

Chung, J., Kang, JS., Jurng, JS., Jung, JH., & Kim, BC. (2015). Fast and continuous microorganism detection using aptamer-conjugated fluorescent nanoparticles on an optofluidic platform. *Biosensors and Bioelectronics*, *67*, 303–308. https://doi.org/10.1016/j.bios.2014.08.039

Coltro, WKT., Cheng, CM., Carrilho, E., & Jesus, DPd. (2014). Recent advances in low-cost microfluidic platforms for diagnostic applications. *Electrophoresis*, *35* (16), 2309–2324. https://doi.org/10.1002/elps.201400006

Crosby, D., Bhatia, S., Brindle, KM., Coussens, LM., Dive, C., Emberton, M., Esener, S., Fitzgerald, RC., Gambhir, SS., Kuhn, P., Rebbeck, TR., & Balasubramanian, S. (2022). Early detection of cancer. *Science*, *375* (6586). https://doi.org/10.1126/science.aay9040

Crulhas, BP., Karpik, AE., Delella, FK., Castro, GR., & Pedrosa, VA. (2017). Electrochemical aptamer-based biosensor developed to monitor PSA and VEGF released by prostate cancer cells. *Analytical and Bioanalytical Chemistry*, *409* (29), 6771–6780. https://doi.org/10.1007/s00216-017-0630-1

deMello, AJ. (2006). Control and detection of chemical reactions in microfluidic systems. *Nature*, *442* (7101), 394–402. https://doi.org/10.1038/nature05062

Ellington, AD. & Szostak, JW. (1990). In vitro selection of RNA molecules that bind specific ligands. *Nature*, *346* (6287), 818–822. https://doi.org/10.1038/346818a0

Fu, Z., Lu, YC., & Lai, JJ. (2019). Recent advances in biosensors for nucleic acid and exosome detection. *Chonnam Medical Journal*, *55* (2), 86. https://doi.org/10.4068/cmj.2019.55.2.86

Gowers, SAN., Rogers, ML., Booth, MA., Leong, CL., Samper, IC., Phairatana, T., Jewell, SL., Pahl, C., Strong, AJ., & Boutelle, MG. (2019). Clinical translation of microfluidic sensor devices: focus on calibration and analytical robustness. *Lab on a Chip*, *19* (15), 2537–2548. https://doi.org/10.1039/C9LC00400A

Han, Z., Lv, W., Li, Y., Chang, J., Zhang, W., Liu, C., & Sun, J. (2020). Improving tumor targeting of exosomal membrane-coated polymeric nanoparticles by conjugation with aptamers. *ACS Applied Bio Materials*, *3* (5), 2666–2673. https://doi.org/10.1021/acsabm.0c00181

He, P., Oncescu, V., Lee, S., Choi, I., & Erickson, D. (2013). Label-free electrochemical monitoring of vasopressin in aptamer-based microfluidic biosensors. *Analytica Chimica Acta*, *759*, 74–80. https://doi.org/10.1016/j.aca.2012.10.038

He, S., Song, B., Li, D., Zhu, C., Qi, W., Wen, Y., Wang, L., Song, S., Fang, H., & Fan, C. (2010). A graphene nanoprobe for rapid, sensitive, and multicolor fluorescent DNA analysis. *Advanced Functional Materials*, *20* (3), 453–459. https://doi.org/10.1002/adfm.200901639

Hiramoto, K., Ino, K., Nashimoto, Y., Ito, K., & Shiku, H. (2019). Electric and electrochemical microfluidic devices for cell analysis. *Frontiers in Chemistry*, *7*. https://doi.org/10.3389/fchem.2019.00396

Huang, Y., Agrawal, B., Sun, D., Kuo, JS., & Williams, JC. (2011). Microfluidics-based devices: New tools for studying cancer and cancer stem cell migration. *Biomicrofluidics*, *5* (1), 013412. https://doi.org/10.1063/1.3555195

Jiang, H., Sun, Z., Guo, Q., & Weng, X. (2021). Microfluidic thread-based electrochemical aptasensor for rapid detection of Vibrio parahaemolyticus. *Biosensors and Bioelectronics*, *182*, 113191. https://doi.org/10.1016/j.bios.2021.113191

Jing, G., Polaczyk, A., Oerther, DB., & Papautsky, I. (2007). Development of a microfluidic biosensor for detection of environmental mycobacteria. *Sensors and Actuators B: Chemical*, *123* (1), 614–621. https://doi.org/10.1016/j.snb.2006.07.029

Jolly, P., Damborsky, P., Madaboosi, N., Soares, RRG., Chu, V., Conde, JP., Katrlik, J., & Estrela, P. (2016). DNA aptamer-based sandwich microfluidic assays for dual quantification and multi-glycan profiling of cancer biomarkers. *Biosensors and Bioelectronics*, *79*, 313–319. https://doi.org/10.1016/j.bios.2015.12.058

Kao, PK. & Hsu, CC. (2014). One-step rapid fabrication of paper-based microfluidic devices using fluorocarbon plasma polymerization. *Microfluidics and Nanofluidics*, *16* (5), 811–818. https://doi.org/10.1007/s10404-014-1347-5

Khan, NI. & Song, E. (2020). Lab-on-a-chip systems for aptamer-based biosensing. *Micromachines*, *11* (2), 220. https://doi.org/10.3390/mi11020220

Kim, J., Olsen, TR., Zhu, J., Hilton, JP., Yang, KA., Pei, R., Stojanovic, MN., & Lin, Q. (2016). Integrated microfluidic isolation of aptamers using electrophoretic oligonucleotide manipulation. *Scientific Reports*, *6* (1). https://doi.org/10.1038/srep26139

Kwa, T., Zhou, Q., Gao, Y., Rahimian, A., Kwon, L., Liu, Y., & Revzin, A. (2014). Reconfigurable microfluidics with integrated aptasensors for monitoring intercellular communication. *Lab Chip*, *14* (10), 1695–1704. https://doi.org/10.1039/c4lc00037d

Lafleur, JP., Jönsson, A., Senkbeil, S., & Kutter, JP. (2016). Recent advances in lab-on-a-chip for biosensing applications. *Biosensors and Bioelectronics*, *76*, 213–233. https://doi.org/10.1016/j.bios.2015.08.003

Lee, T., Kwon, S., Choi, HJ., Lim, H., & Lee, J. (2021). Highly sensitive and reliable microRNA detection with a recyclable microfluidic device and an easily assembled SERS substrate. *ACS Omega*, *6* (30), 19656–19664. https://doi.org/10.1021/acsomega.1c02306

Li, LD., Chen, ZB., Zhao, HT., Guo, L., & Mu, X. (2010). An aptamer-based biosensor for the detection of lysozyme with gold nanoparticles amplification. *Sensors and Actuators B: Chemical*, *149* (1), 110–115. https://doi.org/10.1016/j.snb.2010.06.015

Lin, CS., Tsai, YC., Hsu, KF., & Lee, GB. (2021). Optimization of aptamer selection on an automated microfluidic system with cancer tissues. *Lab on a Chip*, *21* (4), 725–734. https://doi.org/10.1039/d0lc01333a

Lin, X., Leung, KH., Lin, L., Lin, L., Lin, S., Leung, CH., Ma, DL., & Lin, JM. (2016). Determination of cell metabolite VEGF165 and dynamic analysis of protein–DNA interactions by combination of microfluidic technique and luminescent switch-on probe. *Biosensors and Bioelectronics*, *79*, 41–47. https://doi.org/10.1016/j.bios.2015.11.089

Liu, CW., Tsai, TC., Osawa, M., Chang, HC., & Yang, RJ. (2018). Aptamer-based sensor for quantitative detection of mercury (II) ions by attenuated total reflection surface enhanced infrared absorption spectroscopy. *Analytica Chimica Acta*, *1033*, 137–147. https://doi.org/10.1016/j.aca.2018.05.037

Liu, M., Suo, S., Wu, J., Gan, Y., Hanaor, DA., & Chen, CQ. (2019). Tailoring porous media for controllable capillary flow. *Journal of Colloid and Interface Science*, *539*, 379–387. https://doi.org/10.1016/j.jcis.2018.12.068

Liu, R., Huang, Y., Ma, Y., Jia, S., Gao, M., Li, J., Zhang, H., Xu, D., Wu, M., Chen, Y., Zhu, Z., & Yang, C. (2015). Design and synthesis of target-responsive aptamer-cross-linked hydrogel for visual quantitative detection of ochratoxin A. *ACS Applied Materials & Interfaces, 7* (12), 6982–6990. https://doi.org/10.1021/acsami.5b01120

Liu, Y., Lin, Z., Zheng, Z., Zhang, Y., & Shui, L. (2022). Accurate isolation of circulating tumor cells via a heterovalent DNA framework recognition element-functionalized microfluidic chip. *ACS Sensors, 7* (2), 666–673. https://doi.org/10.1021/acssensors.1c02692

Liu, Y., Wang, N., Chan, CW., Lu, A., Yu, Y., Zhang, G., & Ren, K. (2021). The application of microfluidic technologies in aptamer selection. *Frontiers in Cell and Developmental Biology, 9.* https://doi.org/10.3389/fcell.2021.730035

Liu, Y., Zhang, H., Du, Y., Zhu, Z., Zhang, M., Lv, Z., Wu, L., Yang, Y., Li, A., Yang, L., Song, Y., Wang, S., & Yang, C. (2020). Highly sensitive minimal residual disease detection by biomimetic multivalent aptamer nanoclimber functionalized microfluidic chip. *Small, 16* (20), 2000949. https://doi.org/10.1002/smll.202000949

Lu, G., Ocola, LE., & Chen, J. (2009). Reduced graphene oxide for room-temperature gas sensors. *Nanotechnology, 20* (44), 445502. https://doi.org/10.1088/0957-4484/20/44/445502

Mahmoudpour, M., Karimzadeh, Z., Ebrahimi, G., Hasanzadeh, M., & Dolatabadi, JEN. (2022). Synergizing functional nanomaterials with aptamers based on electrochemical strategies for pesticide detection: current status and perspectives. *Critical Reviews in Analytical Chemistry, 52* (8), 1818–1845. https://doi.org/10.1080/10408347.2021.1919987

Martinez, A., Phillips, S., Butte, M., & Whitesides, G. (2007). Patterned paper as a platform for inexpensive, low-volume, portable bioassays. *Angewandte Chemie International Edition, 46* (8), 1318–1320. https://doi.org/10.1002/anie.200603817

Menz, W. & Guber, A. (1994). Microstructure technologies and their potential in medical applications. *min – Minimally Invasive Neurosurgery, 37* (01), 21–27. https://doi.org/10.1055/s-2008-1053444

Ming, T., Luo, J., Liu, J., Sun, S., Xing, Y., Wang, H., Xiao, G., Deng, Y., Cheng, Y., Yang, Z., Jin, H., & Cai, X. (2020). Paper-based microfluidic aptasensors. *Biosensors and Bioelectronics, 170,* 112649. https://doi.org/10.1016/j.bios.2020.112649

Neethirajan, S., Ragavan, V., Weng, X., & Chand, R. (2018). Biosensors for sustainable food engineering: Challenges and perspectives. *Biosensors, 8* (1), 23. https://doi.org/10.3390/bios8010023

Nguyen, NV., Yang, CH., Liu, CJ., Kuo, CH., Wu, DC., & Jen, CP. (2018). An aptamer-based capacitive sensing platform for specific detection of lung carcinoma cells in the microfluidic chip. *Biosensors, 8* (4), 98. https://doi.org/10.3390/bios8040098

Ohno, Y., Maehashi, K., & Matsumoto, K. (2010). Label-free biosensors based on aptamer-modified graphene field-effect transistors. *Journal of the American Chemical Society, 132* (51), 18012–18013. https://doi.org/10.1021/ja108127r

Ozalp, VC., Bayramoglu, G., Erdem, Z., & Arica, MY. (2015). Pathogen detection in complex samples by quartz crystal microbalance sensor coupled to aptamer functionalized core–shell type magnetic separation. *Analytica Chimica Acta, 853,* 533–540. https://doi.org/10.1016/j.aca.2014.10.010

Park, C., Han, YD., Kim, HV., Lee, J., Yoon, HC., & Park, S. (2018). Double-sided 3D printing on paper towards mass production of three-dimensional paper-based microfluidic analytical devices (3D-PADs). *Lab on a Chip, 18* (11), 1533–1538. https://doi.org/10.1039/c8lc00367j

Park, JW., Lee, SJ., Ren, S., Lee, S., Kim, S., & Laurell, T. (2016). Acousto-microfluidics for screening of ssDNA aptamer. *Scientific Reports, 6* (1). https://doi.org/10.1038/srep27121

Pawell, RS., Inglis, DW., Barber, TJ., & Taylor, RA. (2013). Manufacturing and wetting low-cost microfluidic cell separation devices. *Biomicrofluidics, 7* (5), 056501. https://doi.org/10.1063/1.4821315

Pawell, RS., Taylor, RA., Morris, KV., & Barber, TJ. (2014). Automating microfluidic part verification. *Microfluidics and Nanofluidics*, *18* (4), 657–665. https://doi.org/10.1007/s10404-014-1464-1

Pelletier, J., Halvorsen, K., Ha, BY., Paparcone, R., Sandler, SJ., Woldringh, CL., Wong, WP., & Jun, S. (2012). Physical manipulation of the. *Proceedings of the National Academy of Sciences*, *109* (40). https://doi.org/10.1073/pnas.1208689109

Perréard, C., d'Orlyé, F., Griveau, S., Liu, B., Bedioui, F., & Varenne, A. (2017). Aptamer entrapment in microfluidic channel using one-step sol-gel process, in view of the integration of a new selective extraction phase for lab-on-a-chip. *Electrophoresis*, *38* (19), 2456–2461. https://doi.org/10.1002/elps.201600575

Pulikkathodi, AK., Sarangadharan, I., Hsu, CP., Chen, YH., Hung, LY., Lee, GY., Chyi, JI., Lee, GB., & Wang, YL. (2018). Enumeration of circulating tumour cells and investigation of cellular responses using aptamer-immobilized AlGaN/GaN high electron mobility transistor sensor array. *Sensors and Actuators B: Chemical*, *257*, 96–104. https://doi.org/10.1016/j.snb.2017.10.127

Qi, H., Hu, Z., Yang, Z., Zhang, J., Wu, JJ., Cheng, C., Wang, C., & Zheng, L. (2022). Capacitive aptasensor coupled with microfluidic enrichment for real-time detection of trace SARS-CoV-2 nucleocapsid protein. *Analytical Chemistry*, *94* (6), 2812–2819. https://doi.org/10.1021/acs.analchem.1c04296

Qiu, L., Wimmers, F., Weiden, J., Heus, HA., Tel, J., & Figdor, CG. (2017). A membrane-anchored aptamer sensor for probing IFN secretion by single cells. *Chemical Communications*, *53* (57), 8066–8069. https://doi.org/10.1039/c7cc03576d

Ramalingam, S., Collier, CM., & Singh, A. (2021). A paper-based colorimetric aptasensor for the detection of gentamicin. *Biosensors*, *11* (2), 29. https://doi.org/10.3390/bios11020029

Sanghavi, BJ., Moore, JA., Chávez, JL., Hagen, JA., Kelley-Loughnane, N., Chou, CF., & Swami, NS. (2016). Aptamer-functionalized nanoparticles for surface immobilization-free electrochemical detection of cortisol in a microfluidic device. *Biosensors and Bioelectronics*, *78*, 244–252. https://doi.org/10.1016/j.bios.2015.11.044

Santiago, GTd., Flores-Garza, BG., Tavares-Negrete, JA., Lara-Mayorga, IM., González-Gamboa, I., Zhang, YS., Rojas-Martínez, A., Ortiz-López, R., & Álvarez, MM. (2019). The tumor-on-chip: Recent advances in the development of microfluidic systems to recapitulate the physiology of solid tumors. *Materials*, *12* (18), 2945. https://doi.org/10.3390/ma12182945

Sheng, W., Chen, T., Tan, W., & Fan, ZH. (2013). Multivalent DNA nanospheres for enhanced capture of cancer cells in microfluidic devices. *ACS Nano*, *7* (8), 7067–7076. https://doi.org/10.1021/nn4023747

Silva, ACQ., Vilela, C., Santos, HA., Silvestre, AJD., & Freire, CSR. (2020). Recent trends on the development of systems for cancer diagnosis and treatment by microfluidic technology. *Applied Materials Today*, *18*, 100450. https://doi.org/10.1016/j.apmt.2019.100450

Son, KJ., Gheibi, P., Stybayeva, G., Rahimian, A., & Revzin, A. (2017). Detecting cell-secreted growth factors in microfluidic devices using bead-based biosensors. *Microsystems & Nanoengineering*, *3* (1). https://doi.org/10.1038/micronano.2017.25

Song, Y., Shi, Y., Huang, M., Wang, W., Wang, Y., Cheng, J., Lei, Z., Zhu, Z., & Yang, C. (2019). Bioinspired engineering of a multivalent aptamer-functionalized nanointerface to enhance the capture and release of circulating tumor cells. *Angewandte Chemie International Edition*, *58* (8), 2236–2240. https://doi.org/10.1002/anie.201809337

Strong, EB., Schultz, SA., Martinez, AW., & Martinez, NW. (2019). Fabrication of miniaturized paper-based microfluidic devices (microPADs). *Scientific Reports*, *9* (1). https://doi.org/10.1038/s41598-018-37029-0

Su, CH., Tsai, MH., Lin, CY., Ma, YD., Wang, CH., Chung, YD., & Lee, GB. (2020). Dual aptamer assay for detection of Acinetobacter baumannii on an electromagnetically-driven microfluidic platform. *Biosensors and Bioelectronics, 159*, 112148. https://doi.org/10.1016/j.bios.2020.112148

Tai, YL., Chen, KC., Hsieh, JT., & Shen, TL. (2018). Exosomes in cancer development and clinical applications. *Cancer Science, 109* (8), 2364–2374. https://doi.org/10.1111/cas.13697

Thompson, LF. (1983). An introduction to lithography. In LF. Thompson, CG. Willson, & MJ. Bowden (Eds.), *Introduction to microlithography* (pp. 1–13). American Chemical Society. https://doi.org/10.1021/bk-1983-0219.ch001

Tseng, CC., Lu, SY., Chen, SJ., Wang, JM., Fu, LM., & Wu, YH. (2022). Microfluidic aptasensor POC device for determination of whole blood potassium. *Analytica Chimica Acta, 1203*, 339722. https://doi.org/10.1016/j.aca.2022.339722

Tseng, YT., Wang, CH., Chang, CP., & Lee, GB. (2016). Integrated microfluidic system for rapid detection of influenza H1N1 virus using a sandwich-based aptamer assay. *Biosensors and Bioelectronics, 82*, 105–111. https://doi.org/10.1016/j.bios.2016.03.073

Wang, CH., Chang, CP., & Lee, GB. (2016). Integrated microfluidic device using a single universal aptamer to detect multiple types of influenza viruses. *Biosensors and Bioelectronics, 86*, 247–254. https://doi.org/10.1016/j.bios.2016.06.071

Wang, L., Musile, G., & McCord, BR. (2017). An aptamer-based paper microfluidic device for the colorimetric determination of cocaine. *Electrophoresis, 39* (3), 470–475. https://doi.org/10.1002/elps.201700254

Wang, Y., Rink, S., Baeumner, AJ., & Seidel, M. (2022). Microfluidic flow-injection aptamer-based chemiluminescence platform for sulfadimethoxine detection. *Microchimica Acta, 189* (3). https://doi.org/10.1007/s00604-022-05216-6

Weng, X. & Neethirajan, S. (2016). A microfluidic biosensor using graphene oxide and aptamer-functionalized quantum dots for peanut allergen detection. *Biosensors and Bioelectronics, 85*, 649–656. https://doi.org/10.1016/j.bios.2016.05.072

Xue, J., Chen, F., Bai, M., Cao, X., Fu, W., Zhang, J., & Zhao, Y. (2020). Aptamer-functionalized microdevices for bioanalysis. *ACS Applied Materials & Interfaces, 13* (8), 9402–9411. https://doi.org/10.1021/acsami.0c16138

Yamada, K., Henares, TG., Suzuki, K., & Citterio, D. (2015). Paper-based inkjet-printed microfluidic analytical devices. *Angewandte Chemie International Edition, 54* (18), 5294–5310. https://doi.org/10.1002/anie.201411508

Yang, J., Zhu, J., Pei, R., Oliver, JA., Landry, DW., Stojanovic, MN., & Lin, Q. (2016). Integrated microfluidic aptasensor for mass spectrometric detection of vasopressin in human plasma ultrafiltrate. *Analytical Methods, 8* (26), 5190–5196. https://doi.org/10.1039/C5AY02979A

Yildirim, N., Long, F., Gao, C., He, M., Shi, HC., & Gu, AZ. (2012). Aptamer-based optical biosensor for rapid and sensitive detection of 17-estradiol in water samples. *Environmental Science & Technology, 46* (6), 3288–3294. https://doi.org/10.1021/es203624w

Yu, J., Wu, H., He, L., Tan, L., Jia, Z., & Gan, N. (2021). The universal dual-mode aptasensor for simultaneous determination of different bacteria based on naked eyes and microfluidic-chip together with magnetic DNA encoded probes. *Talanta, 225*, 122062. https://doi.org/10.1016/j.talanta.2020.122062

Zamay, AS., Zamay, GS., Kolovskaya, OS., Zamay, TN., & Berezovski, MV. (2017). Aptamer-based methods for detection of circulating tumor cells and their potential for personalized diagnostics. *Advances in Experimental Medicine and Biology, 994*, 67–81. https://doi.org/10.1007/978-3-319-55947-6_3

Zhang, H., Hu, X., & Fu, X. (2014). Aptamer-based microfluidic beads array sensor for simultaneous detection of multiple analytes employing multienzyme-linked nanoparticle amplification and quantum dots labels. *Biosensors and Bioelectronics*, *57*, 22–29. https://doi.org/10.1016/j.bios.2014.01.054

Zhang, J., Lin, B., Wu, L., Huang, M., Li, X., Zhang, H., Song, J., Wang, W., Zhao, G., Song, Y., & Yang, C. (2020). DNA nanolithography enables a highly ordered recognition interface in a microfluidic chip for the efficient capture and release of circulating tumor cells. *Angewandte Chemie International Edition*, *59* (33), 14115–14119. https://doi.org/10.1002/anie.202005974

Zhang, W., Tian, Z., Yang, S., Rich, J., Zhao, S., Klingeborn, M., Huang, PH., Li, Z., Stout, A., Murphy, Q., Patz, E., Zhang, S., Liu, G., & Huang, TJ. (2021a). Electrochemical micro-aptasensors for exosome detection based on hybridization chain reaction amplification. *Microsystems & Nanoengineering*, *7* (1). https://doi.org/10.1038/s41378-021-00293-8

Zhang, X., Wei, X., Men, X., Wu, CX., Bai, JJ., Li, WT., Yang, T., Chen, ML., & Wang, JH. (2021b). Dual-multivalent-aptamer-conjugated nanoprobes for superefficient discerning of single circulating tumor cells in a microfluidic chip with inductively coupled plasma mass spectrometry detection. *ACS Applied Materials & Interfaces*, *13* (36), 43668–43675. https://doi.org/10.1021/acsami.1c11953

Zhang, Y., Gao, D., Fan, J., Nie, J., Le, S., Zhu, W., Yang, J., & Li, J. (2016). Naked-eye quantitative aptamer-based assay on paper device. *Biosensors and Bioelectronics*, *78*, 538–546. https://doi.org/10.1016/j.bios.2015.12.003

Zhang, Y., Wang, Z., Wu, L., Zong, S., Yun, B., & Cui, Y. (2018). Combining multiplex SERS nanovectors and multivariate analysis for in situ profiling of circulating tumor cell phenotype using a microfluidic chip. *Small*, *14* (20), 1704433. https://doi.org/10.1002/smll.201704433

Zhao, W., Cui, CH., Bose, S., Guo, D., Shen, C., Wong, WP., Halvorsen, K., Farokhzad, OC., Teo, GSL., Phillips, JA., Dorfman, DM., Karnik, R., & Karp, JM. (2012). Bioinspired multivalent DNA network for capture and release of cells. *Proceedings of the National Academy of Sciences*, *109* (48), 19626–19631. https://doi.org/10.1073/pnas.1211234109

Zhou, L., Gan, N., Zhou, Y., Li, T., Cao, Y., & Chen, Y. (2017). A label-free and universal platform for antibiotics detection based on microchip electrophoresis using aptamer probes. *Talanta*, *167*, 544–549. https://doi.org/10.1016/j.talanta.2017.02.061

9 Fabrication of aptamer-based electrochemical biosensor for health care monitoring

*Ayushi Singhal, Apoorva Shrivastava,
Arpana Parihar, and Raju Khan*

9.1 INTRODUCTION

The last more than two decades, aptamers and their synthesis technology systematic evolution of ligands by exponential enrichment (SELEX) is gaining immense attention from researchers (Sun et al. 2015). Aptamers are single-stranded short DNA oligonucleotides (RNA) usually 20–85 nucleotides long with a molecular weight of 6–30 kDa. Similar to the antigen-antibody recognition mechanism, aptamers bind with their targets with high affinity through various interactions mainly Vander Waals forces, hydrogen bonding, and electrostatic bonding. Thus, aptamers are also referred to as "chemical antibodies" (Tommasone et al. 2019). Due to the possible modifications chemically, their stability, and modification, aptamers can be fabricated using various supports which serve as artificial receptors in biosensors. Aptamers are the best alternatives to some natural biorecognition elements (BREs) such as enzymes, antigen MIPs, and antibodies (Purohit et al. 2020; Singhal et al. 2022b, a, c, d). As compared to natural BREs, aptamers offer several benefits. Aptamers are non-immunogenic and non-toxic in vivo conditions and do not show any side effects (Gowsalya et al. 2021). Due to their smaller size, aptamers can penetrate the tissue barrier and reach the target cells (Zhao et al. 2020). Aptamers can be synthesized for numerous targets. To date, many aptamers have been synthesized for the targets such as drugs, peptides, polypeptides, cells, or tissues. As they are thermally stable, they can be easily transported, stored, and can be utilized for industrial purposes. Aptamers can be synthesized on a large scale in a short time with minimal batch-to-batch variation (Reverdatto et al. 2015).

The systematic evolution of ligands by exponential enrichment is a common process used to create aptamers (Tuerk and Gold 1990). "SELEX" method involves a merging of selected nucleic acid ligands which interact with the target biomolecule in a desirable manner. The SELEX procedure requires many iterations, exponential oligonucleotide multiplication, and enrichment, which results in aptamers with the

DOI: 10.1201/9781003304227-9

ability to carry the desired tasks like catalysis or target binding and high affinity towards the target. Conceptually, this process is governed by the potential of these small oligonucleotides to fold into their unique three-dimensional structures that can interact with a particular target with high affinity and specificity. Usually libraries of at least 10^{15}–10^{19} independent sequences are utilized, with a variable region of 30 bases flanked by primers of 15–30 bases normally being used. Functionally important sequences, mostly are retrieved and amplified to produce a new group of molecules that has sequences which can do the desired functions. The amplification and selection processes are carried on until there is a clear domination of sequences that have a higher affinity for the selected target in the pool (Yoshikawa et al. 2022). Using computational techniques, the sequence's Watson-Crick base-pairing-capable sections are found, and the aptamers obtained by this systematic technique are checked in order to obtain probable secondary structures. The DNA aptamer's secondary structure which binds to human thrombin is an example of the different secondary structures that aptamers can evolve (Chang and Yeh 2021).

Aptamers which are as small as 20–100 nucleotide short can be created using above above-discussed SELEX and some other related invitro selection techniques (Rose et al. 2019). The original technique has changed and improved since SELEX was introduced in terms of the amount of time, effectiveness, and cost reduction needed to produce powerful aptamers. Recently, a thorough explanation of the most often used techniques was evaluated (Li et al. 2021). The majority of these new selection processes, however, adhere to the fundamental ideas of the SELEX procedure. Polymerase chain reactions (PCR) or primer extension reactions (PEX) are used to produce enormous libraries of oligonucleotides (usually 1014 molecules or more) (Townshend et al. 2022). Only pools with exact and equal distribution patterns of all four nucleotides enhance the quality, the sequence space to be examined and the design of the initial libraries are essential for effective SELEX investigations (Kohlberger and Gadermaier 2021). The number of molecules contained in the beginning- pool (1014 molecules; 0.2–1 nmol) and empirical rules still govern how long the random area can be (Klenov 2020). Short randomized areas (N20) will provide complete coverage of the sequence space in the selection experiment process, despite reducing the number of potential structural motifs. The complexity of potential three-dimensional structures and folds is higher in bigger randomized sections (N40), even though only a small portion of the sequence space will be used in the selection trials (Jumper et al. 2021).

Consequently, despite the fact that aptamers sequences as long as 228 nucleotides and as short as 8 nucleotides have been identified, most of the selection experiments are conducted using randomized sections made up of between 20 and 60 nucleotides (Qi et al. 2022). For physical separation from unattached molecules, the libraries are maybe incubated with targets accumulated on a solid platform or, directly with cells as in the case of SELEX (Saito 2021). The species that can attach to the target molecule are then selected and amplified with the polymerase chain reaction process, and the populations produced are further introduced in the additional selection rounds (Yan et al. 2019). By gradually changing physicochemical factors like the ionic strength, temperature, incubation duration, and the target's concentration, or by also taking a negative-selection phase into account, the selection stringency or pressure can be further enhanced over repetitive cycles (Susaki et al. 2020). The remaining binders are then cloned, and sequenced, and various species are described once no more enrichment is visible (usually after 5–15 cycles) (Komarova et al. 2020). The K_d (equilibrium dissociation constants) of aptamers, which frequently fall in the low nanomolar range, are typically the best indicators of their binding ability (Yan et al. 2019). Biophysical techniques like surface plasmon resonance or microscale thermophoresis are utilized in measuring their K_d values (MST). Aptamers have been used in a broad range of practical applications due to properties such as strong binding affinities along with selectivity, including drug delivery systems, diagnostic applications, and medicines even beginning to penetrate the disciplines of DNA nanotechnology and medical imaging (Nuzzo et al. 2020).

Aptamers are prone to quick nuclease-mediated degradation, like all naturally occurring oligonucleotides. Unmodified nucleic acids typically survive for less than 60 minutes in living cells and around 5 minutes in serum, according to early studies on the therapeutic antisense oligonucleotides and their development (Ni et al. 2020). Similar to modified aptamers, unmodified aptamers perform poorly and are quickly hydrolyzed in vivo by endo- and exonucleases (Helm et al. 2022). Last but not least, temperature is a further variable that might impair aptamer binding effectiveness and hasten the nuclease destruction of aptamers (Lacroix and Sleiman 2021). Aptamers do, in fact, create complex tertiary and secondary structures that allow them to connect to their target. As shown by the cocaine-binding thermolabile aptamer, an increment in temperature (for example, to 40°C) may cause the disintegration of these secondary structures and tertiary structures which prevents binding. Aptamers are susceptible to effective renal clearance along with fast nuclease-mediated metabolic degradation. In fact, aptamers are quickly eliminated by the kidneys, which may remove molecules with a molecular weight of 50 kDa due to their relatively small size (Derin and Inci 2021). The total plasma clearance of unmodified aptamers, which is the result of overall metabolic clearance along with the renal filtration, and irreversible absorption by the tissues, is relatively high and poses a significant problem for therapeutic in vivo applications (Pandey et al. 2022). The fabrication, advantages, and applications of the electrochemical-based aptasensors are shown in Figure 9.1.

In this book chapter, we have described a detailed stance on electrochemical sensing of analytes employing aptasensors.

9.2 APTAMERS-BASED BIOSENSORS FOR POINT-OF-CARE TESTING

A transducer plus a biological recognition component (such as an enzyme, an antibody, a receptor, etc.) make up a standard biosensor (electrochemical, optical, thermal, etc.) Biosensors are straightforward analytical tools, in contrast to other analytical techniques like spectrophotometry or mass spectrometry, which can require multiple steps for a single measurement (Noviana et al. 2021; Ranjan et al. 2022). The term "aptasensors" refers to biosensors that use aptamers as biorecognition components. Aptamers are used in the development of biosensors because of their strong affinity and adaptability, albeit the transducer has a significant impact on their sensitivity (Mahmoudpour et al. 2021). Aptasensors in the form of POCT have attained remarkable consideration in the last decade. The aptamers have significant benefits over the

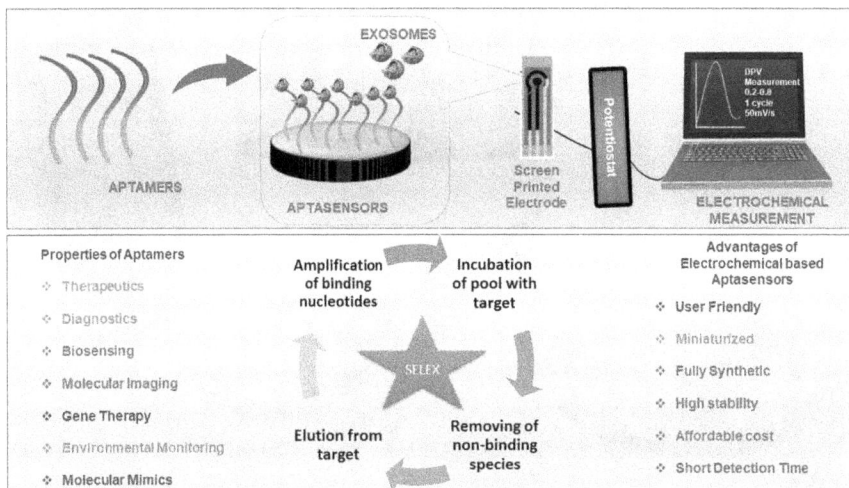

FIGURE 9.1 Fabrication of aptasensors and their integration with a portable potentiostat, steps of SELEX, properties, and advantages of aptamers-based electrochemical sensor.

traditional BREs. Aptasensors are economical, selective, sensitive, and stable, and show very little batch-to-batch variation. Its association with device multiplexing, miniaturization, and its integration with the Internet of Things (IoT)-enabled smart-phones with the combination of other interdisciplinary fields has optimized the system of POCT sensing (Parihar et al. 2022). The aptamer technique for point-of-care testing is not just limited to diagnostics in medical, but may also be utilised for quality control and environmental monitoring. Sandwich-like detection methods have been created for aptamers. After the oligonucleotide has linked to its target, a second aptamer links to a different binding site of the target, forming a "sandwich" structure. Two aptamers directed at different target epitopes or an aptamer and antibody combination can be used to carry out this procedure. Aptamer-target-antibody hybrids are thus possible. It has been effectively demonstrated that such hybrid systems can recognize cardiovas-cular indicators like troponin (Prante et al. 2020).

The conventional SPR-based sensors are heavy and make on-site diagnostics dif-ficult. The primary obstacle for a point-of-care diagnostic is thought to be the size of the conventional SPR-based sensor. Aptamer against the H_5N_1 influenza-causing virus was immobilised over the surface of a streptavidin-coated gold surface in one portable SPR biosensor. A reflecting mirror, a gold-coated SPR surface, and an LED light source are all parts of this portable SPR sensor chip. The proposed SPR assay may be used to identify AIV H_5N_1 on-site in the poultry business (Cennamo et al. 2013; Citartan and Tang 2019; Liu et al. 2017; Verma and Gupta 2015).

It is possible to avoid the requirement to add a quencher to the extremities of an aptamer by using paper that acts as a natural quencher. One such substance is the naturally quenching MoS_2 nanosheet. In a study, a MoS_2 nanosheet was employed to create an aptasensing application for the quick diagnosis of malaria employ-ing an aptamer which is against the malarial biomarker i.e., Plasmodium lactate

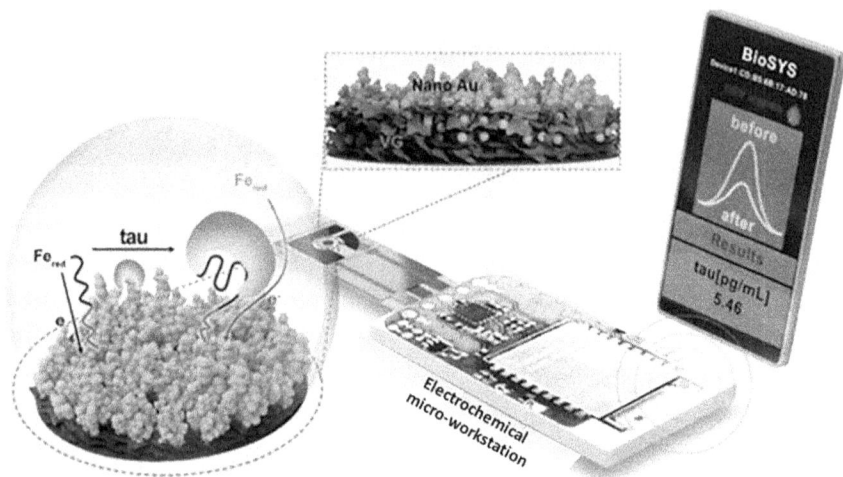

FIGURE 9.2 Fabrication of portable electrochemical aptasensor for Point-of-Care testing of tau protein with integration to a smartphone (Liu et al. 2022).

dehydrogenase. Graphene oxide and multi-walled carbon nanotubes (MWCNT) are further paper-based natural quenchers that were used to detect norovirus (Citartan and Tang 2019; Weng and Neethirajan 2017).

    Another most sought-after portable electrochemical sensor that may be utilized anywhere for identification and detection is a smartphone. A smartphone system uses an aptamer-dependent fluorescence assay to document the creation of aptamer-target complexes, with the help of a fluorescent signal reader to record the signal. Using fluorescent magnetic nanoparticles with aptamer functionality, Staphylococcus aureus could be detected quickly and without the need for culture. The aptamers caught the target cells, and the smartphone camera captured the fluorescence signal caused by the aptamer-target combination (Citartan and Tang 2019; Shrivastava et al. 2018; Zhang and Liu 2016). A portable electrochemical sensor for Point-of-Care identification of Alzheimer's disease (AD) biomarkers found in blood has been developed as shown in Figure 9.2. The sensor was developed using nano-modified graphene as a working electrode to detect tau protein, the key AD biomarker (Liu et al. 2022).

9.3   APPLICATION OF APTASENSORS FOR THE HEALTH CARE MONITORING

To date, there have been studies reported involving the utilization of aptasensors in the health monitoring field, like sensing of disease biomarkers associated with malignancy, cardiovascular diseases, neurodegenerative disorders, etc. There has been the development of aptasensors for environmental pollutant detection too. Moreover, the aptasensors are also available for microbial detection. In this section, various recent studies along with their methodologies have been described (Table 9.1).

TABLE 9.1

Various recent studies involving the application of aptasensors

S. no.	Analyte	Detection method	LOD	Linear range	References
1.	Tetracycline	CV	3.2×10^{-16} M	10^{-15} to 10^{-11} M	Xie et al. (2021)
2.	Penicillin G	CV	~0.3 nM	1.0 nM to 10.0 µM	He et al. (2020)
3.	Cadmium	CV	2.75×10^{-10} M	10^{-3} to 10^{-9} M	Rabai et al. (2021)
4.	Profenofos	CV	0.052 ng mL^{-1}	0.1 to 1×10^5 ng mL^{-1}	Zhang et al. (2020)
5.	Acetamiprid	CV	0.30 pM	1 pM to 1 µM	Shi et al. (2020)
6.	PSA in prostate cancer	SWV	1.24 pg mL^{-1}	10 pg mL^{-1} to 500 ng mL^{-1}	Zhao et al. (2021)
7.	Lead	DPV	312 pM	0.6–50 nM	Taghdisi et al. (2016)
8.	Epidermal growth factor receptor	CV	5 pg mL^{-1}	0.05–200 ng mL^{-1}	Wang et al. (2020)
9.	Ab oligomers	DPV	10 fM	0.0443–443.00 pM	Tao et al. (2021)
10.	Prometryn	CV and DPV	60 pg mL^{-1}	0.16–500 ng mL^{-1}	Zhang et al. (2022)
11.	Acetamiprid residue	CV	71.2 fM	0.1 pM to 0.1 µM	Yi et al. (2020)
12.	Diazinon pesticide	EIS	2.0×10^{-15} mol L^{-1}	1.0×10^{14} to 1.0×10^8 mol L^{-1}	Khosropour et al. (2020)
13.	Aflatoxin B1	CV	3 pg mL^{-1}	0.01–50 ng mL^{-1}	Guo et al. (2021)
14.	Zearalenone	DPV	4.57×10^{-6} ng mL^{-1}	1×10^{-4} to 1×10^3 ng mL^{-1}	Yan et al. (2022)
15.	Cadmium	CV	11.23 ppb	80–150 ppb	Hai et al. (2020)
16.	Streptomycin residues	CV	0.8×10^{-8} M	10^{-8} to 10^{-16} M	Vanani et al. (2021)
18.	Sulfaquinoxaline	DPV	0.547 pg mL^{-1}	1 pg mL^{-1} to 100 ng mL^{-1}	Li et al. (2021)
19.	Tau protein	DPV	0.46 fM	0.5–80 fM	Ameri et al. (2020)
20.	Troponin I	EIS	10 fM	10 fM to 1 nM	Vasudevan et al. (2021)
21.	Platelet-derived growth factor-BB	CV	0.4 pM	0.001–1.0 nM	Liu et al. (2015)
22.	Carcinoembryonic antigen	DPV	11.2 pg mL^{-1}	1.0×10^{-2} to 75.0 ng mL^{-1}	Shekari et al. (2021)
23.	Cancer antigen 15-3	DPV	11.2×10^{-2} U mL^{-1}	1.0×10^{-2} U mL^{-1} to 150.0 U mL^{-1}	Shekari et al. (2021)

In a recent study, the porous N-doped carbon aerogel (NCA) with a large nitrogen atom concentration and a high specific surface area was used to create the SL-AuNPs (Stonelike Au nanoparticles) as shown in Figure 9.3a. The benefits of SL-AuNPs and NCA allow the development of an electrochemical sensing of tetracycline (TET) with a linear range ranging from 10^{-15} to 10^{-11} M and a lower detection limit (LOD) of 3.2×10^{-16} M. Importantly, NCA@SL-AuNPs also function exceptionally well at identifying TET in milk. When the GCE was altered by the NCA@SL-AuNPs, a few distinct reduction-oxidation peaks with modest peak currents were found, but the peak current considerably rose to 60 A. demonstrating that the electroactive surface area of NCA@SL-AuNPs was enlarged and that this facilitated the transmission of an electron in between $[Fe(CN)_6]^{3-/4-}$ and the electrode. The immobilized aptamer over the GCE surface might create a TET/anti-TET combination. The complex TET/anti-TET complex may prevent electrons from moving from the $[Fe(CN)_6]^{3-/4-}$ solution to the electrode, drastically reducing peak currents. The electrochemical aptasensor can therefore be a quick, accurate, and practical platform for sensing TET and possibly another medication (Xie et al. 2021).

An electrochemical aptasensor was fabricated based on the silver-metal organic frameworks (Figure 9.3b and c) and was reported to be the first study using Ag-MOFs for aptasensing. The fabricated electrochemical-based aptasensor showed high stability with a linear detection range of 0.001–0.5 ng mL^{-1} and an LOD of 0.849 pg mL^{-1}. The sensor also exhibited good repeatability with high selectivity and selectivity. The sensor displayed high affinity towards penicillin even in the presence of some other closely related interferents like chloramphenicol, kanamycin, neomycin, etc. As the penicillin antibiotic is widely used for the cow's treatment, the chances of presence of penicillin residue are high in milk and the real sample analysis was carried out in the milk samples. The recovery of the penicillin was found to be ranging between

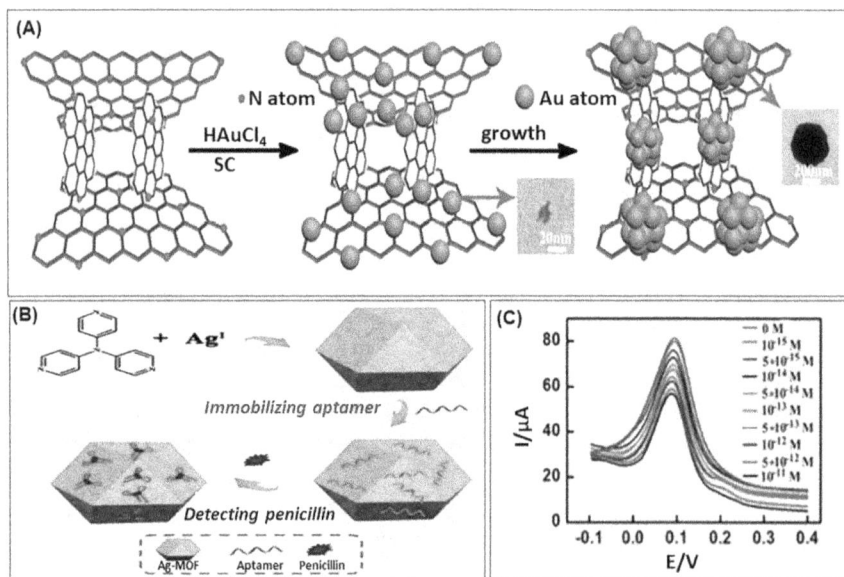

FIGURE 9.3 (a) Formation of SL-AuNPs on the NCA (Xie et al. 2021). (b) Construction of an electrochemical aptasensor based on Ag-MOF for penicillin detection. (c) The NCA@ SL-AuNPs@aptamer aptasensor's DPV plots after being exposed to TET at various concentrations on being scanned at a speed of 50 mV s^{-1} (He et al. 2020).

99.26% and 104.80% with the RSD values below 5%. The outcomes suggest the applicability of this fabricated aptasensor in raw milk samples (He et al. 2020).

A cadmium detection electrochemical aptasensor is created as shown in Figure 9.4A. Through CMA molecules, the aptamer was covalently bound onto gold WE. With a LOD of approximately $2.75'10^{-10}$ M, the investigated aptasensor demonstrated a linear relationship between the logarithm of Cd^{2+} concentration over a wide range from 10^{-3} to 10^{-9} M and impedance change. The bare Gold WE may be seen to have the oxidation-reduction peaks of the redox couple, which are two quasi-reversible peaks typical of the reduction-oxidation with cathodic and anodic current peak ratios of roughly one and peak-to-peak separation of 0.1 V. The current was then found to significantly diminish following the electrochemical grafting of diazonium salt. The current variation during the first cycle revealed a decreasing wave localized at –0.6V. The reduction of diazonium salt in solution, which results in the creation of a radical amine, corresponds to this current. After that, we observed that the reduction current significantly drops after the second scan cycle. This can be attributable to the CMA blocking layer's reduction in the electron transport rate. The reduction of the diazonium salt in solution, which results in the formation of a radical amine, corresponds to this current. After that, we observed that the reduction current significantly drops after the second scan cycle. This can be attributable to the CMA blocking layer's reduction in the rate of electron transfer. Here, the cyclic voltammetry (CV) peaks have once more decreased, indicating that the cadmium ions have successfully been adsorbed onto the gold WE surface (Rabai et al. 2021). A successful fabrication of an aptasensor for the determination of profenofos (PFF) based on $MWCNT_{Gr}$ and Au nanoshell was performed as shown in Figure 9.4B. The test platform was a screen-printed carbon electrode (SPCE) modified with graphitized multi-walled carbon nanotubes ($MWCNT_{Gr}$) and an Au nanoshell, which allowed for a quick detection technique and demonstrated good electrochemical performance. The surface area and electrical conductivity were improved by $MWCNT_{Gr}$ and gold particle nanoshell, which led to an increase in the detection signal. Additionally, CV was used to assess the effects of the aptamers modified with $-NH_2$ and $-SH$ on the current signal. The results revealed that the aptamers modified with $-NH_2$ made the current signal change more noticeable. Based on the information presented above, a high-efficiency electrochemical aptasensor was created under optimal conditions, with a linear range of $0.1-1'10^5$ ng mL^{-1} and a detection limit of 0.052 ng mL^{-1}. CVs were recorded during each fixed stage of the aptasensor's construction as shown in Figure 9.4Ca and Cb). A pair of good reversible redox peaks were seen at the bare SPCE due to the improved redox properties of $[Fe(CN)_6]^{3-/4-}$. The redox peak appears to have increased when the electrode was coated with modified $MWCNT_{Gr}$. The redox peak currents then further rose as the SPCE's Au nanoshell was changed in this manner. Due to their exceptional shape and high electrical conductivity, $MWCNT_{Gr}$ could more tightly modify SPCE. The $MWCNT_{Gr}$ and Au nanoshell in conjunction could significantly boost the aptasensor's electrical activity. SPCE offered a viable platform for sensitively identifying PFF in vegetables due to its advantages in handling convenience and portability for on-site analysis. As a result, the technology can be used to create various sensors with strong conductivity, simple modification, and straightforward operation (Zhang et al. 2020). For instance, the detection of acetamiprid was performed using a novel dual signal amplification method for aptasensors employing reduced graphene with silver nanoparticles and Prussian blue-gold nanocomposites. Reduced graphene oxide-silver nanoparticles (rGo-AgNPs) were changed on a bare glassy carbon electrode surface to increase the sensitivity of aptasensors. This increased the specific surface area for subsequent material immobilization and amplified the current signal. With a detection limit of 0.30 pM (S/N = 3), the analysis experiment demonstrated that it had extremely high sensitivity and satisfied the needs of the vast majority of daily leaf vegetable tests. The suggested aptasensor demonstrated a broad linear detection range from 1 pM to 1 M while operating under optimal conditions. The characterization of the bare electrode and modified electrode was done in 5.0 mM $[Fe(CN)_6]^{3-/4-}$ and 0.1 M KCl in order to describe the conductivity of different electrodes shown in Figure 9.4D. The scan rate was 50 mV/s, and the potential range was between 0.1 and 0.5 V. Two redox maxima for the unadorned GCE. The current peak of rGo-AgNPs/GCE was increased as rGo-AgNPs modified GCE, demonstrating that rGo-AgNPs/GCE exhibited strong electrical conductivity. The current peak of PB-AuNPs/rGo-AgNPs/GCE was dramatically increased after the electrodeposition of B-AuNPs, showing that PB-AuNPs greatly stimulated the redox reaction of the sensor and further enhanced the output of the current signal. After aptamers were immobilized, their electrostatic repulsion stopped the $[Fe(CN)_6]^{3-/4-}$probe's free electron mobility within the reaction system. As a result, the present response was greatly diminished. Free electron transport was impacted and the current peak was further diminished when the BSA was altered on the electrode. Additionally, due to the synergy between the two materials, electron microscopy or electrochemical characterization demonstrated that the rGO-AgNPs/PBAuNPs composites showed improved electrocatalytic properties and electrical conductivity in comparison to PB-AuNPs or rGO-AgNPs. It has good redox reaction catalysis in addition to good conductivity (Shi et al. 2020).

For the detection of Prostate Specific Antigen (PSA), a new, straightforward, and sensitive electrochemical aptasensor based on target-induced resolution has been developed. Two stem-loop structures are formed by a brief, single-stranded DNA pseudoknot as shown in Figure 9.5a. The distance between the electrode surface and MB was extended by an aptamer tagged with MB to the 30-terminal end, which also decreased the transfer of Faraday current. Three conformations of pre-designed DNA aptamers, comprising two stem-loop structures and a double-strand structure, have been looked at and contrasted in order to achieve a satisfactory performance. The maximum signal diversity was discovered in this structure, which was generated by target-induced binding. The suggested aptasensor showed a broad concentration detection range from 10 pg mL^{-1} to 500 ng mL^{-1}, with a LOD as low as 1.24 pg mL^{-1} after the aptamer concentration and incubation time were tuned. It was observed that an MB redox peak pairs with the aptamer-modified gold electrode (AuE) in order to determine the ideal receptor concentration. The peak currents were exactly proportional to the potential scanning rates, suggesting that the electrochemical reaction is surface-confined. It was discovered that the aptasensor responded well to human serum samples, making it simple to use for the detection of the physiological concentration of PSA. For the detection of PSA, the electrochemical aptasensor showed good repeatability, sensitivity, selectivity, and reliability (Zhao et al. 2021). Based

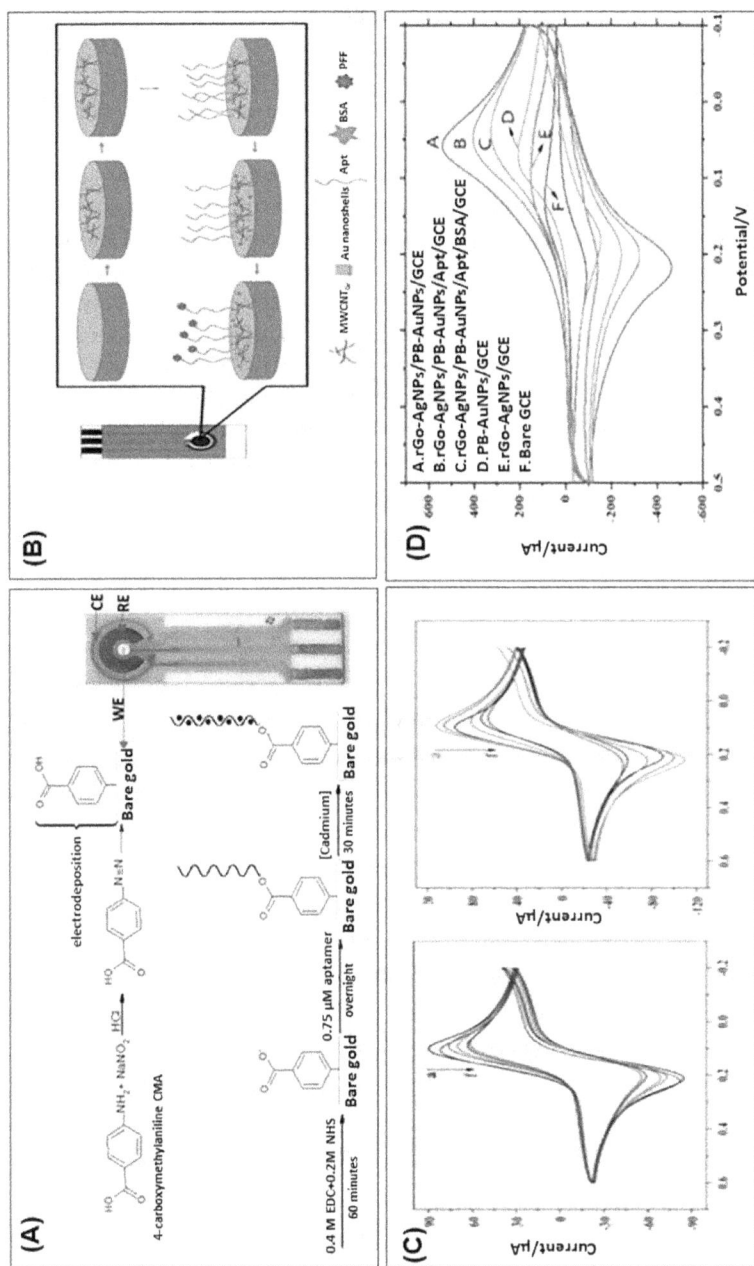

FIGURE 9.4 (A) Shown an example of immobilization of aptamer and immobilization for cadmium detection utilizing combined RE and CE after chemical surface modification of the gold WE by CMA (Rabai et al. 2021). (B) Steps for the fabrication of the aptasensors. (C) Different modified SPCE CV responses (a) Au nanoshell/MWCNTGr/SPCE and (b) Apt2/Au nanoshell/MWCNT$_{Gr}$/SPCE (Zhang et al. 2020). (D) CV characterization of the GCE in an aqueous solution containing 5 mmol L^{-1} of [Fe(CN)$_6$]$^{3/4}$ and 0.1 mol L^{-1} of KCl after it has been modified with various aptamers or, BSA (Shi et al. 2020).

on gold nanoparticles (AuNPs), a hairpin structure of complementary aptamer (CS), and thionine, an electrochemical aptasensor for the sensitive and selective detection of lead ($Pb^{2+)}$ was created. With a limit of detection (LOD) as low as 312 pM, the electrochemical aptasensor that was built demonstrated high selectivity toward Pb^{2+}. Additionally, Pb^{2+} was successfully detected in tap water and serum with LODs of 326 and 537 pM, respectively, using the constructed electrochemical aptasensor. At a concentration of 50 nM lead, the DPV peak started to wane and eventually plateaued, as shown in Figure 9.5b. The experiment revealed a very linear range for lead (0.6–50 nM). The LOD was established to be 312 pM (Taghdisi et al. 2016). By using anti-EGFR aptamers as the biorecognition component, an electrochemical paper-based aptasensor for label-free and ultrasensitive detection of EGFR was created as shown in Figure 9.5c. The device reduced sampling quantities and enhanced operation convenience by utilizing the idea of origami, or the folding of paper, as a valve between sample introduction and detection. In addition to generating the electrochemical signals, amino-functionalized graphene (NH_2-GO)/thionine (THI)/ gold particle (AuNP) nanocomposites were employed to change the working electrode in order to create an environment favourable for aptamer immobilization. In 0.1 M PBS solution (pH of 7.4) both CV and DPV methods were used to characterize

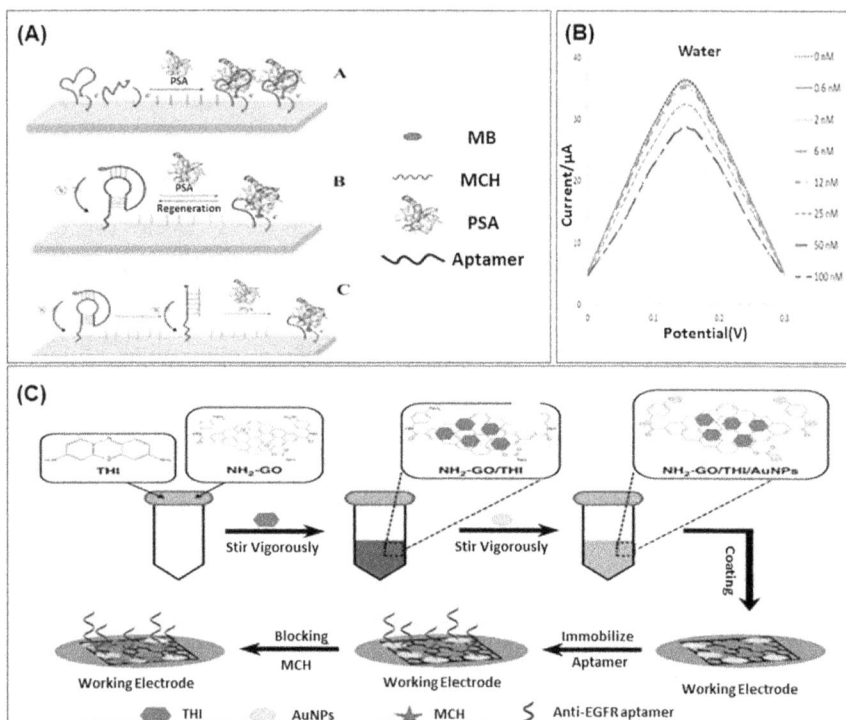

FIGURE 9.5   (a) The process involved in the assembly of electrochemicals for PSA detection (Zhao et al. 2021). (b) DPV peaks of the Apt-CS-modified electrode at varied lead-in-water concentrations (Taghdisi et al. 2016). (c) Modification of the EGFR aptasensor made of origami paper (Wang et al. 2020).

the construction of the origami paper-based EGFR aptasensor and its accompanying electrochemical behaviour. There was no oxidation or reduction activity in the bare WE. In contrast, after treatment with NH_2-GO/THI/AuNP nanocomposites, a well-behaved electrochemical response was found under identical circumstances. At 0.18 and 0.31 V, there were two distinct redox peaks that were attributable to the THI molecules. By incorporating the idea of origami, the gadget was made even simpler and used fewer samples. The rate of electron transfer on the working electrode surface was effectively accelerated by the addition of graphene-based nanocomposites, which also improved the detection signal. The very specific detection was made possible by the aptamer utilized as the recognition element (Wang et al. 2020).

The electrochemical aptasensor, which was made from 3D carbon nanomaterials adsorbed DNA aptamer and was used to analyze the AD biomarkers. Under ideal circumstances, the DPV current responses dropped as AbO concentration increased. The developed AbO aptasensor had a LOD of 10 fM and a large linear range of 0.0443–443.00 pM. AbO aptasensor, meanwhile, demonstrated astounding stability and selectivity. The presence of various quantities of AbO was detected using. Analysis was done on the Th-rGO-MWCNTs aptasensor's analytical capabilities. The aptasensor showed significant promise for AD early diagnosis (Tao et al. 2021).

9.4 CONCLUSION AND FUTURE PERSPECTIVE

Aptasensors have developed remarkably during the past 10 years, and they have sufficiently proven their potential and value in the field of bioanalysis. The market for aptasensors and aptamer-based diagnostics is not being explored in spite of this tremendous progress. Several difficulties should be addressed at industrial and technical aspects in order for aptasensors to continue to gain market share. Due to their clear knowledge and characterization, very few aptamers, including those which bind to adenosine, thrombin, ATP, cocaine, and PDGF, have initially been used in various aptasensors as proof of ideas and principles of innovative aptamer-based sensors. To be used for commercial purposes, however, researchers must focus on analytes that are required by end users in order to be found in the market. Even if aptasensors offer some advantages over immune sensors for the same targets and purposes, it is particularly difficult to change immune sensors that have previously been approved for clinical tests due to regulatory problems. So, one way to compete with immune sensors for commercialization is to build aptasensors for recently discovered targets. Of course, prior to the construction of aptasensors, high-quality aptamers targeting commercially significant targets should be identified. Second, practically all of the aptamer-based sensing techniques that have been published so far are too difficult or sophisticated to utilize as a sensor, which typically increases the coefficient of variation and is not practical for field use. It is crucial that different aptasensors be connected in technically feasible sensor platforms like lateral flow strip. Through effective signal amplification techniques or increasing aptamer affinity to target, the specificity and sensitivity of POC-type aptasensors should also be increased. The aptasensor's sensitivity can be greatly enhanced by the addition of nanomaterials like AuNPs. A few successful instances must show the commercial potential of aptasensors and aid in their commercialization if they are to compete with well-known immuno-sensors or enzyme-based biosensors. Since the subsequent creation of cognate aptamer duos, generated from the immobilization-free technique utilizing graphene oxide, which makes the use of sandwich-type assays conceivable, it is now possible to realize the successful fabrication of aptasensors. Technical developments in the selection procedure, synthesis of aptamers, and analytical capabilities of aptasensors are predicted to support a rapid expansion of the global market for aptamers and aptasensors. Additionally, aptamer businesses have been regularly formed in the bioanalytical and pharmaceutical industries. According to a survey by "Markets and Markets," the aptamer market was worth roughly $200 million worldwide in 2013 and is projected to expand by 49% annually to reach $2.1 billion by 2018 (compound annual growth rate). Although aptamer synthesis and aptamer separation services make up the majority of business, which shows that potentially aptamers will receive greater attention in the near future in the biosensor sector.

ACKNOWLEDGEMENTS

The authors express their sincere thanks to the Director, CSIR-AMPRI for his support and encouragement in this work. Raju Khan would like to acknowledge SERB for providing funds in the form of the IPA/2020/000130 project. Arpana Parihar's fellowship under the DST-WoS-B (DST/WOS-B/HN-4/2021) initiative is gratefully acknowledged.

REFERENCES

Ameri M, Shabaninejad Z, Movahedpour A, et al. (2020) Biosensors for detection of Tau protein as an Alzheimer's disease marker. *Int J Biol Macromol* 162:1100–1108.

Cennamo N, D'Agostino G, Donà A, et al. (2013) Localized surface plasmon resonance with five-branched gold nanostars in a plastic optical fiber for bio-chemical sensor implementation. *Sensors* 13:14676–14686. https://doi.org/10.3390/S131114676

Citartan M, Tang TH (2019) Recent developments of aptasensors expedient for point-of-care (POC) diagnostics. *Talanta* 199:556–566. https://doi.org/10.1016/J.TALANTA.2019.02.066

Guo W, Umar A, Algadi H, et al. (2021) Design of a unique "ON/OFF" switch electrochemical aptasensor driven by the pH for the detection of Aflatoxin B1 in acid solutions based on titanium carbide/ carboxylated graphene oxide-poly(4-vinyl pyridine)/aptamer composite. *Microchem J* 169:106548. https://doi.org/10.1016/J.MICROC.2021.106548

Hai T le, Hung LC, Phuong TTB, et al. (2020) Multiwall carbon nanotube modified by antimony oxide (Sb_2O_3/MWCNTs) paste electrode for the simultaneous electrochemical detection of cadmium and lead ions. *Microchem J* 153:104456. https://doi.org/10.1016/J.MICROC.2019.104456

He H, Wang SQ, Han ZY, et al. (2020) Construction of electrochemical aptasensors with Ag(I) metal–organic frameworks toward high-efficient detection of ultra-trace penicillin. *Appl Surf Sci* 531:147342. https://doi.org/10.1016/J.APSUSC.2020.147342

Khosropour H, Rezaei B, Rezaei P, Ensafi AA (2020) Ultrasensitive voltammetric and impedimetric aptasensor for diazinon pesticide detection by VS2 quantum dots-graphene nanoplatelets/carboxylated multiwalled carbon nanotubes as a new group nanocomposite for signal enrichment. *Anal Chim Acta* 1111:92–102. https://doi.org/10.1016/J.ACA.2020.03.047

Li S, He B, Liang Y, et al. (2021) Sensitive electrochemical aptasensor for determination of sulfaquinoxaline based on AuPd NPs@UiO-66-NH$_2$/CoSe$_2$ and RecJf exonuclease-assisted signal amplification. *Anal Chim Acta* 1182:338948. https://doi.org/10.1016/J.ACA.2021.338948

Liu Q, Liu Y, Chen S, et al. (2017) A low-cost and portable dual-channel fiber optic surface plasmon resonance system. *Sensors* 17:2797. https://doi.org/10.3390/S17122797

Liu X, Shuai HL, Huang KJ (2015) A label-free electrochemical aptasensor based on leaf-like vanadium disulfide-Au nanoparticles for the sensitive and selective detection of platelet-derived growth factor BB. *Anal Methods* 7:8277–8284. https://doi.org/10.1039/C5AY01793A

Liu Y, Liu X, Li M, et al. (2022) Portable vertical graphene@Au-based electrochemical aptasensing platform for point-of-care testing of tau protein in the blood. *Biosensors* 12:564. https://doi.org/10.3390/BIOS12080564

Mahmoudpour M, Ding S, Lyu Z, et al. (2021) Aptamer functionalized nanomaterials for bio-medical applications: recent advances and new horizons. *Nano Today* 39:101177. https://doi.org/10.1016/J.NANTOD.2021.101177

Noviana E, Ozer T, Carrell CS, et al. (2021) Microfluidic paper-based analytical devices: from design to applications. *Chem Rev* 121:11835–11885. https://doi.org/10.1021/acs.chemrev.0c01335

Parihar A, Singhal A, Kumar N, et al. (2022) Next-generation intelligent MXene-based electrochemical aptasensors for point-of-care cancer diagnostics. *Nano-Micro Lett* 14:1–34. https://doi.org/10.1007/S40820-022-00845-1

Prante M, Segal E, Scheper T, et al. (2020) Aptasensors for point-of-care detection of small molecules. *Biosensors* 10:108. https://doi.org/10.3390/BIOS10090108

Purohit B, Vernekar PR, Shetti NP, Chandra P (2020) Biosensor nanoengineering: design, operation, and implementation for biomolecular analysis. *Sens Int* 1:100040. https://doi.org/10.1016/J.SINTL.2020.100040

Rabai S, Benounis M, Catanante G, et al. (2021) Development of a label-free electrochemical aptasensor based on diazonium electrodeposition: application to cadmium detection in water. *Anal Biochem* 612:113956. https://doi.org/10.1016/J.AB.2020.113956

Ranjan P, Singhal A, Sadique MA, et al. (2022) Scope of biosensors, commercial aspects, and miniaturized devices for point-of-care testing from lab to clinics applications. In Khan R, Parihar A, Sanghi SK (Eds.), *Biosensor Based Advanced Cancer Diagnostics: From Lab to Clinics*, pp. 395–410. Academic Press. https://doi.org/10.1016/B978-0-12-823424-2.00004-1

Reverdatto S, Burz DS, Shekhtman A (2015) Peptide aptamers: development and applications. *Curr Top Med Chem* 15:1082. https://doi.org/10.2174/1568026615666150413153143

Shekari Z, Zare HR, Falahati A (2021) Dual assaying of breast cancer biomarkers by using a sandwich-type electrochemical aptasensor based on a gold nanoparticles–3D graphene hydrogel nanocomposite and redox probes labeled aptamers. *Sens Actuators B Chem* 332:129515. https://doi.org/10.1016/J.SNB.2021.129515

Shi X, Sun J, Yao Y, et al. (2020) Novel electrochemical aptasensor with dual signal amplification strategy for detection of acetamiprid. *Sci Total Environ* 705:135905. https://doi.org/10.1016/J.SCITOTENV.2019.135905

Shrivastava S, Lee W-I, Lee N-E (2018) Culture-free, highly sensitive, quantitative detection of bacteria from minimally processed samples using fluorescence imaging by smartphone. *Biosens Bioelectron* 109:90–97. https://doi.org/10.1016/J.BIOS.2018.03.006

Singhal A, Parihar A, Kumar N, Khan R (2022a) High throughput molecularly imprinted polymers based electrochemical nanosensors for point-of-care diagnostics of COVID-19. *Mater Lett* 306. https://doi.org/10.1016/j.matlet.2021.130898

Singhal A, Ranjan P, Sadique MA, et al. (2022b) Molecularly imprinted polymers-based nano-biosensors for environmental monitoring and analysis. In: Singh RP, Ukhurebor KE, Singh J, Adetunji CO, Singh KR (Eds.), *Nanobiosensors for Environmental Monitoring*, pp. 263–278. Springer, Cham. https://doi.org/10.1007/978-3-031-16106-3_14

Singhal A, Sadique MA, Kumar N, et al. (2022c) Multifunctional carbon nanomaterials decorated molecularly imprinted hybrid polymers for efficient electrochemical antibiotics sensing. *J Environ Chem Eng* 10. https://doi.org/10.1016/j.jece.2022.107703

Singhal A, Yadav S, Sadique MA, et al. (2022d) MXene-modified molecularly imprinted polymers as an artificial bio-recognition platform for efficient electrochemical sensing: progress and perspectives. *Phys Chem Chem Phys* 24:19164–19176. https://doi.org/10.1039/d2cp02330j

Sun H, Zu Y, Miller AOA, et al. (2015) A highlight of recent advances in aptamer technology and its application. *Molecules* 20:11959–11980. https://doi.org/10.3390/MOLECULES200711959

Taghdisi SM, Danesh NM, Lavaee P, et al. (2016) An electrochemical aptasensor based on gold nanoparticles, thionine and hairpin structure of complementary strand of aptamer for ultrasensitive detection of lead. *Sens Actuators B Chem* 234:462–469. https://doi.org/10.1016/J.SNB.2016.05.017

Tao D, Xie C, Fu S, et al. (2021) Thionine-functionalized three-dimensional carbon nanomaterial-based aptasensor for analysis of Aβ oligomers in serum. *Anal Chim Acta* 1183:338990. https://doi.org/10.1016/J.ACA.2021.338990

Tommasone S, Allabush F, Tagger YK, et al. (2019) The challenges of glycan recognition with natural and artificial receptors. *Chem Soc Rev* 48:5488–5505. https://doi.org/10.1039/C8CS00768C

Vanani SM, Izadi Z, Hemmati R, Saffar B (2021) Fabrication of an ultrasensitive aptasensor for precise electrochemical detection of the trace amounts of streptomycin in milk. *Colloids Surf B Biointerfaces* 206:111964. https://doi.org/10.1016/J.COLSURFB.2021.111964

Vasudevan M, Tai MJY, Perumal V, et al. (2021) Cellulose acetate-MoS₂ nanopetal hybrid: a highly sensitive and selective electrochemical aptasensor of Troponin I for the early diagnosis of acute myocardial infarction. *J Taiwan Inst Chem Eng* 118:245–253. https://doi.org/10.1016/J.JTICE.2021.01.016

Verma R, Gupta BD (2015) Detection of heavy metal ions in contaminated water by surface plasmon resonance based optical fibre sensor using conducting polymer and chitosan. *Food Chem* 166:568–575. https://doi.org/10.1016/J.FOODCHEM.2014.06.045

Wang Y, Sun S, Luo J, et al. (2020) Low sample volume origami-paper-based graphene-modified aptasensors for label-free electrochemical detection of cancer biomarker-EGFR. *Microsyst Nanoeng* 6:1–9. https://doi.org/10.1038/s41378-020-0146-2

Weng X, Neethirajan S (2017) Aptamer-based fluorometric determination of norovirus using a paper-based microfluidic device. *Microchim Acta* 184:4545–4552. https://doi.org/10.1007/S00604-017-2467-X/TABLES/1

Xie B, Peng H, Zhang R, et al. (2021) Label-free electrochemical aptasensor based on stone-like gold nanoparticles for ultrasensitive detection of tetracycline. *J Phys Chem C* 125:5678–5683. https://doi.org/10.1021/ACS.JPCC.0C10809

Yan, J., Xiong, H., Cai, S., Wen, N., He, Q., Liu, Y., Peng, D. and Liu, Z., 2019. Advances in aptamer screening technologies. *Talanta*, 200, pp.124–144.

Yan H, He B, Zhao R, et al. (2022) Electrochemical aptasensor based on Ce₃NbO₇/CeO₂@Au hollow nanospheres by using Nb.BbvCI-triggered and bipedal DNA walker amplification strategy for zearalenone detection. *J Hazard Mater* 438:129491. https://doi.org/10.1016/J.JHAZMAT.2022.129491

Yi J, Liu Z, Liu J, et al. (2020) A label-free electrochemical aptasensor based on 3D porous CS/rGO/GCE for acetamiprid residue detection. *Biosens Bioelectron* 148:111827. https://doi.org/10.1016/J.BIOS.2019.111827

Zhang D, Liu Q (2016) Biosensors and bioelectronics on smartphone for portable biochemical detection. *Biosens Bioelectron* 75:273–284. https://doi.org/10.1016/J.BIOS.2015.08.037

Zhang H, Sun J, Cheng S, et al. (2020) A dual-amplification electrochemical aptasensor for profenofos detection. *J Electrochem Soc* 167:027515. https://doi.org/10.1149/1945-7111/AB6972

Zhang Z, Luan Y, Ru S, et al. (2022) Selection of highly specific aptamer and its application in fabrication of Ag@Au nanoflowers based signal-enhanced electrochemical aptasensor for ultrasensitive detection prometryn. *SSRN Electron J.* https://doi.org/10.2139/SSRN.4095599

Zhao B, Miao P, Hu Z, et al. (2021) Signal-on electrochemical aptasensors with different target-induced conformations for prostate specific antigen detection. *Anal Chim Acta* 1152:338282. https://doi.org/10.1016/J.ACA.2021.338282

Zhao Z, Ukidve A, Kim J, Mitragotri S (2020) Targeting strategies for tissue-specific drug delivery. *Cell* 181:151–167. https://doi.org/10.1016/J.CELL.2020.02.001

10 Challenges and advances in aptamer-based biosensing approaches

Srikanth Ponnada, Sarita Yadav, Demudu
Babu Gorle, Meghali Devi, Anjali Palariya,
Rapaka S. Chandra Bose, Rakesh K. Sharma

10.1 INTRODUCTION

The accurate and rapid identification of bioanalytes plays a significant role in our life. Currently, the world is experiencing an outbreak of COVID-19, i.e., an infectious disease or pandemic that emerged by a new coronavirus (Severe Acute Respiratory Syndrome Coronavirus 2 or SARS-CoV-2) reminds us of the importance of biosensors that facilitate diagnostic recognition of definite targets viz., coronavirus biomarkers (Remuzzi and Remuzzi 2020, Wu et al. 2020). Till now, no infectious disease has shown greater disasters to mankind than the current pandemic i.e., COVID-19, particularly for diseases that are caused by viruses that create a severe global risk to mankind such as the influenza pandemic (Gram 1919), the human immunodeficiency virus (HIV) infection (Traeger et al. 2018), the severe acute respiratory syndrome (SARS) (Ksiazek et al. 2003), the Middle East respiratory syndrome (MERS) (Zaki et al. 2012)). All these infectious diseases have considerably disturbed the social stability, global health, economy, and ultimately the development of human society. Thus, it is significant to develop novel point-of-care (POC) diagnostics in order to improve early detection and interference of the diseases.

Infectious disease is a type of ailment that exists due to living pathogens including viruses, parasites, and bacteria and is able in the fast-spreading and contamination amongst humans or animals by vaccination, air, or waterway (Johnson et al. 2015). There are three strategies available to manage infectious diseases i.e., control of the infection causes, eliminating communication ways, and defence of vulnerable people. Among these methods, management of the infection cause is of utmost importance and needs early recognition, separation, and treatment of patients followed by the progress of quick, susceptible, and precise recognition techniques and kits (Weigl 2020). The diagnostic techniques alter the existence or concentrations of definite biological analytes to identifiable signals (such as fluorescence, colour, and electrical current) which is further used in the easy and rapid detection of preferred areas in different kinds of samples such as environmental or clinical specimens. The

DOI: 10.1201/9781003304227-10

growth of rapid, precise, and susceptible biosensors could realize timely diagnosis of diseases and can prevent the communication of infectious diseases. Due to these reasons, the application of biosensors has been widened (including the food industry, environmental monitoring, drug discovery, and forensic science) and the economic effects of biosensors have developed considerably (Hernandez-Vargas et al. 2018). The rapid growth in the occurrence of chronic illness (such as diabetes, asthma, and cancer) and infectious diseases has significantly increased in healthcare and POC diagnostics and therefore, helpful in the development of biosensing research. The worldwide biosensors market size is emerging at a speedy pace and is predicted to increase from US$21.1 billion to US$31.5 billion from 2019 to 2024, respectively having 8.3% of compound annual progress. Recently, *in vitro* diagnostic (IVD) methods have created innovative aspects along the start of POC testing that advance the field of diagnostics and biosensing by increasing the pace and precision of diagnoses.

POC diagnostics exhibit various advantages over labour and time-consuming traditional diagnostic techniques including, low manufacturing cost, better sensitivity, high diagnostic speed, specificity, more competence, and capacity for on-site discovery. Owing to their unique characteristics, aptamers are considered biorecognition elements in the advancement of infection diagnostic systems and stand out exclusively in the digital and personalized medicine period. Aptamers are known to be 3D-folded single-stranded nucleic acids and are considered artificial antibodies that particularly connect to target areas. Significant consideration has been provided to aptamers owing to their low production charge, good stability, flexible sequence design, chemical modification, negligible immunogenicity, the binding tendency to monoclonal antibodies (dissociation constant = 0.1–50 Nm), cold-train-free storage, diverse binding capability, reusability, and repeatability. Owing to these properties, aptamers have been frequently considered for POC diagnostics and health care applications in the last 10 years. In 1990, its first application was established (Robertson and Joyce 1990), Systematic Evolution of Ligands by Exponential Enrichment (SELEX) has undergone many transformations. At the current stage of new pandemic outbreaks, particular aptamers for infectious microorganisms can be swiftly obtained via proficient SELEX methodology. Various research groups have made trials to develop signal amplification methodology for the improvement of the sensitivity of aptamer-based technologies. Mainly three methods i.e., cyclic enzymatic, catalytic molecule, and rolling-circle amplification have been utilized for the amplification of signals for improved recognition and advancement have been prepared in the sensitivity of aptamer-based detection techniques (Karunanayake Mudiyanselage et al. 2018, Li et al. 2020, Ma et al. 2018). The particular aptamers of pathogenic microbes and the sensitive and stable aptamer-based detection techniques are responsible for the quick, convenient, and effective diagnosis of infectious agents in any environment.

The current chapter offers information on the new advancement in exploiting aptamer-based biosensors for POC diagnostics and worldwide health care. This chapter begins with the existing aptamer-based methodologies for the recognition of viral, bacterial, and protozoan pathogens for worldwide health care applications. The narration of general aptasensing principles and recent developments in aptamer-based POC will be also discussed. Finally, new insights in developing the aptamer-based POC diagnostics for the management, prevention, and control of infectious diseases and pandemics like COVID-19 are discussed. We herein present the major challenges that rising technology is facing in the search for these novel instruments from the research stage to the society.

10.2 APTAMER SYNTHESIS

In the year 1990, three different research groups shared the outcomes on the progress of a vitro selection and amplification method for the separation of sequences of a specific nucleic acid that join the target molecules having high affinity and specificity (Ellington and Szostak 1990, Robertson and Joyce 1990, Tuerk and Gold 1990). This method was known as SELEX (Systematic Evolution of Ligands by Exponential Enrichment) and the final oligonucleotides are known as aptamers. These are basically ligands of nucleic acid which can be produced against drugs, proteins, amino acids, etc. Aptamers own a high affinity in favour of their targets and connect to them with binding affinity ranging in the lower pico- or nanomolar range. The aptamer can particularly bind with analyte viz., nucleotides, amino acids, peptides, metal ions, enzymes, other proteins, cells and bacteria with high affinity (Chen et al. 2016, Geiger et al. 1996, Hermann and Patel 2000, Idili et al. 2019, Ji et al. 2017, Lee et al. 2017, Li et al. 2021, Liu et al. 2019a, Sun et al. 2019b, Wang et al. 2019). A SELEX method consists of negative and counter-selection steps to choose aptamers having high affinity and specificity. These selections assist in removing the nonspecific nucleotide sequences against structurally nonspecific and analogue targets. During a SELEX process, the affinity of aptamers by which they bind to the target site is reliant on the severity of the target binding and aptamer elution procedure. Severity is increased gradually with the progression of SELEX by varying various factors such as detergent concentration, target concentration, aptamer concentration, elution temperature, and binding conditions.

SELEX comprises repetitive cycles of binding, improvement of bound DNA/ RNA, and amplification. It starts with a nucleic acid collection that comprises of DNA or RNA molecules consisting of an arbitrary area situated on both sides having preset primer sequences for the purpose of amplification. Since hydrogen bonding is responsible for most of the aptamer-target interactions, RNA libraries offer a large variety as compared to DNA; however, the ensuing aptamers are vulnerable to nucleases. The library is incubated with the goal and the binding process is started. The objective can be added on resin, magnetic beads, and affinity columns or be free in solution. Using magnetic or centrifugal force, the DNA or RNA that is not bound to the target should be differentiated from the bound sequences. If the objective is not immobilized, severance through a film filtration has been used for the competent process of separating the bound and unbound DNA or RNA. This is followed by the elution of target bound DNA or RNA which is acquired by washing through an elution buffer. It is functional to utilize the process of negative selection and counter-selection beside the positive selection process for the better improvement of the aptamer specificity. The severity gets raised with each cycle and the amount of DNA or RNA and target become less. Once the maximum affinity is achieved, the enriched documentation is copied and arranged in some pattern, and various techniques viz., surface plasmon resonance (SPR), flow cytometry, and fluorescent binding assays will be used for the investigation of individual sequencing

TABLE 10.1

Different variants of SELEX methodologies (Stanciu et al. 2021)

SELEX method	Advantages	Disadvantage
Bead-based	Rapid selection of aptamers	Immobilization of aptamer: restrictions in surface interaction
	Ease in controlling selection stringency	
	In-solution binding and equilibrium	Density-dependent cooperativity towards nonspecific relations
	Applicable to proteins, cells, small molecules, and peptides	
Microarray-based	Utilized as a binding assay on large scale	Restricted amount of exclusive aptamer sequences
	Stable connection with in-solution target and immobilized aptamer	Aptamer sequences should be prearranged
		Manufacturing microarray having various sequences exclusive for every target
Binding of nitrocellulose filter	Easy selection	Limited to proteins
	No requirement of complex equipment	Numerous selection rounds are essential
Cell-SELEX	Discovery of biomarker	Limited to cell surface's molecules
	Beneficial potential of selected aptamers	Choice of aptamers to an unplanned target is possible
In vivo SELEX	In vivo functional aptamers selection	Selection of aptamers to an unplanned target is so expected

again. The same kind of aptamers can typically generate lots of sequences having the tendency to combine particularly to the objective area of interest and design findings and detailed reports are typically required for the additional characterization of the sequencing of the aptamer and then selecting the sequences having the finest affinity and specificity. The ultimate consequential aptamer is generated in considerable amounts via a chemical process. In literature, three methods i.e., nitrocellulose filtering, affinity chromatography, and magnetic bead technology have been used for the generation of aptamers in bulk by SELEX. In order to select the preferred aptamers having high affinity, advances in SELEX have concentrated on the significant parts of the old SELEX methodology that involves different techniques of objective immobilization, severance, and exclusion of unnecessary aptamer molecules, quantification of DNA or RNA and determination of binding tendency. The information related to a variety of variants of SELEX methodologies is listed in Table 10.1. After the synthesis of aptamers having binding capacity towards a specific target will be finally incorporated into a sensing arrangement so that they can be used to design the POC platforms.

10.3 APTAMER-BASED POC DIAGNOSTIC DEVICES

Rapid and precise diagnosis is a vital aspect of curing contagious diseases. Diagnostics technologies play a vital role in the identification of healthiness at the starting stages, providing cure courses and tracking the result of therapeutic interventions. However, available analytical apparatus is basically planned for laboratory use only and thus is insufficient to complete health demands. Nowadays, the current research in the field of medical diagnostics is gaining popularity i.e., to develop POC techniques for quick testing in distant areas to balance typical medical diagnostics. Aptamers are one of them that exclusively show interesting applications in this latest period of digital and tailored medicine and increases the conversion of old bench-top therapeutic diagnostics to POC tests. Aptamers can differentiate two molecules that are of the same kind including proteins or conformational isomers (Jenison et al. 1998). Aptamers are capable of the same antibodies in terms of their selectivity and sensitivity (Liss et al. 2002). The high density of aptamer packing than antibodies enhances the joining tendency of the sensors and extends their range to detect an analyte. Considering these properties of aptamers, they are used as detection essentials in diagnostic instruments having numerous advantages and bringing a novel aspect to diagnostics.

10.3.1 Aptamer-based Optical Biosensors

The interaction of the analyte with bioreceptors results in the detection via optical signal changes that come under "optical biosensors". Optical biosensors possess a wide range of applications for detecting pathogenic bacteria through combination with aptamers owing to their security and high resolution. These biosensors comprise two main modes i.e., label-free and label-based biosensors. The first category i.e., Label-free sensors give optical signals through the communication between the analyte and the transducer. However, a label-based sensor utilizes a label to produce optical signals that can be luminescent, colorimetric, or fluorescent (Damborský et al. 2016).

10.3.2 Aptamer-based Colorimetric Biosensors

Colorimetric aptamers sense analyte on the basis of rapid colour development depending on cationic polymers, structural colours, catalyzed oxidation of nanomaterials, oxidation of substrate by enzyme, or the behaviour of nanoparticles (Bala et al. 2016, Hu et al. 2015, Mondal et al. 2018, Sivakumar et al. 2005, Wu et al. 2015). No complicated analytical instruments are required in this method, which makes colorimetric aptamers much simpler than other methods. These aptamers usually use sandwich geometry for capturing and identifying bacteria. For instance, the gold nanoparticle-based enzyme coupled antibody-aptamer sandwich technique has been used to detect *Salmonella typhimurium* (Wu et al. 2014). Then, magnetic microparticles (MMP) were customized with *S. typhimurium* specific aptamers. This is followed by the subsequent sandwiching of MMP-aptamers and detection antibodies. This sandwich composite further reacts with nanoprobes with an antibody and horseradish peroxidase leads to a change in colour. The sensitivity of this aptamer is much higher as compared to the colorimetric ELAAS and chemiluminescent enzyme-linked antibody-aptamer sandwich (ELAAS). A similar kind of sandwich structure has been used to detect Listeria monocytogenes (Liu et al. 2018a).

Aptamer-based colorimetric biosensors together with polymerase chain reaction (PCR) can moreover be used to detect bacteria. The combination of PCR and

G-quadruplex DNAzyme catalytic reaction has been studied (Liu et al. 2019b) to detect L. monocytogenes and Helicobacter pylori (Figure 10.1).

In order to develop the competence of aptamers in colorimetric biosensors, aptamers have been used to detect bacteria. For instance, optimal truncated aptamer has been generated having high affinity once the original aptamer sequence has been used for Vibrio parahaemolyticus. After that, the truncated aptamers have been combined with magnetic nanoparticles for the construction of capture probes and G-quadruplex DNAzyme that can be utilized for the catalysis of chromogenic reaction of 3,3′,5,5′-tetramethylbenzidine (TMB). This technique is helpful in the detection of V. parahaemolyticus that ranges from 102 to 107 CFU mL^{-1} (Sun et al. 2019). Additionally, truncated aptamers have been used for the enhanced adsorption onto gold nanoparticles (AuNPs) in order to identify Campylobacter in chicken carcass samples by the clustering of AuNPs that results in the change in colour (Kim et al. 2018).

In the consecutive research of aptamer-based colorimetric biosensors, a few methods viz., colorimetric analysis and multicolour detection linked with further techniques have also been raised. For example, gold nanorods (AuNRs) have been used to detect *L. monocytogenes* (Figures 10.1 and 10.2) (Liu et al. 2019b). A sandwich-kind compound is produced by Apt-MNPs and nanoenzyme in the existence of L. monocytogenes that can oxidize TMB to TMB^{2+} captured the goal and imprinted AuNRs having different concentrations so that the method shows signals in multicolour for

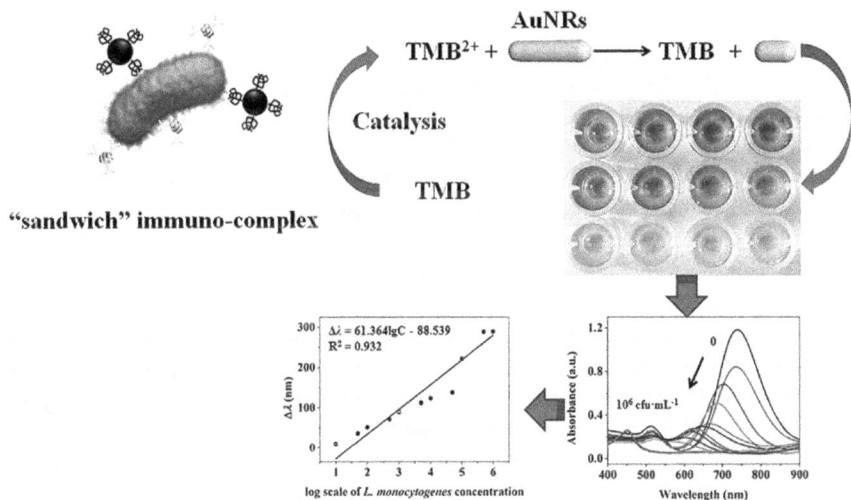

FIGURE 10.1   The Apt-MNP is used as capture probe for *L. monocytogenes*. The Apt-MNP (black), *L. monocytogenes* (blue), and oxidase-like nano-artificial enzyme (green) form a sandwich-type immunocomplex that can catalyze TMB to TMB^{2+}. With the concentration of *L. monocytogenes* increased, more TMB^{2+} is generated and then etched the AuNRs with various aspect ratios, resulting in vivid colour change in the solution.

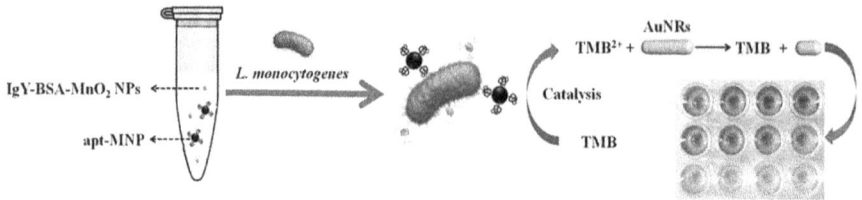

FIGURE 10.2   Illustration of multicolorimetric assay for detection of *L. monocytogenes.*
Image adapted with permission (Liu et al. 2019b) Copy right © 2018 Elsevier B.V. All
rights reserved.

detection. Likewise, more sensitive and accurate detection of pathogenic bacteria
has been performed (Das et al. 2019, Wu et al. 2018) using colorimetric signals with
Surface-enhanced Raman scattering (SERS) signals and electrochemical signals.

10.3.3 APTAMER-BASED FLUORESCENCE BIOSENSORS

When the fluorophore material interacts with the light having a higher wavelength
as compared to the excitation wavelength, the emission of photons takes place. This
resulting indication is very susceptible to the surroundings and therefore, can be used
to determine parameters including binding of the analyte and fluorescence biosensors. Aptamer-based fluorescence biosensors exhibit different properties including
low cost, sensitivity, and fast response. The aptamers can modify their conformation while connecting the target that resulting into the variation in the properties of
fluorescence and therefore, enabling the plan of POC instruments for a large range
of targets.

Aptamer-based fluorescence biosensors attain quantitative analyte detection with
the change in fluorescence by combining aptamers and fluorophores or fluorescent
nanomaterials. The sensitive and specific signal detection is easier to attain in fluorescent biosensors as compared to colorimetric biosensors. In aptamer-based fluorescent biosensors, the same sandwich geometry can be functional that is used in
aptamer-based colorimetric biosensors. For instance, vancomycin-stabilized fluorescent gold nanoclusters (AuNCs@Van) and aptamer-coated magnetic beads have been
prepared for the identification and capturing of *Staphylococcus aureus* (Cheng et al.
2016). This double identification approach significantly enhanced the sensitivity and
specificity of the detection and can be used to identify *S. aureus* in complex samples. Similarly, an identification approach with AuNCs@Van and aptamer-modified
nanoparticles (Apt-AuNPs) has been done (Yu et al. 2017). Here, the sensitive and
selective identification of *S. aureus* can be easily made in 30 min.

Aptamer-based fluorescent biosensors are also useful for identifying various
pathogenic bacteria concurrently. For example, aptamers designated with fluorescent
dyes to carbon nanoparticles have been used for the sensitive and steady concurrent
recognition of *S. typhimurium, V. parahaemolyticus,* and *S. aureus* via multiple fluorescence resonance energy transfer system (FRET) system (Duan et al. 2016). Recent
aptamer-based fluorescence recognition methods follow simple and fast processes

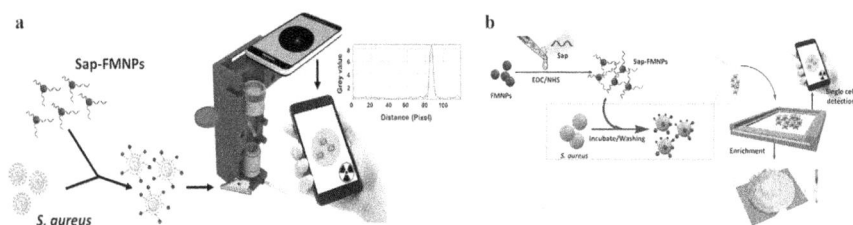

FIGURE 10.3 (a) Quantitative detection of *S. aureus* by smartphone with aptamer-based fluorescent. (b) The *S. aureus* specific aptamer (Sap) was covalently attached to fluorescent magnetic nanoparticles (FMNPs). The Sap-conjugated FMNPs (Sap-FMNPs) were used to tag target bacteria, and those fluorescently tagged bacteria were then spiked in a minimally processed, complex liquid sample.

and ease to fulfil the demands of medical analysis, food safety, and ecological monitoring. For instance, a FRET assay has been developed and can be used in medical specimens to detect methicilin-resistant *S. aureus* (MRSA) based on a PBP2a protein aptamer (Qiao et al. 2018). In comparison to the conventional antimicrobial vulnerability test, this method reduces the time consumption for detection and is not required for the separation and purification of bacteria from experimental samples. In another study, pathogenic bacteria can be sensitively detected by quantitative imaging using smartphones wherein aptamer-conjugated fluorescent MNPs have been utilized to capture target bacteria and the light-emitting diode is present in a smartphone that functions as an excitation basis for fluorescence imaging (Shrivastava et al. 2018) (Figure 10.3a). This technique is very useful in the quick on-site detection of *S. aureus* and can be useful in distant areas. This development shows the use of smart mobile phones in manufacturing aptamer-based POC analytical systems for potential new applications (Shrivastava et al. 2018) (Figure 10.3b).

10.3.4 SERS-BASED APTAMERS

The third category of optical aptamers has been broadly investigated utilizes SERS principles. In spite of the outstanding applications of the aptamer-based fluorescence biosensors; partial sensitivity, high background signals, and incapability to attain several detections are always present. SERS has been proven as a great sensing system wherein enhanced inelastic light scattering takes place by the adsorption of molecules on either plasmonic nanostructures or corrugated metallic surfaces. Owing to high sensitivity, well multiplexing tendency, narrow bandwidth of the Raman peaks, no photobleaching, and low background noise, this technique can overcome the disadvantages of aptamer-based fluorescence biosensors. The foremost benefit of SERS-based aptamers is that these sensors can attain single molecule detection via coinage metal nanostructures.

SERS-based aptamers have been broadly explored to detect pathogens of contagious diseases at the POC (bacteria and viruses), proteins, toxins, and nucleic acids with high sensitivity and specificity. For instance, magnetically assisted SERS-based biosensors using aptamer or antibiotic molecules to recognize bacterial cells have been developed (Pang et al. 2019). Here, aptamerFe$_3$O$_4$@Au magnetic nanoparticles have been prepared in the form of magnetic and SERS-activated substrate for particular bacteria enrichment whereas vancomycin-SERS tags were synthesized for the susceptible quantification of the pathogenic bacteria. This aptamer showed high sensitivity and specificity against the marked pathogenic bacteria with 3 cells mL^{-1} ultra-low detection value and 10–107 cells mL^{-1} wide dynamic linear range, which is much better than the available biosensors. In the case of biological samples, a fast SERS-based lateral flow immunoassay biosensor for the responsive POC recognition of *Escherichia coli* O157:H7 has been studied (Shi et al. 2020). In one recent research, PCR coupled paper-based SERS biosensor composed of silver-nanowires (AgNWs) has been used for quick and responsive determination of Mycoplasma pneumonia DNA at the POC has been developed (Lee et al.) (Figure 10.4). Here, a DNA intercalating molecule i.e., EvaGreen dye has been used for the low-cycled PCR product,

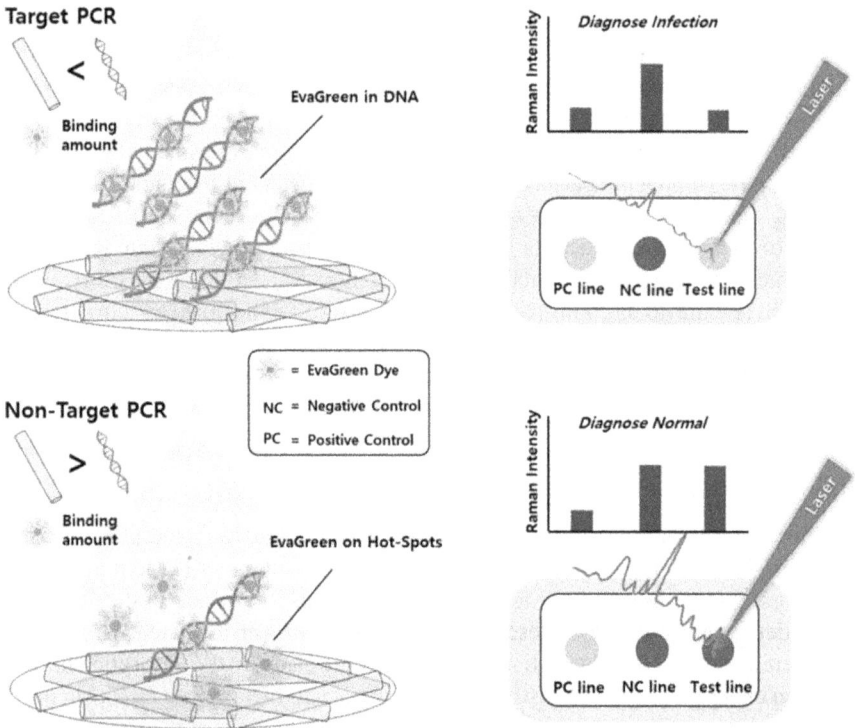

FIGURE 10.4 In the presence of the target, EvaGreen dye intercalation is dominant in DNA structure while in the presence of non-target or no-target, the majority of EvaGreen adheres on the hot-spots area of the AgNWs. The diagnosis can be made by comparing the Raman intensity between the test line and the control lines.

where variation in the intercalation of DNA arrangement could be identified using Raman spectroscopy. This SERS substrate has been arranged as a fast kit comprising of a test, positive and negative control lines that can attain particular prejudice of the target and non-target DNA i.e., valid after 10 cycles of augmentation. The whole evaluation time through the prototype SERS biosensor has been found to be 30 min that shows potential to be utilized as a novel identification technique for the POC diagnostics of a variety of bacteria and viruses.

10.3.5 APTAMER-BASED ELECTROCHEMICAL BIOSENSORS

Aptamer-based electrochemical (EC) biosensors use the tendency of aptamers to purposely connect to a target and their finer constancy than other biorecognition elements. They merge these enviable aptamer properties through the portability, more sensitivity, tendency for miniaturization, and quantitative recognition of EC systems. In these biosensors, one aptamer should be there that can selectively join systematic target and is chemically immobilized on a conductive working electrode and then further can be utilized in an impedimetric, amperometric voltammetry pattern for the selective detection and determine the required target.

Aptamer-based EC biosensors were first discovered in 2004 wherein sandwich-type biosensors were constructed that can be used for the quantitative analysis of thrombin through current in the form of the signal via aptamers having glucose dehydrogenase (Ikebukuro et al. 2004). This discovery results in the extensive usage of aptamer-based EC biosensors in different areas (including environment pollution, food safety, and health monitoring). For instance, *Pseudomonas aeruginosa* can be detected in serum by using aptamer-based EC biosensors (Roushani et al. 2019). In this study, Roushani et al. deposited silver nanoparticles (AgNPs) on a glassy carbon electrode so that the surface area could be increased, and thus, significant acceleration of electron transfer takes place which finally improves EC signal proficiently. *P. aeruginosa* has been collected by NH^{2-} aptamer which is strongly bonded to the surface of AgNP/GCE and detected on the basis of charge transfer resistance in the existence of the target. This method is helpful for the detection of *P. aeruginosa* in the limit lie between 102 and 107 CFU mL^{-1}. Likewise, an rGO-TiO$_2$/GCE has been constructed by the coating of reduced graphene oxide-titanium dioxide (rGO-TiO$_2$) nanocomposite on the surface of GCE (Muniandy et al. 2019). Then, aptamers can be combined with the rGO-TiO$_2$ for the capturing of *S. typhimurium*. The complex having aptamer and bacteria i.e., *S. typhimurium*/Apt/rGO-TiO$_2$/GCE creates a physical obstacle that controls the electronic dynamics at the surface of GCE. In this technique, a smaller number of samples are required that are sufficient for the rapid measurement through a portable device. Hence, this method exhibits a vast potential in on-site detection.

Aptamer-based EC biosensors have applications in monitoring bacterial proliferation. For example, an aptamer-functionalized capacitance sensor array has been developed to examine the growth and death of the bacteria and to evaluate the behaviour of bacteria towards antibiotics (Jo et al. 2018). The aptamer has been immobilized on the surface of the sensor and the count of feasible bacteria bound to the sensor surface has been directly associated with the capacitance. Thus, by measuring the change of capacitance, the growth of bacteria can be easily controlled in real-time. Similarly, Zhang et al. (2019) have utilized aptamers connected to magnetic beads to encapsulate target pathogenic bacteria and then after magnetic separation, the bacteria were cultured in conductometric sensors. The time-dependent conductivity differences among the culture media can be used to measure the growth kinetics of bacteria. As a result, the graph between normalized apparent conductivity values and incubation time can be plotted that showing the development of bacteria (Figure 10.5).

MXenes i.e., a group of 2D materials, 3D carbides, and nitrides having astonishing electrical conductivity and have been used in an EC aptamer to identify the breast cancer marker mucin 1 for the very first time (Wang et al.). The main aim behind these kinds of new electrode materials is to examine different ways to augment the sensitivity and selectivity and lower the detection limit. Reports show the development of the electrode materials design in EC sensors with the aim of improved detection performance, sensitivity, and linear range, together with the development of targets that can be detected using technologies based on aptamers.

10.3.6 APTAMER-BASED MICROFLUIDIC BIOSENSORS

One of the recommended methods for controlling the flow of fluids (microfluidic channels) at micro levels is to design the aforementioned devices with micro-channels

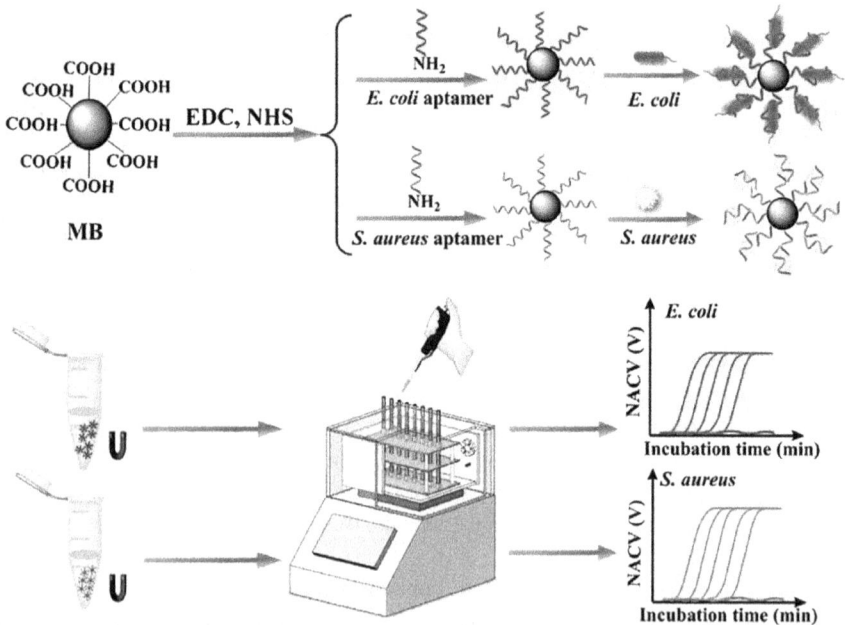

FIGURE 10.5   The procedure of aptamer-based multichannel conductometric sensor for the determination of viable bacteria.

Image adapted with permission from (Zhang et al. 2019) Copyright © 2019, Springer-Verlag GmbH Austria, part of Springer Nature.

(Mark et al. 2010, Nolte 2009). When samples are scarce or need to be handled carefully to prevent the disease from spreading, micro-channels are required (Mark et al. 2010, Nomura et al. 2013). Additionally, typical fluid samples like blood may contain unknown illnesses, necessitating careful handling. Micro-channels help in sample transportation, mixing, separating/sorting, and more procedures.

For on-site blood testing, an array of interconnected microfluidic channels on a chip employing a multilayered aptamer was fabricated (Inoue et al. 2011). For the purpose of determining the blood glucose level during the previous months, the detection of glycosylated haemoglobin (HBA1C) is crucial (approximately 3 months). For diabetics, taking this measurement is strongly recommended to safeguard their internal organs. To measure HBA1C, a portable microfluidic device backed by aptamers has been developed. This device could provide a thorough measurement in 25 minutes (Chang et al. 2015) (Figure 10.6). In light of the fact that microcystin decreases pancreatic function due to an increase in cytotoxicity and an increase in liver glucokinase activity, identification of microcystin-leucine-arginine (a biotoxin that induces apoptosis) is essential (Ji et al. 2011, Saad et al. 2012). When microcystin-leucine-arginine levels are abnormally high, HBA1C levels rise in diabetics. Recently, a fluidic system was used to create an immunoassay that uses aptamers in a microchannel

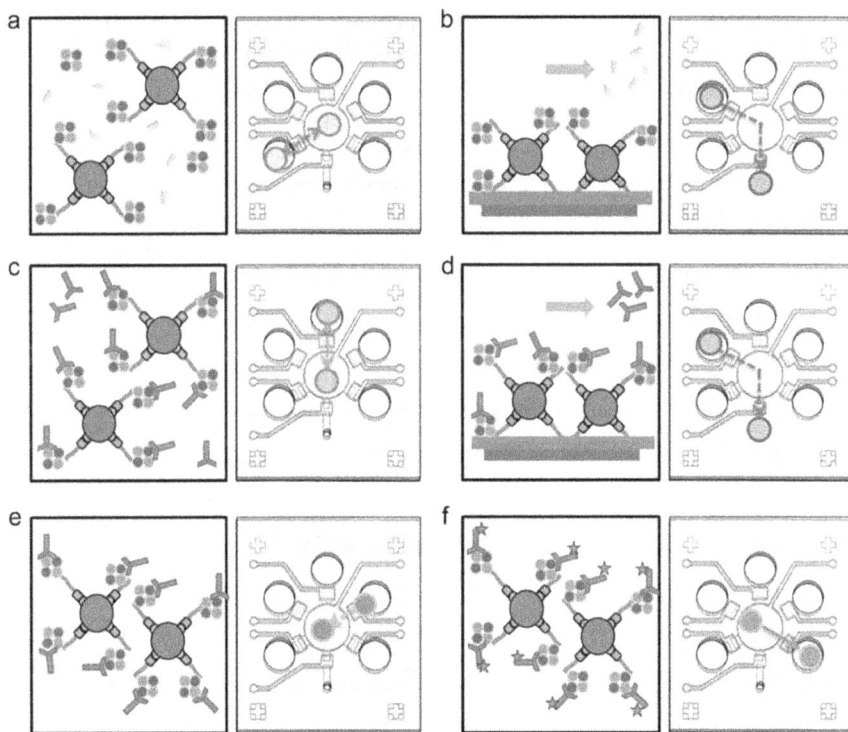

FIGURE 10.6 The experimental procedure was performed on the integrated microfluidic chip.

as a portable analyzer to detect microcystin-leucine-arginine (Xiang et al. 2014). To detect microcystine-leucine-arginine, they employed an aptamer and antibody sandwich pattern in their method. In this study, aptamers were trapped on a glass substrate. Aptamers can be altered and immobilized on various substrates. With this configuration, an aptamer-based online monitoring system was developed to assess environmental contaminants at a sensitivity threshold of 0.3 g L^{-1}. The portable detection of microbial and viral pathogens has also been demonstrated using aptamers and microfluidic channels (Torres-Chavolla and Alocilja 2009). On a microfluidic paper-based analytical system for cocaine detection, an aptamer-based POCT has also been shown (Tian et al. 2016). Because multiplex analyses may be performed on a single microfluidic system with less sample consumption, they are currently quite popular (Ashiba et al. 2016; Nolte 2009).

10.3.7   3D PRINTING-BASED APTAMERS

Till now, commercially accessible POC test show much dependency on the lateral flow formats. Nevertheless, the current arrangement of 3D printing and microfluidics technology is on the way to revolutionize this example. In 3D printing, polymers have been deposited progressively in the form of layers for the formation of solid objects via computer programming designs. The combination of the 3D printing technology and lab-based device progress results in the "design-test-optimize-redesign" of numerous ideas in a quite lesser time period. The detection of bacteria and virus analysis using 3D-printed biochips clearly shows the benefit of simple alteration to other applications without major changes. Recently, 3D printer technology has been employed to plan and optimization of two novel prototypes for the analysis of malaria through the samples of patient's blood (Dirkzwager et al. 2016). They had also produced a specific aptamer to Plasmodium falciparum biomarker lactate dehydrogenase. For the

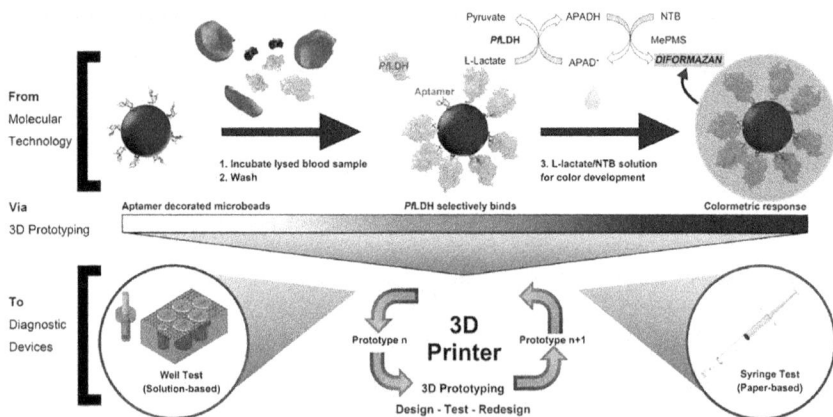

FIGURE 10.7   Using 3D printing to aid rapid prototyping and redesign, this microbead-based assay was incorporated into two new prototypes for point-of-care testing: a good test and a syringe test.

Image adapted with permission from (Dirkzwager et al. 2015) Copyright © 2016, American Chemical Society.

purpose of diagnosis, they discovered a 96-well format colorimetric format for their aptamer-tethered enzyme capture assay. No additional enzymes or antibodies were needed in the test for the function, so it is appropriate for POC implementation if tailored to a suitable design. Tanner's group has quickly prototyped and again planned the aptamer-tethered enzyme capture (APTEC) microbead format as a POC and syringe test by using the stereolithography-type 3D printer (Figure 10.7). The syringe test comprises of syringe attachable spin column assembly having syringe filter device packed with cotton wool that is followed by PfLDH aptamer-functionalized Whatmann 3MM punched paper. The syringe has been used to apply all reagents including samples and buffers. The most interesting fact that has been observed in this method was that test sensitivity was not changed even after the variation of the 96-well APTEC to paper-based visual format which is a significant concern in the growth of POC tests. Using 3D printing technology, both devices have been fabricated and optimized which is permitted for quick prototype synthesis during the whole procedure and aided in transforming the wet lab into a simplistic bedside test layout (Dirkzwager et al. 2015).

10.4 POC DIAGNOSTIC APPLICATIONS OF APTAMER-BASED BIOSENSOR

10.4.1 PROTEIN BIOMARKER IDENTIFICATION

Various protein biomarker aptamer-based biosensor has been synthesized to discover the protein biomarkers in a variety of natural fluids. For instance, an aptsensor has been manufactured to detect the tumour necrosis factor-α (TNF-α) i.e., a main inflammatory cytokine present in total blood. The sensitivity of the assay was susceptible to the detection of 58-pM TNF-α by 6 nM linear range. An EC aptasensor system has been manufactured to detect lung cancer interrelated to protein present in blood plasma samples wherein iron oxide MBs coated with silica have been utilized to improve the detection limit of aptasensor to 0.023 ng mL^{-1} (Zamay et al. 2016). The same principles of EC aptasensing have been used to detect lysozyme, prostate-specific antigen, vascular endothelial growth factor, C-reactive protein, and interleukin-6 (Kumar et al. 2016). Bhardwaj et al. (2019) employed a DNA aptamer that targets the stem area of hemaglutinin for subtyping the influenza A H1 N1 virus. In a recent study, an aptasensor has been used to detect tuberculosis biomarker MPT64 i.e., a protein released by Mycobacterium tuberculosis. EC sensor using an aptamer-gated zeolitic imidazolate framework-derived porous carbon nanocontainer has been developed (Ren et al. 2020) for the better recognition of thrombin at 0.57 fM. In an additional study, an aptamer-antibody sandwich assay with methylene blue as an EC indicator has been documented to detect the mucin 16 protein that is also recognized as cancer antigen 125 (Lu et al. 2020) (Figure 10.8).

10.4.2 SMALL-MOLECULE BIOMARKER DETECTION

Small molecules consist of a numerous biologically active compounds that participate in human well-being. However, they are difficult to sense owing to their minute size, which decreases the accessibility of requisite places for the targeting ligand, such as aptamer. In the past few years, aptamers have been greatly used for the

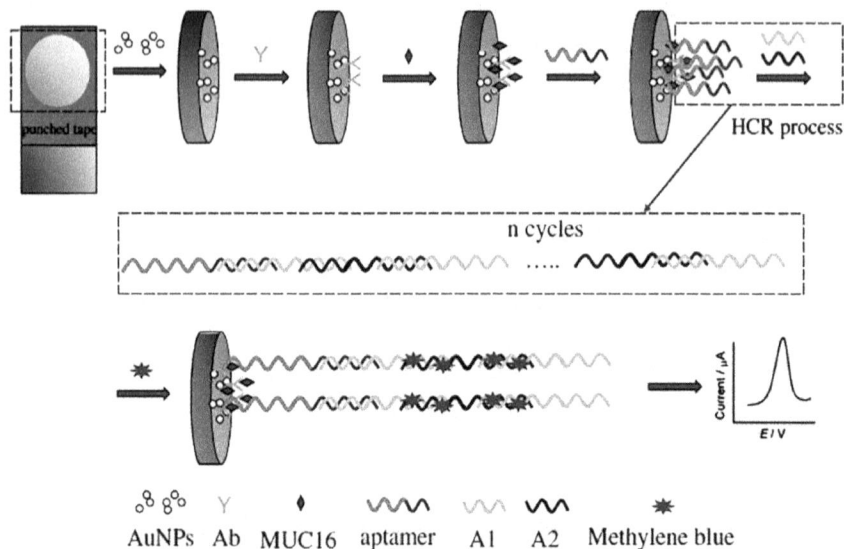

FIGURE 10.8   The fabrication procedure of the biosensor.

Image adapted with permission from (Lu et al. 2020) Copyright © 2020, Springer.

TABLE 10.2
Aptasensing strategy and limit of detection of few important small molecules (Stanciu et al. 2021)

Target compound	Aptasensing strategy	Limit of detection
Antibiotics and drugs		
Aminoglycosidic antibiotics	Colorimetric	1–100 nM
Chloramphenicol	Photoelectrochemical	3.1 nM
Kanamycin	Electrochemical	5.8 nM
Lincomycin	Chemiluminescent	1.6×10^{-13} mol L^{-1}
Tetracycline	Colorimetric	45.8 nM
Heavy metals		
Cu^{2+}	Electrochemical	0.1 pM
As^{3+}	Colorimetric	5.3 ppb
Hg^{2+}	SPR spectroscopy	10 fM
Pesticides and insecticides		
Acetamiprid	Electrochemical	0.33 pM
Carbofuran	Chemiluminescent	88 pM
Chloramphenicol	Colorimetric	18.3 pM
Isocarbophos	Electrochemical	0.01 nM
Microbial toxins		
Aflatoxin B1	Spectrophotometry	0.1 ng mL^{-1}
Ochratoxin A	Colorimetric	20 nM
Tetracycline	Colorimetric	266 pM
Zearalenone	Colorimetric	10 ng L^{-1}

growth of diagnostics for toxins, antibiotics, drug molecules, pesticide residues, and heavy metals. Table 10.2 lists an aptasensing strategy and limit of detection of some important small molecules.

10.4.3 INTACT PATHOGENS DETECTION

Various quick and susceptible diagnostics technologies for different intact pathogens have been developed. The aptasensors have been found to have different merits over the conventional antibody-based assays viz., easy usage, cheap, constancy, and less batch-to-batch inconsistency. These merits led to a wide range of applications of aptasensors for diagnostics progress. The recognition limits for whole-cell pathogens along with aptasensors attained very low levels close to the single-cell level. Nonetheless, most part of the investigation is not changing clinically or still getting the patent phase. The comparatively high steadiness of aptamers besides antibodies provides a chance for combining aptasensors into large inventions and bringing whole-cell pathogen findings from the lab scale to the market.

10.4.4 CIRCULATING TUMOUR CELLS

Cancer is the second major reason of death worldwide (Garcion et al. 2009). Cancer is a kind of non-communicable disease that is an unusual development due to the mutation of human genes. This disease can affect the nearest tissues and organs. Numbers of conventional analytical methods are available to detect cancer cells for example, immunohistochemistry, PCR, and flow cytometry (Schamhart et al. 2003, Singh et al. 2004, Xenidis et al. 2006). However, these methods do not show suitable sensitivity and need expensive tools and a lengthy healing period. Thus, novel tools are much needed to improve early diagnosis and therapeutic results. Biosensors are cheap, effective, sensitive, and fast analytical devices that are used to detect cancer cells at an early stage. Additionally, the integration of recognition element through cancer cells or biomarkers results in the enhancement of selectivity and sensitivity of detection techniques. Biomarkers exist in different types wherein protein is known to be the most valuable biomarker type on the surface of cancer cells.

Aptamers have been considered as ligands to confine and separate circulating tumour cells (CTCs) via targeting a variety of epidermal growth factor receptors, cell membrane proteins, and epithelial cell adhesion molecules (Kordasht and Hasanzadeh 2020). Two POC-friendly platforms i.e., nanomaterials and microfluidic devices are surface functionalized through aptamer-based binding ligands to collect CTCs via clinical or cultural samples. For example, gold surfaces conjugated with aptamers offer a DNA-based nanotetrahedron bio scaffold to augment human hepatocellular carcinoma CTC binding tendency for the utmost convenience of aptamers to target CTCs. In addition to this, cell-SELEX-derived aptamers for the separation of CTC on microchips are gaining popularity for quick testing. For instance, aptamer-based microfluidic chips to capture cells with specific aptamers have been utilized (Xu et al. 2009). In order to increase the CTC capturing competence, irregular surfaces, and multivalent relations have been introduced into the microchip models. Aptamers have been integrated to imaging contrast parameters viz., NPs and fluorophores act as chosen optical probes to target imaging of CTCs. Numerous aptamer-conjugated

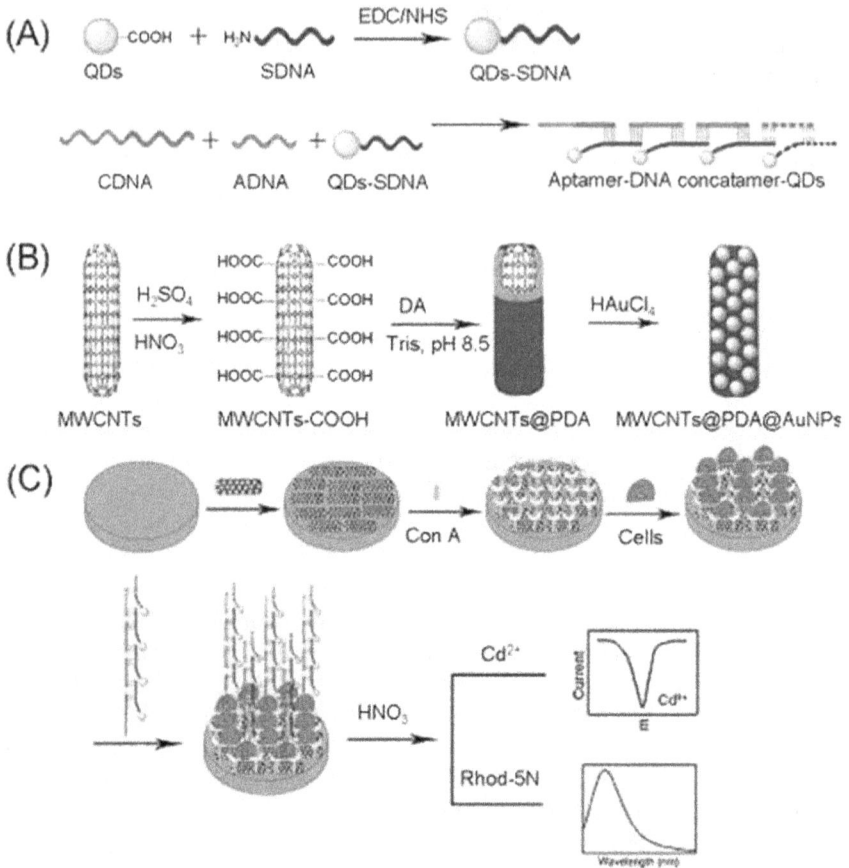

FIGURE 10.9 (a) Procedures for the fabrication of aptamer-DNA concatamer-QDs, (b) MWCNTs@PDA@AuNPs composites, and (c) super sandwich Cyto sensor.

NPs have been produced for quick CTC detection and analysis. For instance, an aptamer-functionalized gold nanofilm chip for the discovery of CTCs from gastric, breast, and ovarian cancer cells has been constructed (Chiu et al. 2015).

In addition to above-mentioned aptamers, EC aptasensors have been also developed to detect CTC. For instance, EC aptasensors has been used to identify CTCs in serum samples that exhibit an LOD of 1–100 cells mL^{-1} and via clinical samples with an LOD of 3 cells mL^{-1}. Moreover, super sandwich EC cytosensors exploiting quantum dots as electroactive types for the amplification of signals have been developed (Liu et al. 2013) (Figure 10.9).

10.5   DRAWBACKS OF APTAMER-BASED BIOSENSORS

Aptamers have gained popularity in the exposure of pathogenic bacteria (Dhimana et al. 2017, Hyebin et al. 2020, Li et al. 2021, Stanciu et al. 2021, Wang et al.). Due to the specificity and similarity, aptamers reduce the detection time and simplify the enrichment processes. However, few limitations exist in aptamer-based techniques to detect pathogenic bacteria that limit the progress of their applications. Generally, aptamers resulting through SELEX consist of 60–100 nucleotides. Lengthy aptamers can result in self-folding which results in a reduction in connection between the aptamer and its target. Though the aptamers in vitro are more stable than the natural antibodies, aptamers are simply ruined by nuclease in vivo. The high affinity between aptamer and its target occur simply under appropriate circumstances but that can be hard to apply in vivo. Further, no efficient methodology is available for the advancement of aptamer that may obstruct the purpose of aptamer. Thus, it is essential for the optimization of SELEX methods that are more appropriate for the circumstances in complex samples or in vivo.

10.6 FUTURE PROSPECTS AND CONCLUSIONS

Aptamer-based biosensors have gained significant popularity in the past few decades. They have a wide range of merits over old antibody-based recognition. The functions of aptamer-based biosensors in the perspective of POC diagnostics or human well-being have also been quickly investigated in the last few years. They have exceptional characteristics including low cost, high sensitivity and selectivity, and negligible batch-to-batch variation. The current chapter highlights some major aptamer-based biosensor devices for the recognition of a range of clinically relevant biomarkers.

In literature, aptamers have been used as affective binding ligands for the particular recognition of targeted analytes. However, few reports are available wherein the 3D arrangement of aptamers has been used for the signal transduction mechanism. Aptamers are also connected with microfluidic models or nanomaterials to facilitate high throughput screening or new signal production procedures. Though there are so many advantages of aptamers present, however, several major challenges aptamers face today. For instance, more clinical studies are required for the further validation of their act in evaluating samples of real patients. The validity of various aptamer-based techniques is needed in more complex biofluid sample matrices including saliva, whole blood, serum, or urine. Additionally, premature analysis of diseases exhibits an important part in the advancement of medical intervention, thus treatment of health situation changes or beginning of disease on time will be needed for the upcoming aptamers. Considering this, aptamer-based biosensors providing real-time and constant monitoring tendencies have been anticipated to fulfil future progress. Regardless of the remaining challenges, the current advancement of POC-friendly aptamer-based biosensors has revealed a great potential to enhance modified diagnostics and worldwide well-being on a great level. Through extra medical justification, scaling up, and commercialization, aptamers can offer more insightful effects in the future of digital and precision medicine.

ACKNOWLEDGEMENTS

All authors would like to thank the Indian Institute of Technology Jodhpur-Rajasthan, India, Indian Institute of Science-Bengaluru, India; and Centre for Materials for Electronics Technology-Thrissur, India, for resources and technical support. Dr. Srikanth Ponnada would like to thank the Department of Science and Technology-India and University Grants Commission for funding and support.

COMPETING INTEREST

Authors declare no competing of interest.

REFERENCES

Ashiba, H., M. Fujimaki, K. Awazu, T. Tanaka, and M. Makishima. 2016. Microfluidic chips for forward blood typing performed with a mulitichannel waveguide-mode sensor. *Sens Bio-Sens Res.* 7:121–126.

Bala, R., M. Kumar, K. Bansal, R.K. Sharma and N. Wangoo. 2016. Ultrasensitive aptamer biosensor for malathion detection based on cationic polymer and gold nanoparticles. *Biosens. Bioelectron.* 85:445–449.

Bhardwaj, J., N. Chaudhary, H. Kim and J. Jang. 2019. Subtyping of influenza A H1N1 virus using a label-free electrochemical biosensor based on the DNA aptamer targeting the stem region of HA protein. *Anal. Chim. Acta.* 1064:94–103.

Chang, K.-W., J. Li, C.-H. Yang, S.-C. Shiesh and G.-B. Lee. 2015 An integrated microfluidic system for measurement of glycated hemoglobin levels by using an aptamer–antibody assay on magnetic beads. *Biosens. Bioelectron.* 68:397–403.

Chang, C.C., Yeh, C.Y. 2021. Using simple-structured split aptamer for gold nanoparticle-based colorimetric detection of estradiol. *Analytical Sciences.* 37(3):479–83.

Chen, H., A. Das, L. Bi, N. Choi, J.I. Moon, Y. Wu and S. Park. 2020. Recent advances in surface-enhanced Raman scattering-based microdevices for point-of-care diagnosis of viruses and bacteria. *Nanoscale.* 12:21560–21570.

Chen, Y., N. Deng, C. Wu, Y. Liang, B. Jiang, K. Yang, et al. 2016. Aptamer functionalized hydrophilic polymer monolith with gold nanoparticles modification for the sensitive detection of human α-thrombin. *Talanta.* 154:555–559.

Cheng, D., Yu, M., Fu, F., Han, W., Li, G., Xie, J., Song, Y., Swihart, M.T., and Song, E. 2016. Dual Recognition Strategy for Specific and Sensitive Detection of Bacteria Using Aptamer-Coated Magnetic Beads and Antibiotic-Capped Gold Nanoclusters. *E. Anal. Chem.* 88:820–825.

Chiu, W.J., T.K. Ling, H.P. Chiang, H.J. Lin and C.C. Huang. 2015. Monitoring cluster ions derived from aptamer-modified gold nanofilms under laser desorption/ionization for the detection of circulating tumor cells. *ACS Appl. Mater. Interfaces.* 7:8622.

Damborský, P., J. Švitel and J. Katrlík. 2016. Optical biosensors. *Essays Biochem.* 60:91–100.

Das, R., A. Dhiman, A. Kapil, V. Bansal and T.K. Sharma. 2019. Aptamermediated colorimetric and electrochemical detection of *Pseudomonas aeruginosa* utilizing peroxidase-mimic activity of gold NanoZyme. *Anal. Bioanal. Chem.* 411:1229–1238.

Dhimana, A., P. Kalraa, V. Bansal, J.G. Bruno and T.K. Sharma. 2017. Aptamer-based point-of-care diagnostic platforms. *Sens. Actuators B.* 246:535–553.

Dirkzwager, R.M., A.B. Kinghorn, J.S. Richards and J.A. Tanner. 2015. APTEC: aptamer-tethered enzyme capture as a novel rapid diagnostic test for Malaria. *Chem. Commun.* 51(22):4697–4700.

Dirkzwager, R.M., S. Liang and J.A. Tanner. 2016. Development of aptamer-based point-of-care diagnostic devices for malaria using three-dimensional printing rapid prototyping. *ACS Sens.* 1(4):420–426.

Duan, N., W.H. Gong, Z.P. Wang, S.J. Wu. 2016. An aptasensor based on fluorescence resonance energy transfer for multiplexed pathogenic bacteria determination. *Anal. Methods.* 8:1390–1395.

Ellington, A.D. and J.W. Szostak. 1990. In vitro selection of RNA molecules that bind specific ligands. *Nature*. 346:818–822.

Garcion, E., P. Naveilhan, F. Berger and D. Wion. 2009. Cancer stem cells: beyond Koch's postulates. *Canc. Lett.* 278(1):3–8.

Geiger, A., P. Burgstaller, H.v.d. Eltz, A. Roeder and M. Famulok. 1996. RNA aptamers that bind L-arginine with submicromolar dissociation constants and high enantioselectivity. *Nucl Acids Res.* 24:1029–1036.

Gram, F.C. 1919. The influenza epidemic and its after-effects in the city of Buffalo: detailed survey. *JAMA*. 73:886–891.

Hermann. T and D.J. Patel. 2000. Adaptive recognition by nucleic acid aptamers. *Science (New York, NY)* 287:820–825.

Hernandez-Vargas, G., J.E. Sosa-Hernandez, S. Saldarriaga-Hernandez, A.M. Villalba-Rodríguez, R. Parra-Saldivar and H. Iqbal. 2018. Electrochemical biosensors: a solution to pollution detection with reference to environmental contaminants. *Biosensors*. 8(2):29.

Hu, J., P. Ni, H. Dai, Y. Sun, Y. Wang, S. Jiang and Z. Li. 2015. Aptamer-based colorimetric biosensing of abrin using catalytic gold nanoparticles. *Analyst*. 140:3581–3586.

Hyebin, Y., H. Jo and S.S. Oh. 2020. Detection and beyond: challenges and advances in aptamer-based biosensors. *Mater. Adv.* 1:2663.

Idili, A., J. Gerson, C. Parolo, T. Kippin and K.W. Plaxco. 2019. An electrochemical aptamer-based sensor for the rapid and convenient measurement of l-tryptophan. *Anal. Bioanal. Chem.* 411:4629–4635.

Ikebukuro, K., C. Kiyohara and K. Sode. 2004. Electrochemical detection of protein using a double aptamer sandwich. *Anal. Lett.* 37:2901–2909.

Inoue, S., M. Seyama, T. Miura, T. Horiuchi, Y. Iwasaki, J.-I. Takahashi and E. Tamechika. 2011. Multi-layered aptamer array integrated in microfluidic chip for on-site blood analysis. *15th International Conference on Miniaturized Systems for Chemistry and Life Sciences*. Seattle, Washington, DC: pp. 1876–1878.

Jenison, R.D, S.D. Jennings, D.W. Walker, R.F. Bargatze and D. Parma. 1998. Oligonucleotide inhibitors of P-selectin-dependent neutrophil-platelet adhesion. *Antisense Nucleic Acid Drug Dev.* 8:265–279.

Ji, D., H. Wang, J. Ge, L. Zhang, J. Li, D. Bai, et al. 2017. Label-free and rapid detection of ATP based on structure switching of aptamers. *Anal. Biochem.* 526:22–28.

Ji, Y., G. Lu, G. Chen, B. Huang, X. Zhang, K. Shen and S. Wu. 2011. Microcystin-LR induces apoptosis via NF-κB /iNOS pathway in INS-1 cells. *Int. J. Mol. Sci.* 12:4722–4734.

Jo, N., B. Kim, S.M. Lee, J. Oh, I.H. Park, K.J. Lim, et al. 2018. Aptamer-functionalized capacitance sensors for realtime monitoring of bacterial growth and antibiotic susceptibility. *Biosens. Bioelectron*. 102:164–170.

Johnson, P.T.J., J.C. De Roode and A. Fenton. 2015. Why infectious disease research needs community ecology. *Science*. 349:1259504.

Karunanayake Mudiyanselage, A.P., Q. Yu, M.A. Leon-Duque, B. Zhao, R. Wu and M. You. 2018. Genetically encoded catalytic hairpin assembly for sensitive RNA imaging in live cells. *J. Amer. Chem. Soc.* 140(28):8739–8745.

Kim, Y.J., H.S. Kim, J.W. Chon, D.H. Kim, J.Y. Hyeon and K.H. Seo. 2018. New colorimetric aptasensor for rapid on-site detection of *Campylobacter jejuni* and *Campylobacter coli* in chicken carcass samples. *Anal. Chim. Acta*. 1029:78–85.

Kohlberger, M. and G. Gadermaier. 2022. SELEX: Critical factors and optimization strategies for successful aptamer selection. *Biotechnology and Applied Biochemistry* 69(5):1771–1792.

Kordasht, H.K. and M. Hasanzadeh. 2020. Aptamer based recognition of cancer cells: recent progress and challenges in bioanalysis. *Talanta*. 220:121436.

Ksiazek, T.G., D. Erdman, C.S. Goldsmith, S.R. Zaki, T. Peret, S. Emery, et al. 2003. A novel coronavirus associated with severe acute respiratory syndrome. *N. Engl. J. Med.* 348:1953–1966.

Kumar, L.S., X. Wang, J. Hagen, R. Naik, I. Papautsky and J. Heikenfeld. 2016. Label free nano-aptasensor for interleukin-6 in protein-dilute bio fluids such as sweat. *Anal. Methods.* 8:3440–3444.

Lee, H.G., W. Choi, S.Y. Yang, D.H. Kim, S.G. Park, M.Y. Lee, et al. 2021. PCR-coupled paper-based surface-enhanced Raman scattering (SERS) sensor for rapid and sensitive detection of respiratory bacterial DNA, *Sens. Actuators. B. Chem.* 326:128802.

Lee, K.H. and H. Zeng. 2017. Aptamer-based ELISA assay for highly specifc and sensitive detection of Zika NS1 protein. *Anal. Chem.* 89:12743–12748.

Li, D., L. Liu, Q. Huang, T. Tong, Y. Zhou, Z. Li, et al. 2021. Recent advances on aptamer-based biosensors for detection of pathogenic bacteria. *World J. Microbiol. Biotechnol.* 37(3):1–20.

Li, H.Y., W.N. Jia, X.Y. Li, L. Zhang, C. Liu and J. Wu. 2020. Advances in detection of infectious agents by aptamer-based technologies. *Emerg Microb Infect.* 9:1, 1671–1681.

Li, J., H.E. Fu, L.J. Wu, A.X. Zheng, G.N. Chen and H.H. Yang. 2012. General colorimetric detection of proteins and small molecules based on cyclic enzymatic signal amplification and hairpin aptamer probe. *Anal. Chem.* 84(12):5309–5315.

Li, Y.K, W.T. Li, X. Liu, T. Yang, M.L. Chen and J.H. Wang. 2019. Functionalized magnetic composites based on the aptamer serve as novel bio-adsorbent for the separation and preconcentration of trace lead. *Talanta.* 203:210–219.

Liss, M., B. Petersen, H. Wolf and E. Prohaska. 2002. An aptamer-based quartz crystal protein biosensor. *Anal. Chem.* 74:4488–4495.

Liu, H, S. Xu, Z. He, A. Deng and J.J. Zhu. 2013. Supersandwich cytosensor for selective and ultrasensitive detection of cancer cells using aptamer-DNA concatamer-quantum dots probes. *Anal. Chem.* 85:3385–3392.

Liu, X., K. Deng, H. Wang, C. Li, S. Zhang and H. Huang. 2019a. Aptamer based ratiometric electrochemical sensing of 17β-estradiol using an electrode modifed with gold nanoparticles, thionine, and multiwalled carbon nanotubes. *Mikrochim. Acta.* 186:347.

Liu, Y., J. Wang, C. Zhao, X. Guo, X. Song, W. Zhao, et al. 2019b. A multicolorimetric assay for rapid detection of Listeria monocytogenes based on the etching of gold nanorods. *Anal. Chim. Acta.* 1048:154–160.

Liu, Y., J. Wang, X. Song, K. Xu, H. Chen, C. Zhao and J. Li. 2018a. Colorimetric immunoassay for Listeria monocytogenes by using core gold nanoparticles, silver nanoclusters as oxidase mimetics, and aptamer-conjugated magnetic nanoparticles. *Mikrochim. Acta.* 185:360.

Liu, Z., C. Yao, Y. Wang and W. Zheng. 2018b. Visual diagnostic of *Helicobacter pylori* based on a cascade amplifcation of PCR and G-quadruplex DNAzyme as a color label. *J. Microbiol. Methods.* 146:46–50.

Lu, L., B. Liu, J. Leng, X. Ma and H. Peng. 2020. Electrochemical mixed aptamer-antibody sandwich assay for mucin protein 16 detection through hybridization chain reaction amplification. *Anal. Bioanal. Chem.* 412:7169–7178.

Ma, C., K. Wu, H. Zhao, H. Liu, K. Wang and K. Xia. 2018. Fluorometric aptamer-based determination of ochratoxin A based on the use of graphene oxide and RNase H-aided amplification. *Microchimica Acta.* 185(7):1–7.

Mark, D., S. Haeberle, G. Roth, F. von Stetten and R. Zengerle. 2010 Microfluidic lab-on-a-chip platforms: requirements, characteristics and applications. *Chem. Soc. Rev.* 39:1153–82.

Mondal, B., S. Ramlal, P.S. Lavu and J. Kingston. 2018. Highly sensitive colorimetric biosensor for staphylococcal enterotoxin B by a label-free aptamer and gold nanoparticles. *Front. Microbiol.* 9:179.

Muniandy, S., S.J. Teh, J.N. Appaturi, K.L. Thong, C.W. Lai, F. Ibrahim and B.F. Leo. 2019. A reduced graphene oxide-titanium dioxide nanocomposite based electrochemical aptasensor for rapid and sensitive detection of Salmonella enterica. *Bioelectrochemistry (Amsterdam, Netherlands).* 127:136–144.

Nolte, D.D. 2009. Invited review article: review of centrifugal microfluidic and bio-optical disks. *Rev. Sci. Instrum.* 80:101101.

Nomura, K.-I., S.C.B. Gopinath, T. Lakshmipriya, N. Fukuda, X. Wang and M. Fujimaki. 2013. An angular fluidic channel for prism-free surface-plasmon-assisted fluorescence capturing. *Nat. Commun.* 4:2855.

Pang, Y.F., N. Wan, L.L. Shi, C.W. Wang, Z.W. Sun, R. Xiao, et al. 2019. Dual-recognition surface-enhanced Raman scattering (SERS) biosensor for pathogenic bacteria detection by using vancomycin-SERS tags and aptamer-Fe_3O_4@Au. *Anal. Chim. Acta.* 1077:288–296.

Qiao, J., X. Meng, Y. Sun, Q. Li, R. Zhao, Y. Zhang, et al. 2018. Aptamer-based fluorometric assay for direct identification of methicillin-resistant *Staphylococcus aureus* from clinical samples. *J. Microbiol. Meth.* 153:92–98.

Remuzzi, A and G. Remuzzi. 2020. COVID-19 and Italy: what next. *Lancet.* 395:1225–1228.

Ren, Q., J. Mou, Y. Guo, H. Wang, X. Cao, F. Zhang, et al. 2020. Simple homogeneous electrochemical targetresponsive aptasensor based on aptamer bio-gated and porous carbon nanocontainer derived from ZIF8. *Biosens. Bioelectron.* 166:112448.

Robertson, D.L. and G.F. Joyce. 1990. Selection in vitro of an RNA enzyme that specifically cleaves single-stranded DNA. *Nature.* 344(6265):467–468.

Roushani, M., M. Sarabaegi and F. Pourahmad. 2019. Impedimetric aptasensor for Pseudomonas aeruginosa by using a glassy carbon electrode modifed with silver nanoparticles. *Mikrochim. Acta.* 186:725.

Saad, A., R. Murabat, A. Omari and S. Al-Jassabi. 2012. Protective role of anthocyanain and taurine against microcystin induced pancreatic and testicular toxicity in balb/C mice. *American-Eurasian J. Toxicol. Sci.* 4:72–79.

Schamhart, D., J. Swinnen, K.H. Kurth, A. Westerhof, R. Kusters and H. Borchers. 2003. Numeric definition of the clinical performance of the nested reverse transcription-PCR for detection of hematogenous epithelial cells and correction for specific mRNA of non-target cell origin as evaluated for prostate cancer cells. *Clin. Chem.* 49(9):1458–1466.

Shi, L.L., L. Xu, R. Xiao, Z.H. Zhou, C.W. Wang, S.Q. Wang, et al. 2020. Rapid, quantitative, high-sensitive detection of Escherichia coli O157:H7 by gold-shell silicacore nanospheres-based surface-enhanced Raman scattering lateral flow immunoassay. *Front. Microbiol.* 11:596005.

Shrivastava, S., W.I. Lee and N.E. Lee. 2018. Culture-free, highly sensitive, quantitative detection of bacteria from minimally processed samples using fluorescence imaging by smartphone. *Biosens. Bioelectron.* 109:90–97.

Singh, S.K., C. Hawkins, I.D. Clarke, J.A. Squire, J. Bayani, T. Hide, et al. 2004. Identification of human brain tumour initiating cells. *Nature.* 432(7015):396–401.

Sivakumar, M., R. Tominaga, T. Koga, T. Kinoshita, M. Sugiyama and K. Yamaguchi. 2005. Studies on visual sensor from self-assembled polypeptides. *Sci. Technol. Adv. Mater.* 6:91–96.

Stanciu, L.A., Q. Wei, A.K. Barui and N. Mohammad. 2021. Recent advances in aptamer-based biosensors for global health applications. *Annu. Rev. Biomed. Eng.* 23:433–459.

Sun, D., J. Lu, L. Zhang and Z. Chen. 2019a. Aptamer-based electrochemical cytosensors for tumor cell detection in cancer diagnosis: a review. *Anal. Chim. Acta.* 1082:1–17.

Sun, Y., N. Duan, P. Ma, Y. Liang, X. Zhu and Z. Wang. 2019b. Colorimetric aptasensor based on truncated aptamer and trivalent DNAzyme for *Vibrio parahemolyticus* determination. *J. Agric. Food. Chem.* 67:2313–2320.

Tian, T., X. Wei, S. Jia, R. Zhang, J. Li, Z. Zhu, H. Zhang, Y. Ma, Z. Lin and C.J. Yang. 2016. Integration of target responsive hydrogel with cascaded enzymatic reactions and microfluidic paper-based analytic devices (mPADs) for point-of-care testing (POCT). *Biosens. Bioelectron.* 77:537–542.

Torres-Chavolla, E. and E.C. Alocilja. 2009. Aptasensors for detection of microbial and viral pathogens. *Biosens. Bioelectron.* 24:3175–3182.

Traeger, M.W., S.E. Schroeder, E.J. Wright, M.E. Hellard, V.J. Cornelisse, J.S. Doyle, et al. 2018. Effects of pre-exposure prophylaxis for the prevention of human immunodeficiency virus infection on sexual risk behavior in men who have sex with men: a systematic review and meta-analysis. *Clin. Infect. Dis.* 67:676–686.

Tuerk, C. and L. Gold. 1990. Systematic evolution of ligands by exponential enrichment: RNA ligands to bacteriophage T4 DNA polymerase. *Science.* 249:505–510.

Wang, C., M. Liu, Z. Wang, S. Li, Y. Deng and N. He. 2021. Point-of-care diagnostics for infectious diseases: from methods to devices. *Nano Today.* 37:101092.

Wang, H., J. Sun, L. Lu, X. Yang, J. Xia, F. Zhang, et al. 2020. Competitive electrochemical aptasensor based on a cDNA-ferrocene/MXene probe for detection of breast cancer marker Mucin1. *Anal. Chim. Acta* 1094:18–25.

Wang, H.X, Y.W. Zhao, Z. Li, B.S. Liu and Zhang D. 2019. Development and application of aptamer-based surface-enhanced Raman spectroscopy sensors in quantitative analysis and biotherapy. *Sensors (Basel, Switzerland).* 19:3806.

Weigl, J. 2020. Challenges in infectious disease control and the current pandemic by skewed distributions. *Pravent. Gesundheit.* 15:97–101.

Wu, S., Y. Wang, N. Duan, H. Ma and Z. Wang. 2015. Colorimetric aptasensor based on enzyme for the detection of Vibrio parahemolyticus. *J. Agric. Food. Chem.* 63:7849–7854.

Wu, W., J. Li, D. Pan, J. Li, S. Song, M. Rong, et al. 2014. Gold nanoparticle-based enzyme-linked antibody-aptamer sandwich assay for detection of *Salmonella typhimurium. ACS Appl. Mater. Interfaces.* 6(19):16974–16981.

Wu, Y.C., C.S. Chen and Y.J. Chan. 2020. The outbreak of COVID-19: an overview. *J. Chin. Med. Assoc.* 83:217–220.

Wu, Z., D. He, B. Cui and Z. Jin. 2018. A bimodal (SERS and colorimetric) aptasensor for the detection of *Pseudomonas aeruginosa. Mikro. Chim. Acta.* 185:528.

Xenidis, N., M. Perraki, M. Kafousi, S. Apostolaki, I. Bolonaki, A. Stathopoulou, et al. 2006. Predictive and prognostic value of peripheral blood cytokeratin-19 mRNA-positive cells detected by realtime polymerase chain reaction in node-negative breast cancer patients. *J. Clin. Oncol.* 24(23):3756–3762.

Xiang, A., X. Lei, F. Ren, L. Zang, Q. Wang, J. Zhang, Z. Lu and Y. Guo. 2014. An aptamer-based immunoassay in microchannels of a portable analyzer for detection of microcystinleucine-arginine. *Talanta.* 130:363–369.

Xu, Y., J.A. Phillips, J. Yan, Q. Li, Z.H. Fan and W. Tan. 2009. Aptamer-based microfluidic device for enrichment, sorting, and detection of multiple cancer cells. Anal. Chem. 81:7436–7442.

Yu, M., H. Wang, F. Fu, L. Li, J. Li, G. Li, et al. 2017. Dual-recognition förster resonance energy transfer based platform for one-step sensitive detection of pathogenic bacteria using fluorescent vancomycin–gold nanoclusters and aptamer–gold nanoparticles. *Anal. Chem.* 89(7):4085–4090.

Zaki, A.M., S.V. Boheemen, T.M. Bestebroer, A.D.M.E. Osterhaus and R.A.M. Fouchier. 2012. Isolation of a novel coronavirus from a man with pneumonia in Saudi Arabia. *N. Engl. J. Med.* 367:1814–1820.

Zamay, G.S., T.N. Zamay, V.A. Kolovskii, A.V. Shabanov, Y.E. Glazyrin, D.V. Veprintsev, et al. 2016. Electrochemical aptasensor for lung cancer-related protein detection in crude blood plasma samples. *Sci. Rep.* 6:1–8.

Zhang, X., X. Wang, Q. Yang, X. Jiang, Y. Li, J. Zhao and K. Qu. 2019. Conductometric sensor for viable Escherichia coli and *Staphylococcus aureus* based on magnetic analyte separation via aptamer. *Mikrochim. Acta.* 187:43.

11 Current perspectives of aptasensors as diagnostic tools for oncological diseases

Suman Kumar Ray and Sukhes Mukherjee

11.1 INTRODUCTION

Cancer is the world's second most common (Siegel et al. 2022) non-communicable disease. Despite increased public health attention to early detection and a dedication to 'best practice' treatment tactics, millions of people die each year from cancer, and expected incidence trends continue to rise, implying the need for more effective cancer management measures. Chemotherapy, radiation, and surgery are all traditional tumor treatment modalities, but each has its own set of limitations in clinical practice. Chemotherapy is a popular way to treat malignancies these days (Arruebo et al. 2011). However, because this therapy strategy is not selective, it will harm normal tissues as well as malignant tissues, resulting in non-specific damage. Long-term usage of chemotherapeutic medications can also lead patients to acquire drug resistance, reducing therapy efficacy. Radiation osteonecrosis, radiation pneumonia, and systemic responses are common side effects of systemic and local irradiation (Chen et al. 2020, Crosby et al. 2020). As a result, it is critical to investigate effective cancer diagnosis, early detection, and treatment options to drastically reduce cancer mortality. As a result, there is a growing need to create an accurate, cost-effective, sensitive, and initial-stage cancer detection approach for several cancer types to prevent it. As a result of this pressing need for better cancer therapies, precision medicine has received more attention to prevent off-target effects and improve patient quality of life during treatment.

'Aptasensors' was created by combining aptamers and biosensing platforms. Numerous new and promising point-of-care cancer diagnostics are now possible because of the development of highly sensitive aptasensors (Shabalina et al. 2021). Short RNA or DNA molecules or oligomers known as aptasensors can bind various targets, including proteins, peptides, medicines, and cells. When a tiny molecule is bound, it causes conformational modifications such as folding and forming a double-strand structure. The most appropriate aptasensor's recognition element is a short oligonucleotide chain isolated in vitro by SELEX (Shaban and Kim 2021, Zhang et al. 2019), employing various screening procedures and modulation of selection

DOI: 10.1201/9781003304227-11

conditions to tightly regulate the target binding affinity and specificity of the aptamer (Chen et al. 2019). The aptamer sequence is typically 30–70 nucleotides long, folded into a three-dimensional structure, and attached to certain biological components via specificity and affinity, for instance, metal ions, tumor protein markers, small chemicals, or circulating tumor cells (Labib et al. 2012, Lee et al. 2019, Niu et al. 2021, Safarpour et al. 2020, Wang et al. 2019).

For instance, Li and his colleagues (2020) assembled fluorescent aptasensors from nanomaterials to identify tumor-associated proteins on exosomes derived from prostate and breast cancer. They successfully differentiated healthy specimens from tumor specimens due to their high sensitivity (Li et al. 2020). Biosensors utilizing enzymes as identifying components have been employed for prompt detection of tumor patients, for example detecting circulating tumor cells, prostate antigen, and so on (Abardía-Serrano et al. 2020, Yang et al. 2019). On the other hand, enzymes are temperature and pH-sensitive and have short shelf-life. The production and characterization of novel antibodies for antibody sensors is time-consuming and complex (Rossetti et al. 2020, Verdian et al. 2019). In addition, other processes, for instance, induction by target preparations, animal immunization, antibody purification, and others, are hard and time and material-intensive (Amritkar et al. 2020, Huang et al. 2020). It's also difficult for freshly created antibodies to manage their binding qualities and bind to comparable structures to cause non-target interference (Yu et al. 2021), and they're easily influenced by immunosuppressive medications (Xu et al. 2020) for some small compounds and proteins with lesser immunogenicity. Sensors for enzymes and antibodies are not the same and it is possible to synthesize the precise aptasensor sequence. For tumor marker identification and therapy in vitro with cheap cost, repeatable mass manufacturing, and is easily changed by nanomaterials. They can also withstand a wide range of pH and salt concentrations as well as have high thermal stability (Zhang et al. 2019). These characteristics make maptasensors, rather than enzymes or antibodies, an excellent recognition element for biosensors for tumor surveillance.

Biological information is generally translated to fluorescent, electrochemical signals, or color changes (Dinarvand et al. 2019, Rauf et al. 2021, 24, Wei et al. 2019), which may be separated into fluorescence, electrochemistry, and colorimetric aptasensors (Chen et al. 2019), according to the signal conversion elements of different types of aptasensors. Traditional electrochemistry is still the most widely utilized in building aptasensors because of its portability, superior signal theory along compatibility with biological components (Figure 11.1). Electrochemical aptasensors have several benefits over conventional transducers, including downsizing and automation, turbidity insensitiveness or quenching effects, and eliminating laborious sample preparation nearly entirely (Abd-Ellatief and Abd-Ellatief 2021). Electrochemical aptasensors also have lower detection limits than conventional sensors. The diffusion efficiency, electron transfer, and the final measured signal are all affected by the transduction mediums of electrochemical sensors. The selection of appropriate electroactive chemicals is critical for developing electrochemical sensors. In this book chapter, we review the most recent signs of progress and current aspects of various detection strategies for electrochemical, colorimetric, and fluorescent aptasensors, as well as assess the future application drift of aptasensors to achieve tumor diagnosis and treatment integration.

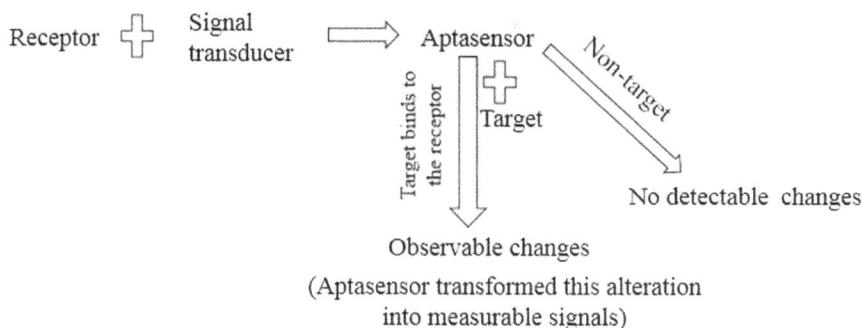

FIGURE11.1 Simplest schematic presentation regarding the working principle of an aptasensor.

11.2 APTASENSOR TRANSDUCTION MECHANISMS

Aptasensor in a typical aptasensing system (Figure 11.2) will selectively bond to the target and provide a signal output. This signal may either be physical or chemical, and it may be transduced into a readout that can be evaluated, interpreted, and frequently amplified for increased sensitivity. Aptamers are synthetic nucleic acid ligands with particular binding qualities to their targets that may be chosen from combinatorial libraries of synthetic nucleic acids. Aptamers may be extracted and created from pools of randomly synthesized RNA or DNA using the systematic evolution of ligands (SELEX) technique (Figure 11.3). Aptasensors are biosensors that use aptamers as a recognition element (O'Sullivan 2002).

Aptasensors can also be designed to resist multiple denaturation and renaturation cycles, allowing immobilized biocomponent function to be regenerated for reuse (Jayasena 1999). Furthermore, they are simple to label in cancer diagnostics (Ulrich and Wrenger 2009). A variety of detection schemes have been used in the development of aptasensors, ranging from label-free methods like surface plasmon resonance (SPR) (Ostatna et al. 2008) and quartz crystal microbalance (QCM) measurements to more label-intensive methods like electrochemistry (Willner and Zayats 2007), fluorescence (Rupcich et al. 2006), chemiluminescence (Wang et al. 2007), and field-effect transistors (Zayats et al. 2006), all of which have been reported and aided the field's electrochemical and optical aptasensors are the two most common types of aptasensors used.

11.2.1 ELECTROCHEMICAL APTASENSORS

An electrochemical aptasensor uses an electrode surface to immobilize biological sensing, and the analyte binding event is monitored using electrochemical current changes (Figure 11.4). Electrochemical transduction benefits better sensitivity, which can be increased by adding biocatalytic labels to the apta-target complexes to amplify signal detection, miniaturization, and inexpensive manufacturing costs because it does not require expensive optical instruments (Lee et al. 2008, Willner and Zayats 2007). Additionally, label-free and reusable detecting methods are available.

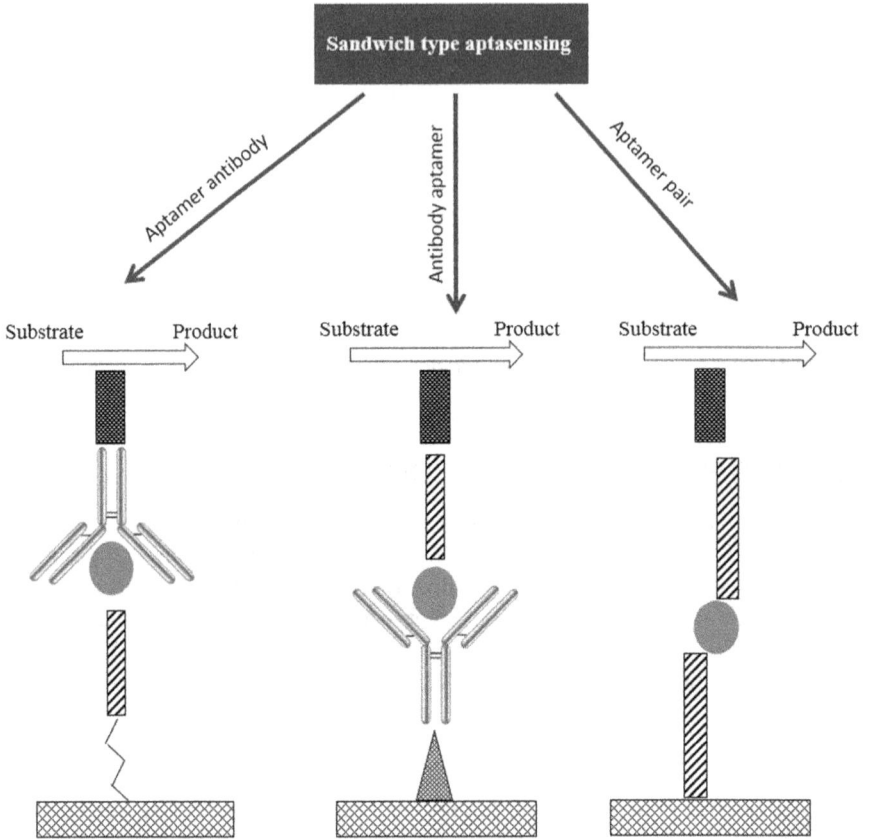

FIGURE 11.2 Formation of sandwich-type aptasensing.

11.2.2 OPTICAL APTASENSORS

Optical aptasensors include fluorescence-labeled aptamers, luminophore-labeled aptamers, enzyme-labeled aptamers, nanoparticles, and label-free detection techniques (e.g., SPR, optical resonance) (Sassolas et al. 2011). The majority of approaches rely heavily on labeling. Colorimetry, chemiluminescence, and utmost advanced fluorescence mode can all be used to identify some targets, as can more modern non-conventional optical approaches like surface plasmon coupled directional emission (SPCDE) (Sassolas et al. 2011). SPR, diffraction grating, evanescent field coupled (EFC) waveguide mode, optical resonance, and Brewster angle straddle interferometry (BASI) have all recently been proven to be useful for creating aptasensors (Sassolas et al. 2011). SPR biosensors made using optical fibers may monitor biomolecular interactions in situ or in vivo and are a cost-effective and relatively easy-to-implement alternative to thriving established biosensor systems (Shevchenko et al. 2011).

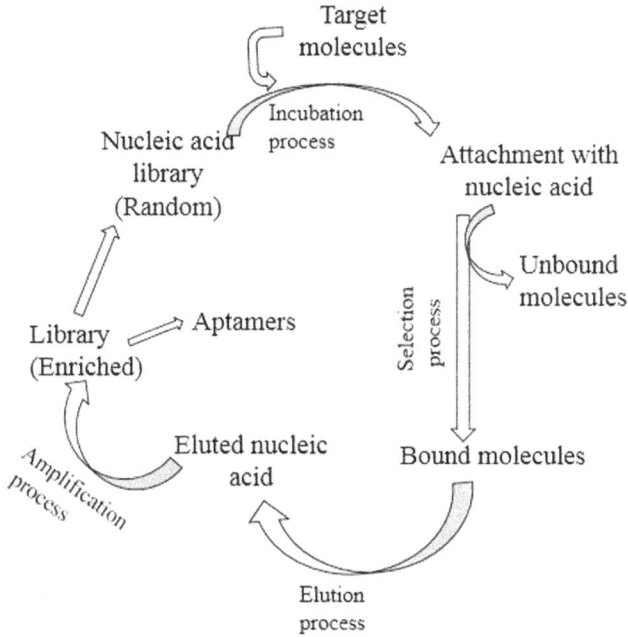

FIGURE 11.3 Flow diagram of SELEX process.

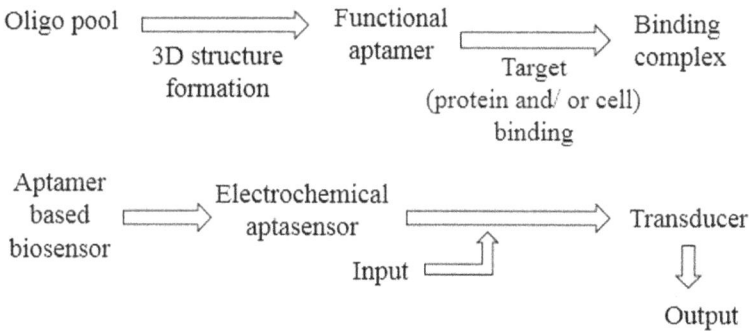

FIGURE 11.4 Electrochemical aptasensor.

11.3 APTASENSORS AND DETECTION OF CANCER BIOMARKERS

Many aptasensors, including human epidermal growth factor receptor-2 (HER2), vascular endothelial growth factor (VEGF), epidermal growth factor receptor (EGFR), PDGF, Mucin 1 (MUC-1), prostate-specific antigen (PSA), and carcinoembryonic antigen (CEA), have been found as biomarkers and cells for many cancers in the last decade (Liu et al. 2021). The following are several aptasensor-based biomarkers.

11.3.1 PROTEIN BIOMARKERS FOR CANCER

Lung, colon, pancreas, breast, and ovarian malignancies are all linked to MUC1 overexpression. As a result, it's thought to be a key protein biomarker in the early detection of human malignancies. Li et al. presented a colorimetric dual-mode surface-enhanced Raman scattering (SERS) aptasensor to detect MUC1 (Li et al. 2020). For invasive breast tumors, HER-2 is an important prognostic factor. Malecka et al. (2019) established a sensitive electrochemical cellulase-based sandwich test using magnetic beads for HER-2 protein, that is overexpressed in most breast tumors (Malecka et al. 2019). Tabrizi et al. (2015) described the use of an aptasensor to detect VEGF in a lung cancer patient's serum.

11.3.2 BIOMARKERS FOR ANTIGENS

CEA is a glycoprotein present in the embryonic endodermal epithelium that might be used to track colorectal cancer treatment as well as identify breast, gastrointestinal, liver, lung, ovarian, and pancreatic cancers. Paniagua and his colleagues (2019) built an aptasensor using NPs with silica and gold on opposing sides (Paniagua et al. 2019).

11.3.3 CIRCULATING TUMOR CELLS

Circulating tumor cells (CTCs) are a kind of tumor cell released from primary tumor tissue and circulated in the bloodstream and lymph nodes. Because they infect multiple parts of the body and establish metastatic sites, they are considered a significant indicator of tumor metastasis. As a result, CTC migration is a precursor to cancer development. MCF-7 cells were directly detectable by Shen et al. (2016). Immobilized EpCAM-binding aptamers were immobilized on the Au electrode, and the impedance value changed when EpCAM on the MCF-7 cell membrane was bound to it (Shen et al. 2016). By adding SYL3C binding aptamers, Liu and his colleagues (2018) used a sandwich-type construction to produce amperometric aptasensors (Liu et al. 2018). For the in situ characterization of cell membrane proteins of CTCs and classifying their cancer subpopulations, Zhang and his colleagues (2018) used an on-chip technique combining SERS analysis with size-based microfluidic cell separation (Zhang et al. 2018). Breast cancer cells of various subtypes may be detected with excellent sensitivity and selectivity. For very sensitive detection of CTCs, colorimetric platforms based on G-quadruplexDNAzymes with peroxidase activity as signal-amplifying components were created (Norouzi et al. 2018).

11.3.4 EXOSOMES

They are extracellular vesicles in the human circulatory system that transport molecular proteins and/or nucleic acids between cells for cell-to-cell communication. They range in size from 30 to 150 nm in diameter. Exosomes are regarded as one of the most significant cancer biomarkers due to their participation in tumor microenvironment modification (Raimondo et al. 2011). Exosome detection aptasensors based on fluorescence or colorimetry have recently been developed. Yu et al. (2019) employed a competitive method to detect an exosome transmembrane protein, CD63, on the surface of exosomes using fluorescence-based aptasensors. Apart from the CD63 protein on exosome surfaces, miRNAs within exosomes are also useful. Lee and his colleagues (2016) showed this for the first time in exosomes from MCF-7 cells employing molecular aptamer beacons for in situ simultaneous detection of three targets miR-21, miR-27a, and miR-375 (Lee et al. 2016). Exosome detection has also been developed using colorimetric aptasensors. Jiang et al. (2017) developed an AuNP-based sensing device that analyses exosome surface protein CD63 (Jiang et al. 2017). The procedure takes only a few minutes, and the outcome may be seen with the naked eye. Aptamerexosome binding caused AuNPs to aggregate in the presence of exosomes, resulting in a dark blue solution claiming that AuNPs-based aptasensors can distinguish and profile fine exosome surface protein variations in a short amount of time (Jiang et al. 2017). Exosome detection using electrochemical aptasensors based on potential, existing, or impedance changes has also been created. Different types of aptasensor used in cancer testing are listed in Table 11.1.

TABLE 11.1
Examples of aptasensor applications in cancer clinical testing (Hong et al. 2012).

Types of aptamsensor based on signal transduction	Cancer marker detected	Detection type
Electrochemical aptasensor	HeLa cells, K562 cells, MDA-231 cells	Label-free detection
	Mucin 1	Single step electrochemical deposition method
	Vascular endothelial growth factor	FET-type biosensor based on CPNTs aptamer
SPR aptasensor	Glutathione	SPR analysis plus isocratic affinity chromatography
Electrogeneratedchemiluminescence (ECL) aptasensor	Platelet-derived growth factor B chain	Sandwich conjugate with modified electrode
	Ramos cancer cell	Label-free detection
	Ramos cancer cell, CEM cells	ECL array with a novel cycle-amplifying technique
Quartz crystal microbalance-based aptasensor	Leukemia cells	A magnet-QCM system
Fluorescence aptasensor	Multi-marker or Ramos cells, CCRF-CEM cells, Toledo Cells	Simultaneous multiplexed analysis
	Mucin 1	Aptamer-based detection using quantum-dot-based fluorescence readout
Chemiluminescenceaptasensor	prostate-specific antigen	Aptamer blotting assay

11.4   APTASENSORS FOR DETECTION OF THE PSA IN PROSTATE CANCER

The predominant prostate cancer marker found in patient blood samples is PSA; in a study, Jolly et al. attempted to construct an aptasensor for PSA (Tahmasebi and Noorbakhsh 2016); their findings were evaluated using the EIS approach. Low analyte detection ability is a critical goal for all aptasensors and diagnostic procedures. PSA detection was studied using a nanoaptasensor that contained gold nanoparticles encapsulated in graphitized mesoporous carbon (Cha et al. 2014). The electrochemical detection technique used in this study was differential pulse voltammetric (DPV), and the aptasensor may detect PSA in the range of 0.25 to 2×10^2 ng mL^{-1} in the patient's blood. Rahi and his colleagues (2016) have designed an electrochemical aptasensor against PSA antigen utilizing goldnanospears. Carbon nanotubes functionalize the carboxylic acid (CNTs(COOH)), chitosan (Chit), carbon nanotubes-chitosan (CNTs-Chit along with CNTs(COOH)-Chit) (Chang et al. 2014) were used to design an electrochemical PSA aptasensor.

11.5   APTASENSORS FOR DETECTION OF MCF-7 CELLS, RAMOS CELLS, AND TUMOR NECROSIS FACTOR-α

Cai et al. (2015) have investigated breast cancer diagnosis and developed an aptasensor that could detect breast cancer MCF-7 cells in the range of $0–5\times10^2$ cells mL^{-1}. Khoshroo and his colleagues (2022) proposed an aptasensor for detecting MCF-7 cells in another study. In all aptasensors, selecting a particular aptamer against analytes is critical. A fluorescent aptasensor was developed to detect MCF-7 cells in a study (Borghei et al. 2016). Cai et al. (2015) employed fluorescence analysis as the primary detection method, and the MCF-7 cells were detected using this aptasensor (Cai et al. 2015). A graphene oxide-based aptasensor was developed in another study to detect MCF-7, HL-60, and K562 cancer cells (Yan et al. 2013). The mesoporous silica nanoparticles (MSNs) were utilized in this aptasensor, and all analyses were monitored using visual fluorescence measurements. The aggregation of gold nanoparticles was used to create a colorimetric nanoaptasensor, which was then used to identify MCF-7 cells after the absorption spectra were investigated. A fluorescent aptasensor based on mesoporous carbon nanospheres is recently developed. MUC1 tumor marker molecules and MCF-7 cells were detected using a unique method. Using gold and silica nanoparticles as well as magnetic beads, an electro-chemiluminescence aptasensor was designed to detect Ramos cells (B-cell, CRL-1596, human Burkitt's lymphoma) (Liu et al. 2013). Liu et al. (2013) studied the experimental design of an aptasensor to detect tumor necrosis factor-α (TNF-α), an anticancer drug utilized in cancer treatment (Liu et al. 2013). Methylene blue was employed as a redox marker in all electrochemical investigations in this study (Figure 11.5).

11.6   APTASENSORS FOR DETECTION OF LEUKEMIA CELLS

Cao and his colleagues (2012) investigated a signal on aptasensor to identify T-cell acute lymphoblastic leukemia cells; they employed graphene oxide-based fluorescence

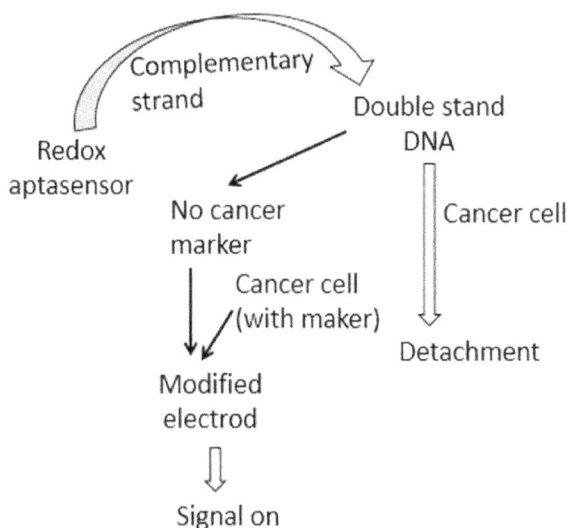

FIGURE 11.5 Flow diagram of aptasensor-based dsDNA conformation and detection.

resonance energy transfer (FRET) in the sensing approach and cell detection (Cao et al. 2012). An electro-chemiluminescence aptasensor utilizing a wireless indium tin oxide bipolar electrode was described in another study to detect adenosine in cancer cells. HeLa cells (human cervical carcinoma), MDA-MB-231 cells (human breast cancer), K562 cells (leukemia line), and NIH3T3 cells (mouse embryonic fibroblast cell line) were detected using graphene in an electrochemical aptasensor (Nezakati et al. 2014). An electrochemical aptasensor was also developed to detect HeLa cells, and this aptasensor was built on grapheme nanocomposites, which caused the detectable signal produced by the analyte to be amplified (Abd-Ellatief and Abd-Ellatief 2021). Based on cell-triggered cyclic enzymatic signal amplification a visual colorimetric aptasensor was developed to identify T-cell acute lymphoblastic leukemia cells (Zhang et al. 2014).

11.7 APTASENSORS FOR DETECTION OF MUC1 CELLS AND CEA

Overexpression of the MUC1 glycoprotein is a key indicator and diagnostic for cancer detection. A fluorescent aptasensor was developed to detect MUC1 with graphene oxide as the signal quencher (Zhang et al. 2018). In another study, Ulucan-Karnak and Akgöl (2021) developed an aptasensor to detect the MUC1 tumor marker using nanomaterials. Researchers also attempted to develop an early detection approach for colon cancer by detecting the MUC1 glycoprotein on the cellular membrane.

Cadmium sulfide graphene nanocomposites are used as co-reactant, and an electro-chemiluminescence aptasensor was constructed to detect the CEA in genuine human blood samples (Liu et al. 2015).

In another study, a nano-aptasensor incorporating nanocomposites (ZnS-CdS nanoparticles (NPs)-decorated molybdenum disulfide (MoS2) was used to test electro-chemiluminescence CEA assay (Verberne et al. 2013). With the inclusion of carbon nanoparticles, a FRET-based aptasensor was created to detect CEA, where an electrochemical aptasensor was developed to detect CEA, and a nanocomposite of gold nanoparticles, hemin, and graphene was used.

11.8 APPLICATION OF APTASENSORS IN CLINICAL DIAGNOSIS OF CANCER

Aside from all of these benefits, using aptasensors as bio-components opened up exciting possibilities in cancer diagnostic tests. Due to the increasing number of cancer cases being identified worldwide, cancer is now the second leading cause of death and morbidity globally. Early detection is critical in all malignancies to enhance patient survival and illness prognosis, and may even lead to cancer prevention – which is why sensitive and precise approaches for early cancer diagnosis are essential. Tumor cell detection and identification rely on identifying specific markers found only on tumor cells, such as lymphoma (Ramos) cells and leukemia cells.

Specialized probes must bind to the cancer markers to detect the probable risk factor. Plasma proteins or free DNA in blood cells might be tumor indicators. Aptasensors have been effectively employed to detect tumor markers in several recent investigations. Based on the first clinical oncology trial II, Feng and his colleagues (2011) gave an example of label-free cancer cell detection utilizing an electrochemical sensor using aptasensor AS1411 and graphene-modified electrode (Feng et al. 2011). The electrochemical aptasensor can tell the difference between cancer and normal cells and can detect as few as 1,000 cells. Different electrochemical aptasensors for cancer detection applications are shown in Table 11.2.

11.9 APPLICATIONS OF APTASENSORS IN THE CANCER FOLLOW-UP

Hashemian and his colleagues (2016) have developed an aptasensor to detect cytochrome c and the screening mechanism was related to the diagnosis of cytochrome c. The B-cell lymphoma 2 (Bcl-2) regulatory protein triggers the release of cytochrome c from the mitochondria, which in turn causes caspase-9 and caspase-3 to activate. Ultimately, this pathway results in cell apoptosis (Hashemian et al. 2016). Thus aptasensor cytochrome c detection is very important for the cancer follow-up process. In another electroanalytical application, researchers have developed an aptasensor for detecting adenocarcinoma (Negahdary et al. 2019). Researchers also followed up by designing a particular aptasensor to detect human hepatoma SMMC-7721 cells (Negahdary et al. 2019). The LC-18 tumor markers are detected using an electrochemical aptasensor in lung cancer patients. Qureshi and his colleagues (2015) attempted to provide a novel approach for detecting human epidermal growth factor receptor 2 (HER2) cancer biomarkers by altering the dielectric parameters of the aptasensor (Qureshi et al. 2015). HepG2 cells are used to develop an aptasensor for liver cancer detection (Chen et al. 2016). This aptasensor's analytical part was built using a commercial cantisens sensor platform and microcantilevers.

TABLE 11.2

Various aptasensors for the detection of cancer (Omage et al. 2022)

Types of cancer	Aptasensor-based detection technique	Target
Breast	Differential pulse voltammetry	Estrogen receptor, human epidermal growth factor receptor 2, breast cancer cell MCF-7, Mucin1 (MUC1), Nucleolin
	CV	Exosomes, human epidermal growth factor receptor 2, breast cancer cell MCF-7, Nucleolin, OPN
	Electrochemical impedance spectroscopy	human epidermal growth factor receptor 2, breast cancer cell MCF-7, MUC1, Nucleolin
	Square wave voltammetry	Breast cancer cell MCF-7, osteopontin (OPN)
	Photoelectrochemical	Exosomes, breast cancer cell MCF-7
	Electro-chemiluminescence	Nucleolin
Prostate cancer	Electrochemical impedance spectroscopy	PSA
	Differential pulse voltammetry	PSA
	Electrochemical impedance spectroscopy	PSA
	Photoelectrochemical	PSA
	Electro-chemiluminescence	PSA
Lung cancer	Differential pulse voltammetry	CEA, VEGF
	Electrochemical impedance spectroscopy	CEA
	Square wave voltammetry	Lung cancer tumor
Blood cancer	linear sweep voltammetry	Ramos cell
Liver cancer	Electrochemical impedance spectroscopy	Human liver hepatocellular carcinoma (HepG2), BNL 1ME A.7R.1 liver cancer cell line (MEAR), Alpha-fetoprotein (AFP)
	Differential pulse voltammetry	HepG2, MEAR
	CV	HepG2.
	Photoelectrochemical	HeLa, breast cancer cell MCF-7, HepG2
Prostate	LSW	CTC HER2, PSMA, and MUC1
	Differential pulse voltammetry	Platelet-derived growth factor-BB (PDGF-BB)
	Electrochemical impedance spectroscopy	PDGF-BB
Cervical cancer	Electrochemical impedance spectroscopy	HeLa
Colon cancer	Electrochemical impedance spectroscopy, CV	MUC-1
	Photoelectrochemical	CEA
	PES	CEA

11.10   APTASENSOR AND POINT-OF-CARE DIAGNOSIS IN CANCER

Aptasensors have grown in popularity during the last few decades. Their benefits over traditional antibody-based recognition have been well researched and documented. Researchers have been investigating the possibility of aptasensors in cancer point-of-care diagnostics in recent years. Their distinctive characteristics, such as dry reagent stability, little batch-to-batch fluctuation, cost-effectiveness, and better detection sensitivity and specificity, make them desirable for field deployment or adoption in low-resource environments. The following two instances are representative of several noteworthy patterns.

First, most research employs aptasensors as binding or targeting ligands for selective identification of specified analytes, however, a few studies used the 3D structure of aptasensors as a signal transduction mechanism.

Second, aptasensors are commonly coupled with microfluidic devices or nanomaterials to enable high-throughput screening or different signal-generating processes, resulting in a field-deployable point-of-care (POC) sensing or diagnostic podium.

More clinical research is needed to confirm their accuracy in assessing cancer patient samples.

Many previous findings were based on small model systems like pure cell cultures or spiked samples of standard buffer solutions. Because early illness detection is critical for better medical intervention, the new generation of aptasensors will be required to indicate changes in health conditions in real time. Aptasensors with real time and continuous monitoring capabilities are predicted to dominate future progress in cancer in this area. Despite the obstacles ahead, the recent development of POC-friendly aptasensors has promised to enhance customized cancer diagnosis (Forouzanfar et al. 2020). Aptasensors might influence the approaching era of digitized and customized onco-medicine with further clinical validation, scaling-up, and commercialization.

11.11   CONCLUSION AND FUTURE OUTLOOK

Aptasensors have been dubbed "smart molecular probes" since they can recognize particular molecular targets like biomarkers. Aptasensors have higher selectivity and sensitivity for detecting tiny compounds and proteins than antibody-based detection techniques. Even though aptasensors have been employed in a wide range of sensing platforms, numerous important technological issues and limitations remain: (a) manufacturing DNA/RNA-based aptasensors on a large scale is expensive, (b) the aptasensors' sensitivity is a key source of worry and (c) despite the availability of several aptasensor systems, their commercial diagnostic uses in clinical settings have yet to be completely realized.

Portable electrode-based, paper-based, lateral flow assay-based, portable SPR-based, and smartphone-based aptasensors have been recently researched to meet the criteria for POC diagnostics. Aptasensors are expected to be the market leader in biosensors, particularly in biomedicine and POC diagnostics. To build aptasensors with outstanding selectivity, linearity, repeatability, and stability for real-world applications, researchers must investigate and understand the aspects that influence their analytical performance. Future research and development in surface function-alization procedures and molecule binding event reporting systems will pave the way for high-performance aptasensors. Because the aptasensors' specificity and sensitivity are better, they are suitable commercial diagnostic instruments for cancer early detection. It is envisaged that the research would lessen the impacts of interfering elements in cancer aptasensors, as well as generate more accurate and portable diagnostic cancer instruments like commercial aptasensors, by merging other technologies. Aptasensors might influence the approaching era of digital and precision onco-medicine with further clinical validation, scaling-up, and commercialization.

CONSENT FOR PUBLICATION

Not applicable.

FUNDING

None.

CONFLICT OF INTEREST

No

ACKNOWLEDGMENTS

Declared none.

ABBREVIATION LIST

AuNPs	Gold nanoparticles
BASI	Brewster angle straddle interferometry
CD63	Cluster of differentiation 63
CEA	Carcinoembryonic antigen
CNT	Carbon nanotubes
CPNT	Conjugated carboxylated polypyrrole nanotubes
CTC	Circulating tumor cell
CV	Cyclic voltammetry
DNA	*Deoxyribonucleic acid*
DPV	Differential pulse voltammetric
ECL	Electrogenerated chemiluminescence
EFC	Evanescent field coupled
EGFR	Epidermal growth factor receptor
EIS	Electrochemical impedance analysis
EpCAM	Epithelial cellular adhesion molecule
FET	Field-effect transistor
FRET	Fluorescence resonance energy transfer
HER2	human epidermal growth factor receptor-2

miR	Micro RNA
MSN	Mesoporous silica nanoparticles
MUC-1	Mucin 1
PDGF	Platelet-derived growth factor
POC	Point-of-care
PSA	Prostate-specific antigen
PSA	Prostate-specific antigen
QCM	Quartz crystal microbalance
RNA	Ribonucleic acid
SELEX	Systematic evolution of ligands by exponential enrichment
SERS	Surface-enhanced Raman scattering
SPCDE	Surface plasmon coupled directional emission
SPR	Surface plasmon resonance
SYL3C	Anti-EpCAM aptamer
TNF-α	Tumor necrosis factor-α
VEGF	Vascular endothelial growth factor

REFERENCES

Abardía-Serrano C, Miranda-Castro R, de-los-Santos-Álvarez N, et al. New uses for the personal glucose meter: Detection of nucleic acid biomarkers for prostate cancer screening. *Sensors*. 2020;20(19):5514.

Abd-Ellatief R, Abd-Ellatief MR. Electrochemical aptasensors: Current status and future perspectives. *Diagnostics (Basel)*. 2021;11(1):104.

Amritkar V, Adat S, Tejwani V, et al. Engineering staphylococcal protein A for high-throughput affinity purification of monoclonal antibodies. *Biotechnol Adv*. 2020;44:107632.

Arruebo M, Vilaboa N, Sáez-Gutierrez B, et al. Assessment of the evolution of cancer treatment therapies. *Cancers (Basel)*. 2011;3(3):3279–3330.

Borghei YS, Hosseini M, Dadmehr M, et al. Visual detection of cancer cells by colorimetric aptasensor based on aggregation of gold nanoparticles induced by DNA hybridization. *Anal Chim Acta*. 2016;904:92–97.

Cai S, Li G, Zhang X, et al. A signal-on fluorescent aptasensor based on single-stranded DNA-sensitized luminescence of terbium (III) for label-free detection of breast cancer cells. *Talanta*. 2015;138:225–230.

Cao L, Cheng L, Zhang Z, et al. Visual and high-throughput detection of cancer cells using a graphene oxide-based FRET aptasensing microfluidic chip. *Lab Chip*. 2012;12(22): 4864–4869.

Cha T, Cho S, Kim YT, Lee JH. Rapid aptasensor capable of simply diagnosing prostate cancer. *Biosens Bioelectron*. 2014;62:31–37.

Chang CC, and Yeh CY. Using simple-structured split aptamer for gold nanoparticle-based colorimetric detection of estradiol. *Analytical Sciences* 2021;37(3):479–83.

Chang K, Pi Y, Lu W, et al. Label-free and highsensitive detection of human breast cancer cells by aptamer based leaky surface acoustic wave biosensor array. *Biosens Bioelectron*. 2014;(60):318–324.

Chen C, Feng S, Zhou M, et al. Development of a structureswitchingaptamer-based nanosensor for salicylic acid detection. *Biosens Bioelectron*. 2019;140:111342.

Chen X, Gole J, Gore A, et al. Non-invasive early detection of cancer four years before conventional diagnosis using a blood test. *Nat Commun*. 2020;11(1):1–10.

Chen X, Pan Y, Liu H, et al. Label-free detection of liver cancer cells by aptamer-based micro-cantilever biosensor. *Biosens Bioelectron*. 2016;79:353–358.

Crosby D, Lyons N, Greenwood E, et al. A roadmap for the early detection and diagnosis of cancer. *Lancet Oncol.* 2020;21(11):1397–1399.

Derin E, and Inci F. Advances in biosensor technologies for acute kidney injury. *ACS Sensors,* 2021;7(2), 358–385.

Dinarvand M, Neubert E, Meyer D, et al. Near-infrared imaging of serotonin release from cells with fluorescent nanosensors. *Nano Lett.* 2019;19(9):6604–6611.

Feng L, Chen Y, Ren J, Qu X. A graphene functionalized electrochemical aptasensor for selective label-free detection of cancer cells. *Biomaterials.* 2011;32:2930–2937.

Forouzanfar S, Alam F, Pala N, et al. Highly sensitive label-free electrochemical aptasensors based on photoresist derived carbon for cancer biomarker detection. *Biosens Bioelectron.* 2020;170:112598.

Gowsalya K, Yasothamani V, and Vivek R. Emerging indocyanine green-integrated nanocarriers for multimodal cancer therapy: a review. *Nanoscale Advances* 2021; 3(12):3332-3352

Hashemian Z, Khayamian T, Saraji M, et al. Aptasensor based on fluorescence resonance energy transfer for the analysis of adenosine in urine samples of lung cancer patients. *Biosens Bioelectron.* 2016;79:334–340.

Helm J, Schöls L, and Hauser S. Towards personalized allele-specific antisense oligonucleotide therapies for toxic gain-of-function neurodegenerative diseases. *Pharmaceutics,* 2022;14(8):1708.

Hong P, Li W, Li J. Applications of aptasensors in clinical diagnostics. *Sensors (Basel).* 2012;12(2):1181–1193.

Huang D, Tran J, Olson A, et al. Vaccine elicitation of HIV broadly neutralizing antibodies from engineered B cells. *Nat Commun.* 2020;11(1):5850.

Jayasena SD. Aptamers: An emerging class of molecules that rival antibodies in diagnostics. *Clin Chem.* 1999;45:1628–1650.

Jiang Y, Shi M, Liu Y, et al. Aptamer/AuNP biosensor for colorimetric profiling of exosomal proteins. *Angew Chem Int Ed.* 2017;56(39):11916–11920.

Jumper J, Evans R, Pritzel A, et al. Highly accurate protein structure prediction with AlphaFold. *Nature* 2021;596(7873):583–589.

Khoshroo A, Fattahi A, Hosseinzadeh L. Development of paper-based aptasensor for circulating tumor cells detection in the breast cancer. *J Electroanal Chem.* 2022;910:116182.

Klenov A. Development of a pokeweed mosaic virus vector as a molecular tool to study host protein function in Phytolacca americana. 2020.

Kohlberge M, and Gadermaier G. SELEX: Critical factors and optimization strategies for successful aptamer selection. *Biotechnology and Applied Biochemistry* 2022;69(5):1771–1792.

Komarova N, Barkova, D, and Kuznetsov, A. Implementation of high-throughput sequencing (HTS) in aptamer selection technology. *International Journal of Molecular Sciences,* 2020; 21(22):8774.

Labib M, Zamay A, Muharemagic D, et al. Aptamer-based viability impedimetric sensor for viruses. *Anal Chem.* 2012;84(4):1813–1816.

Lacroix A, and Sleiman HF. DNA nanostructures: current challenges and opportunities for cellular delivery. *ACS Nano,* 2021;15(3):3631–3645.

Lee JH, Kim JA, Jeong S, et al. Simultaneous and multiplexed detection of exosome microRNAs using molecular beacons. *Biosens Bioelectron.* 2016;86:202–210.

Lee JO, So HM, Jeon EK, et al. Aptamers as molecular recognition elements for electrochemical nanobiosensors. *Anal Bioanal Chem.* 2008;390:1023–1032.

Lee K, Lee J, Ahn B. Design of refolding dnaaptamer on singlewalled carbon nanotubes for enhanced optical detection of target proteins. *Anal Chem.* 2019;91(20):12704–12712.

Li B, Liu C, Pan W, et al. Facile fluorescent aptasensor using aggregation-induced emission luminogens for exosomal proteins profiling towards liquid biopsy. *Biosens Bioelectron.* 2020;168:112520.

Li N, Zong S, Zhang Y, Wang Z, et al. A SERS-colorimetric dual mode aptasensor for the detection of cancer biomarker MUC1. *Anal Bioanal Chem.* 2020;412:5707–5718.

Liu JX, Bao N, Luo X, et al. Nonenzymatic amperometric aptamer cytosensor for ultrasensitive detection of circulating tumor cells and dynamic evaluation of cell surface NGlycan expression. *ACS Omega.* 2018;3(8):8595–860.

Liu LS, Wang F, Ge Y, et al. Recent developments in aptasensors for diagnostic applications. *ACS Appl Mater Interfaces.* 2021;13(8):9329–9358.

Liu Y, Zhou Q, Revzin A. An aptasensor for electrochemical detection of tumor necrosis factor in human blood. *Analyst (Lond).* 2013;138(15):4321–4326.

Liu Z, Wang Y, Guo Y, Dong C. Label-free electrochemical aptasensor for carcino-embryonic antigen based on ternary nanocomposite of gold nanoparticles, hemin and graphene. *Electroanalysis.* 2015;28:1023–1028.

Malecka K, Pankratov D, Ferapontova EE. Femtomolar electroanalysis of a breast cancer biomarker HER-2/neu protein in human serum by the cellulase-linked sandwich assay on magnetic beads. *Anal Chim Acta.* 2019;1077:140–149.

Negahdary M, MoradiA, Heli H. Application of electrochemical aptasensors in detection of cancer biomarkers. *Biomed Res Ther.* 2019;6(7):3315–3324.

Nezakati T, Cousins BG, Seifalian AM. Toxicology of chemically modified graphene-based materials for medical application. *Arch Toxicol.* 2014;88(11):1987–2012.

Ni S, Zhuo Z, Pan Y, et al. Recent progress in aptamer discoveries and modifications for therapeutic applications. *ACS Applied Materials & Interfaces* 2020:13(8):9500–9519.

Niu C, Wang C, Li F, et. al. Aptamer assisted CRISPR-Cas12a strategy for small molecule diagnostics. *Biosens Bioelectron.* 2021;183:113196.

Nuzzo S, Brancato V, Affinito A, et al. The role of RNA and dna aptamers in glioblastoma diagnosis and therapy: a systematic review of the literature. *Cancers* 2020: 12(8); 2173.

Norouzi A, Ravan H, Mohammadi A, et al. Aptamer-integrated DNA nanoassembly: A simple and sensitive DNA framework to detect cancer cells. *Anal Chim Acta.* 2018;1017:26–33.

O'Sullivan CK. Aptasensors—the future of biosensing. *Anal Bioanal Chem.* 2002;372:44–48.

Omage JI, Easterday E, Rumph JT, et al. Cancer diagnostics and early detection using electrochemical aptasensors. *Micromachines (Basel).* 2022;13(4):522.

Ostatna V, Vaisocherova H, Homola J, et al. Effect of the immobilisation of DNA aptamers on the detection of thrombin by means of surface plasmon resonance. *Anal Bioanal Chem.* 2008;391:1861–1869.

Pandey, A., Chauhan, P. and Singhal, A. Potential electrochemical biosensors for early detection of viral infection. In *Advanced Biosensors for Virus Detection*. Academic Press. 2022; pp. 133–154.

Paniagua G, Villalonga A, Eguílaz M, et al. Amperometric aptasensor for carcinoembryonic antigen based on the use of bifunctionalized janus nanoparticles as biorecognition-signaling element. *Anal Chim Acta.* 2019;1061:84–91.

Qi S, Duan N, Khan IM, et al. Strategies to manipulate the performance of aptamers in SELEX, post-SELEX and microenvironment. *Biotechnology Advances* 2022; 55:107902.

Qureshi A, Gurbuz Y, Niazi JH. Label-free capacitance based aptasensor platform for the detection of HER2/ErbB2 cancer biomarker in serum. *Sens Actuators B Chem.* 2015;220:1145–1151.

Rahi A, Sattarahmady N, Heli H. Label-free electrochemical aptasensing of the human prostate-specific antigen using gold nanospears. *Talanta.* 2016;156–157:218–224.

Raimondo F, Morosi L, Chinello C, et al. Advances in membranous vesicle and exosome proteomics improving biological understanding and biomarker discovery. *Proteomics.* 2011;11(4):709–720.

Rauf S, Lahcen A, Aljedaibi A, et al. Gold nanostructured laserscribedgraphene: A new electrochemical biosensing platform for potential point-of-care testing of disease biomarkers. *Biosens Bioelectron.* 2021;180:113116.

Rose KM, Alves Ferreira-Bravo I, Li M, et al. Selection of 2´-deoxy-2´-fluoroarabino nucleic acid (FANA) aptamers that bind HIV-1 integrase with picomolar affinity. *ACS Chemical Biology* 2019;14(10):2166–75.

Rossetti M, Brannetti S, Mocenigo M, et al. Harnessing effective molarity to design an electrochemical DNA-based platform for clinically relevant antibody detection. *Angew Chem Int Ed Engl.* 2020;59(35):14973–14978.

Rupcich N, Nutiu R, Li Y, et. al. Solid-phase enzyme activity assay utilizing an entrapped fluorescence-signaling DNA aptamer. *Angew Chem Int Ed Engl.* 2006;45:3295–3299.

Safarpour H, Dehghani S, Nosrati R, et al. Optical and electrochemical-based nano-aptasensing approaches for the detection of circulating tumor cells (CTCs). *Biosens Bioelectron.* 2020;148:111833.

Saito, S. SELEX-based DNA aptamer selection: a perspective from the advancement of separation techniques. *Analytical Sciences* 2021; 37(1):17–26.

Sassolas A, Blum LJ, Leca-Bouvier BD. Optical detection systems using immobilized aptamers. *Biosens Bioelectron.* 2011;26:3725–3736.

Shabalina AV, Sharko DO, Glazyrin YE, et al. Development of electrochemical aptasensor for lung cancer diagnostics in human blood. *Sensors (Basel).* 2021;21(23):7851.

Shaban SM, Kim DH. Recent advances in aptamer sensors. *Sensors (Basel).* 2021;21(3):979.

Shen H, Yang J, Chen Z, et al. A novel label-free and reusable electrochemical cytosensor for highly sensitive detection and specific collection of CTCs. *Biosens. Bioelectron.* 2016;81:495–502.

Shevchenko Y, Francis TJ, Blair DA, et al. In situ biosensing with a surface plasmon resonance fiber grating aptasensor. *Anal Chem.* 2011;83:7027–7034.

Siegel RL, Miller KD, Fuchs HE, et al. Cancer statistics, 2022. *CA Cancer J Clin.* 2022; 72:7–33.

Susaki EA, Shimizu C, Kuno A, et al. Versatile whole-organ/body staining and imaging based on electrolyte-gel properties of biological tissues. *Nature Communications* 2020; 11(1);1982.

Tabrizi MA, Shamsipur M, Farzin L. A high sensitive electrochemical aptasensor for the determination of VEGF165 in serum of lung cancer patient. *Biosens Bioelectron.* 2015;74:764–769.

Tahmasebi F, Noorbakhsh A. Sensitive electrochemical prostate specific antigen aptasensor: Effect of carboxylic acid functionalized carbon nanotube and glutaraldehyde linker. *Electroanalysis.* 2016;28(5):1134–1145.

Townshend B, Kaplan M, and Smolke CD. Highly multiplexed selection of RNA aptamers against a small molecule library. *Plos One* 2022;17(9):e0273381.

Tuerk C, and Gold L. Systematic evolution of ligands by exponential enrichment: RNA ligands to bacteriophage T4 DNA polymerase. *Science* 1990;249(4968):505–510.

Ulrich H, Wrenger C. Disease-specific biomarker discovery by aptamers. *Cytometry A.* 2009;75:727–733.

Ulucan-Karnak F, Akgöl S. A new nanomaterial based biosensor for MUC1 biomarker detection in early diagnosis, tumor progression and treatment of cancer. *Nanomanufacturing.* 2021;1(1):14–38.

Verberne CJ, Wiggers T, Vermeulen KM, de Jong KP. Detection of recurrences during follow-up after liver surgery for colorectal metastases: Both carcinoembryonic antigen (CEA) and imaging are important. *Ann Surg Oncol.* 2013;20(2):457–463.

Verdian A, Fooladi E, Rouhbakhsh Z. Recent progress in the development of recognition bioelements for polychlorinated biphenyls detection: Antibodies and aptamers. *Talanta.* 2019;202:123–135.

Wang J, Wang Y, Hu X, et al. Dual-aptamer-conjugated molecular modulator for detecting bioactive metal ions and inhibiting metalmediated protein aggregation. *Anal Chem.* 2019;91(1):823–829.

Wang X, Zhou J, Yun W, et al. Detection of thrombin using electro generated chemilumines-cence based on Ru(bpy)3(2+)-doped silica nanoparticle aptasensor via target protein-induced strand displacement. *Anal Chim Acta.* 2007;598:242–248.

Wei Y, Wang D, Zhang Y, et al. Multicolor and photo thermal dual read out biosensor for visual detection of prostate specific antigen. *Biosens Bioelectron.* 2019;140:111345.

Willner I, Zayats M. Electronic aptamer-based sensors. *Angew Chem Int Ed Engl.* 2007;46:6408–6418.

Xu L, Bai X, Tenguria S, et al. Mammalian cell-based immunoassay for detection of viable bacterial pathogens. *Front Microbiol.* 2020;11:575615

Yan M, Sun G, Liu F, et al. An aptasensor for sensitive detection of human breast cancer cells by using porous GO/Au composites and porous PtFe alloy as effective sensing platform and signal amplification labels. *Anal Chim Acta.* 2013;798:33–39.

Yang J, Huang X, Gan C, et al. Highly specific and sensitive pointof-care detection of rare cir-culating tumor cells in whole blood via a dual recognition strategy. *Biosens Bioelectron.* 2019;143:111604.

Yan J, Xiong H, Cai S, et al. Advances in aptamer screening technologies. *Talanta,* 2019;200:124–144.

Yoshikawa AM, Wan L, Zheng L, et al. A system for multiplexed selection of aptamers with exquisite specificity without counterselection. *Proceedings of the National Academy of Sciences* 2022;119(12):e2119945119.

Yu H, Alkhamis O, Canoura J, et al. Advances and challenges in small-molecule DNA aptamer isolation, characterization, and sensor development. *Angew Chem Int Ed Engl.* 2021;60(31):16800–16823.

Yu X, He L, Pentok M, et al. An aptamer-based new method for competitive fluorescence detection of exosomes. *Nanoscale.* 2019;11(33):15589–15595.

Zayats M, Huang Y, Gill R, et al. Label-free and reagentlessaptamer-based sensors for small molecules. *J Am Chem Soc.* 2006;128:13666–13667.

Zhang G, Zhong L, Yang N, et al. Screening of aptamers and their potential application in targeted diagnosis and therapy of liver cancer. *World J Gastroenterol.* 2019;25(26):3359–3369.

Zhang J, Ran F, Zhou W, et al. Ultrasensitive fluorescent aptasensor for MUC1 detection based on deoxyribonuclease I-aided target recycling signal amplification. *RSC Adv.* 2018;8:32009–32015.

Zhang X, Xiao K, Cheng L, et al. Visual and highly sensitive detection of cancer cells by a colorimetric aptasensor based on cell-triggered cyclic enzymatic signal amplification. *Anal Chem.* 2014;86:11:5567–5572.

Index

Note: **Bold** page numbers refer to tables and *italic* page numbers refer to figures.

Abd-Ellatief, M.R. 183
Abd-Ellatief, R. 183
Acinetobacter baumannii 218
adenosine 5'-monophosphate (AMP) 182
Aeon 21
aflatoxin B1 (AFB1) 181
AFM-SELEX 175
AIDS 114
Akgöl, S. 279
alkaline phosphatase placental-like 2 (ALPPL2)
    153
α-l-threofuranosyl nucleic acid (TNA) 185
Alzheimer's disease (AD) biomarkers 236
amplification methods 107, 194
    catalytic hairpin assembly 183
    development 191
    dual-signal 11, 240
    hybridization chain reaction 147, *147,* 214
    polymerase chain reaction 26, 32, 112
    rolling circle 8, 193, 249
    square wave voltammetry 118
anthrax 112
anti-angiogenic aptamers 38
antibody 57, 64, 74, 75, 81–82, *130,* 179
    advantages 25
    aptamer and *50,* 77, **77,** 252, 260, 265
    artificial 77, 249
    benefits over 3–4
    biological molecules 99
    chemical 232
    IgG1 101
    Immuno-SELEX 118
    infectious diseases 221
    monoclonal 32, 33, 185, 249
    production and characterization of 272
    proteinaceous 56
    secondary 33
    selectivity 32
    sensors for 272
anticoagulation 38
antigen-antibody recognition mechanism 232
anti-inflammation 38
aptafluidics microdevices 211–24
aptamer-drug conjugates (ApDCs) 39
aptamer-linked immobilised sorbent assay
    (ALISA) 106, 110, 111
aptamers 1, 2, 100, 127, 133, 232, 250
    advantages 50–51, 64, *64*

and antibodies *50,* 77, **77**
application 57–62, *63,* 179–85
aptamer-based regionally protected PCR 32
aptamer-conjugated nanoparticles 8
aptamer-drug conjugates 39
beacon probes 171–99
benefits over antibodies/enzymes 3–4
bioimaging 28–30
biomarkers 21–42
biosensors (*see* biosensors)
cancer therapy 10, *10*
characterization of 177–78
chemiluminescence immunosorbent assay
    116–17
circulating tumour cells 7–10
colorimetric biosensor 127–57
commercially available **198**
configurations 129–30, *130*
current status of **199**
design 49–66
detection 30, *31,* 116–18
in diagnostics 27–36, 57–61, **62**
distinctive attributes of 25
DNA and RNA 24
electrochemical biosensor, for health care
    monitoring 232–44, **237,** *241, 242*
in emerging diagnostic applications 33–36,
    34, *36*
exosomes 196, *197,* **198**
extracellular vesicles detection 11–13
history and market trend of 2, *3*
in immunohistochemistry 32–33
intact pathogens **6,** 6–7
ligand-binding RNA 131
microfluidic platforms 211–24
and microRNA for therapy 195–96
multichannel conductometric sensor 258, *258*
nanoparticles 27–28
passive immunity using 51
peptide 185
point-of-care (*see* point-of-care testing
    (POCT) technology)
in polymerase chain reaction 31–32
protein biomarkers 4–5
rapid testing with 7, 217
small-molecule biomarkers 4, **5**
synthesis method 49–66, 101, 250–51
therapeutic approach 36–39, 61–62, **62**

tissue samples 13
trends in 128–29, *129*
types of 24–25
against viral diseases *60*
in western blot 30–31
withdrawn from clinical trials **198**
Aptamer Science Inc. 34
aptasensors 29, 179–80, 271, 282–83
    application of *86,* 86–88
    biological analyte detection 83–85, *84,* **85**
    biomarker detection 74–79, 86–88, **87**
    of cancer biomarkers 85–88, **89,** 275–77, **277**
    colorimetric (*see* colorimetric biosensor)
    electrochemical 79–81, 88, *88*
    fabrication 132, 156, 239, 244
    fluorescence-based 115
    health care monitoring 236–43, **237,** *238,*
        241, 242
    leukemia cells 278–79
    MCF-7 cells 278
    MC-LR 77, *78*
    microfluidics-enabled (*see* microfluidics-
        enabled aptasensors (MeAS))
    MUC1 cells 279–80
    MXene-enabled electrochemical 65
    oncological diseases 271–83
    prostate cancer 278
    Ramos cells 278
    recognition element 271
    regeneration of 78
    sandwich-type 273, *274*
    smart phone-based 151
    substantial focus of 83
    transduction mechanisms 273–75
    tumor necrosis factor-α 278
    working principle of *273*
apt blotting 31
aptoprecipitation 34
artificial antibodies 77
artificial intelligence (AI) 66, 119, 219, 224
Artificially Expanded Genetic Information
    System (AEGIS) 55
AuNPs *see* gold nanoparticles (AuNPs)

bacterial infections
    beacon probes 180–81
    point-of-care technology 109–12
beacon probes
    aptamer 171–99
    molecular aptamer 188–94
    nucleic acid aptamer synthesis 173–76
    therapeutic outcomes 194–98
bead-based SELEX 174
Beta, M. 192
Bhardwaj, J. 4, 261
biofluids, exosomes 11
bioimaging, aptamer in 28–30

biomarkers
    for antigens 276
    aptamer 21–42
    aptasensor *vs.* immunosensor 72–91
    cancer 85–88, **89,** 90, 220–21, 275–77, **277**
    detection of 75
    electrochemical detection 75, 79
    exposure 21–22
    limitations and future prospective 40–41
    malarial 235–36
    microfluidics-enabled aptasensors 219
    point-of-care (*see* point-of-care testing
        (POCT) technology)
    protein 4–5, 261, *262*
    small-molecule 4, **5,** 261–63, **262**
biomolecule detection
    microfluidics-enabled aptasensors 219–20
    molecular aptamer beacon probes 189
bioreceptors 81, 83, 91, 116
biorecognition elements (BREs) 73–76, 79, 80,
    82, 232, 235, 249, 257
biosensors 272
    antibody-based 77
    aptamer 1–14, 264–65
    biomarker detection 73–77
    challenges and advances in 248–65
    colorimetric (*see* colorimetric biosensor)
    as diagnostic tool 81–83
    drawbacks 264–65
    electrochemical 80, 82–83, *83,* 232–44, **237,**
        241, 242, 257–58
    fluorescence 254–55, *255*
    future prospects 265
    mechanical 82
    microfluidic 258–60, *259*
    optical 82, 252
    point-of-care technology 234–36, *236,* 251–61
    for tumour imaging purposes 80
Birader, K. 155
bisphenol A (BPA) 180
blocker 13
Bogus, M. 187
Brent, R. 185
BREs *see* biorecognition elements (BREs)
Bui, T.T.T. 187

cadmium telluride quantum dots (QDs) 118
Cai, S. 278
calmodulin protein binding 187
cancer
    aptasensors 85–88, **89,** 275–77, **277**
    biomarkers 85–88, **89,** 90, 220–21, 275–77,
        277
    cell detection 280
    clinical diagnosis of 280
    detection of **281**
    follow-up 280

microfluidics-enabled aptasensors for 220–21, *221*
point-of-care diagnosis 282
SOMAScan technology 27
therapy 10, *10,* 280
voltammetric immunosensors 90
cancer stem cells (CSCs) 182
Cao, L. 278
capillary electrophoresis SELEX (CE SELEX) 52, 175–76
carbon dots 150–51
carbon nanotube field-effect transistors (CNTFETs) 179
carboxytetramethylrhodamine (TAMRA) 30, 192
carcinoembryonic antigen (CEA) 119, 276
catalytic hairpin assembly (CHA) 183–84
cell detection 279, 280
    cancer 220
    nanovescicles secreted from 184
cell-SELEX technology 25, 26, *27,* 36, 53–54, *54,* 102, 174–75, 263
cell surface protein aptamers **197,** 199
Chagas disease 36, 112
Chang, C.C. 151
chemical antibodies *see* aptamers
chemically synthesized antibodies *see* aptamers
chemical toxins detection 180
chemiluminescence immunosorbent assay 116–17
chemotherapy 27, 194, 271
Chen, X. 190
Chen, Y. 183
chloramphenicol (CAP) 134, 151
cholera 111
chromatographic purification 63
chronic disease 2, 249
Chung, J. 216
Chu, Y. 216
circulating tumor cells (CTCs) 7–10, 263–64
    cancer biomarkers 276
    cancer therapy 10, *10*
    detection and analysis 8–9, *9*
    identifying and characterizing 183
    isolation 7–8
    microfluidics-enabled aptasensors 220, *221*
    targeted imaging 8
Cohen, B.A. 185
Colas, P. 185
colorimetric biosensor 127–57, 252–54, *253, 254*
    assay as point-of-care testing 154–56, *156*
    competitive replacement mode 133–34
    limit of detection **136–46**
    material-based (*see* material-based colorimetric biosensors)
    mode of detection and analytical applications **136–46**
    profiling tests 11
    sandwich/sandwich-like mode 132–33

target-induced dissociation/displacement mode 133
target-induced reassembly mode *134,* 134–35
target-induced structure switching mode 130–32, *131*
combination of antiretroviral therapy (cART) 114
compact analytical device *see* biosensors
competitive replacement (CR) mode 133–34
complementary DNA (cDNA) 132, 172, 192
conventional SELEX 51–52, *53*
Corda, E. 187
COVID-19 pandemic 35, 37, 155
    beacon probes 172, 187, 190
    impact of 107
    outbreak 248, 250
    point-of-care tool 116
C-reactive protein (CRP) 153
CTCs *see* circulating tumor cells (CTCs)
cyclic voltammetry (CV) 239, *242,* 242–43

Dausse, E. 57
deep learning methods 176
Deng, X. 114
DeStefano, J.J. 181
differential pulse voltammetric (DPV) *238,* 242, 243, 278
3,5-difluoro 4-hydroxybenzylidene imidazolinone (DFHBI) 114
digital light processing (DLP) printing 213
DNA-based aptamer-magnetic bead sandwich technique 113
Dong, H. 11
Dot Blot analysis 110
downstream molecular analysis 11
drug delivery systems 185
dual-signal amplification aptasensor 11

electrochemical aptasensors 116, 273, *275*
    microfluidics-enabled aptasensors 214
    oncological diseases 272
electrochemical (EC) biosensors 82–83, *83,* 257–58
    biomarkers 75, 79
    cadmium detection 239, *241*
    for health care monitoring 232–44, **237,** *241, 242*
electrochemical immunoassay 75
electrochemical immunosensors 74
electrochemical impedance spectroscopy (EIS) 81, 115, 214, 278
electrochemical sensor (ECS) 111
Ellington, A.D. 2, 23, 171
enzyme-linked aptamer antibody (ELAA) 132–33, 153
enzyme-linked immunosorbent assay (ELISA) 34, 100, 132
enzymes

benefits over 3–4
material-based colorimetric biosensors
153–54, *154*
sensors for 272
epidermal growth factor receptor 2 (EGFR2)
proteins 220
epigenetics approach 22
epithelial cell adhesion molecules (EpCAM) 7, 8,
13, 33, 183, 184
Escherichia coli
colorimetric biosensor 147, 149–51
point-of-care technology 109
Esposito, C.L. 184
EvaGreen dye 256
exosomes 150–51, 276–77
beacon probes 172, 184, 196, *197,* 198
biofluids 11
microfluidics-enabled aptasensors 221
extension SELEX (ExSELEX) 49–66
extracellular vesicles (EVs) 11–13, *12*

fabrication
aptamer-based biosensors 130
aptasensors 132, 156, 239, 244
biosensor *262*
cocaine-encapsulated liposome 86, *86*
electrochemical aptasensor 88, 119
for microbial detections 180
microfluidics-enabled aptasensors 222–23
polymer/resin used for 213
Fact.MR 2
Fang, X. 171
Feng, L. 280
field effect transistor (FET)-based aptafluidics
device 214
flow amplifiers/resistors 215
flow cytometry 33, 178
fluorescein amidite (FAM) 30, 117, 181,
189, 192
fluorescence anisotropy 177
fluorescence-based aptasensor 115
fluorescence biosensors 254–55, *255*
fluorescence energy transfer (FRET) 117–18
fluorescence in situ hybridization (FISH) 30
fluorescence polarization (FP) 177, 179
fluorescence resonance energy transfer (FRET)
30, *31,* 279
beacon probe 171, 188, 189, 193, 194
biosensing approaches 254–55
fluorescence biosensors 255
point-of-care diagnostic device 117–18
fluorescent nanoparticles (FNPs) 8
fluorogenic RNA aptamer (FRA) 192
Food and Drug Administration (FDA) 10, 38,
112, 115, 199
Francisella tularensis 110
fungi detection, beacon probes 181–82

gas-liquid chromatography (GLC) 100
Gerasimova, Y.V. 189
Ghanbari, K. 115
glass microchips 215–16
global health 1
Gold, L. 23, 51
gold nanoparticles (AuNPs) 117, 131, 176, 194,
196, 253, 278
Au-nano-bipyramids 148–49
AuNP-quenched fluorescent probe (GNP-
DNA-FAM) 11
AuNPs-herringbone microchip 7
biotin-streptavidin complexation binds
to 179
colorimetric biosensor 135, 148
lateral flow immunoassays 114
material-based colorimetric biosensors 135,
146–49, *147, 149*
Mycobacterium tuberculosis 111
Salmonella enterotoxin 111
with single-stranded DNA 106
stonelike 237–38, *238*
surface plasmon resonance 135
gold nanorods (AuNRs) 253
Gopinath, S.C. 135
G-quadruplex 10, 129, 153–54, 171–72,
179, 219
graphene oxide (GO) 149–50
graphene quantum dots (GQDs) 115
gravimetric method 215
green fluorescent protein (GFP) 114, 115, 188

hairline 213
hairpin allosteric molecular beacon probes 191
hairpin DNA cascade hybridization reaction
(HD-CHR) 13
Hamaguchi, N. 171
Hashemian, Z. 280
health care monitoring
aptasensors 236–43, **237,** *238, 241, 242*
electrochemical biosensor for 232–44, **237,**
241, 242
hepatitis 115
high-throughput aptamer identification (HAPI)
screen technology 57
HIV 114
hormones 219–20
Huang, L. 11
human cell type detection 182–84
human epidermal growth factor receptor 2
(HER2) 90, 280
human neutrophil elastase (HNE) 178
Hussain, B. 199
Hwang, G.L. 189
hybridization chain reaction (HCR) amplification
147, *147,* 214
hybridoma technology 21, 33

immobilized aptamers, SELEX variants 174, 175
immune cells 33, 183–84
immunoassay 99–100, 116, 256
   conventional 75
   fluidic system 259
   HAPI screen technology 57
   paper-based lateral flow 114
immunohistochemistry (IHC) 32–33
immunosensors
   for alpha-fetoprotein 90, *90*
   β-LG 77, *78*
   biomarker detection 75–79, 81, **91**
   electrochemical 74, 79–81
   voltammetric 90
induced pluripotent stem cells (iPSCs) 183
infectious diseases 248, 249
   aptamer 36–37
   molecular aptamer beacon 190
   point-of-care technology for 99–101, 109–16,
      110
influenza virus 114, 218
   influenza A H1N1 virus 4, 37, 218, 261
inkjet printing 213
Insilco tools 176
in silico molecular dynamics 185
intact pathogens
   aptamer-based biosensors **6,** 6–7
   detection 263
in vivo-based SELEX technique *54,* 55, 175
isothermal titration calorimetry (ITC) 177–78

Jiang, Y. 277
Joshi, R. 181

Kashima, D. 187
Kaur, H. 199
Kawahara, M. 187
Khoshroo, A. 278
Kiel, J.L. 110
Kim, B.H. 189
Kimoto, M. 56
Kolpashchikov, D.M. 189
Kost, G.J. 103, 104
Kumar Kulabhusan, P. 199

label-free sensor 76, 187, 252
   adenosine detection 182
   cancer cell detection 280
   carbon nanotube field-effect transistors 179
   colorimetric sensing 153
   EC impedance spectroscopy 119
   isothermal titration calorimetry 177
Labib, M. 8
lab-on-a-chip (LOC) 214, 216, 218, 220, 224
Lai, Y.-T. 181
Landry, D.W. 154
latent membrane protein 1 (LMP-1) 118

lateral flow assays (LFAs) 59, 111
lateral flow immunoassays (LFIA) 114
Lau, P.S. 131
lead exposure 22
Lee, J.H. 277
leukemia cells 278–79
Li, B. 272
Li, H. 148
Li, J.J. 171
Li, N. 276
Li, P. 13
Li, W.M. 13
ligand-binding RNA aptamers 131
limit of detection (LOD)
   colorimetric biosensor **136–46**
   microfluidics-enabled aptasensors 216, 218
Lin, B. 184
Listeria monocytogenes 60, 112, 252–53, *253–54*
lithography 213–14
Liu, B. 152
Liu, C. 11
Liu, J.X. 276
Liu, Y. 5, 278
Locked Nucleic Acids (LNAs) 56–57
Lu, Y. 182

MAB probes *see* molecular aptamer beacon
      (MAB) probes
Maehashi, K. 179
magnetic beads (MBs)
   DNA-based aptamer-magnetic bead sandwich
      technique 113
   for HER-2 protein 276
   material-based colorimetric biosensors 152
   SELEX 53, 174
   waxberry-like 184
magnetic nanoparticles (MNPs) 8
Malachite green (MG) 134, 182, 194
malaria 113, 235–36
Malecka, K. 276
Manandhar, Y. 187
material-based colorimetric biosensors 135–54
   carbon dots 150–51
   enzymes 153–54, *154*
   gold nanomaterials 135, 146–49, *147, 149*
   graphene 149–50
   magnetic beads 152
   metal-organic framework 152–53
   nanotubes 150–51
   silica beads 152
   silica nanoparticles 152
   2D metal nanoplates 151
matrix metalloproteinase-2 (MMP2) 33
mature beacon, to mature miRNA target 191–92
MBSpinChip 109–10
McCauley, T.G. 179
MCF-7 cells 278

MeAS *see* microfluidics-enabled aptasensors
    (MeAS)
mechanical biosensors 82
medical industry, point-of-care (POC) technology
    107–9, **108**
metabolic disorders 38
metabolites, microfluidics-enabled aptasensors
    (MeAS) 219, *219*
metal-organic framework (MOF) 152–53
methicilin-resistant *Salmonella aureus* (MRSA)
    255
M-fold software tools 116
microbial diseases 36–37
microchips
    glass/plastic-based 215–16
    paper 215
microcystin-leucine-arginine 259, 260
microfluidic biosensors 258–60, *259*
microfluidic SELEX (M-SELEX) approach 55,
    103, 174
microfluidics-enabled aptasensors (MeAS)
    211–24
    advantages 216–18
    analytical methods 214–15
    applications 218–22
    biomarkers and metabolites detection 219
    for cancer 220–21, *221*
    components of *212*
    detection 214–15, 221
    digital light processing printing 213
    electrochemical method 214
    fabrication challenges 222–23
    glass/plastic-based microchips 215–16
    gravimetric method 215
    growth factors 219–20
    high sensitivity and selectivity 216
    hormones and biomolecules 219–20
    inkjet printing 213
    lithography 213–14
    medical laboraory diagnostic techniques 217,
        217
    miniaturized design *212,* 216–17
    multiple analyte detection 218
    multiplexing of multiple signals 216
    optical method 214
    paper microchips 215
    patents 223–24
    patterning methods 212–14
    plasma printing 213
    quantitative and qualitative detection 218
    rapid detection 216
    reusability and disposability 218
    toxins 220
    transistor-based method 214
    wax printing 212–13
    whole-cell detection and separation 218–19
microlithography 213

microRNA (miRNA)
    and aptamers for therapy 195–96
    beacon probes 189
    chemical modification 195
    mature beacon to 191–92
    molecular aptamer beacon probes 190–94,
        191, 193
microscale thermophoresis, for health care
    monitoring 234
micro total analysis systems (µTAS) 215
microvesicles 11
Middle East respiratory syndrome (MERS) 115,
    248
Minimal Residual Disease (MRD) 221
miR-10b antagomir 195
miRNA *see* microRNA (miRNA)
molecular aptamer beacon (MAB) probes 171,
    188–94
    biomolecule detection 189
    mature beacon to mature miRNA target
        191–92
    microRNAs detection methods 190–94, *191,*
        193
    pathogen detections 189–90
    principle of 188–89
    quencher-free 189
    RNA detections, in living cellS 190
    therapeutic outcomes 194–98
molecular biology 21, 29, 30, 218
molecular docking 57, 60
molecular dynamics 57, 60, 185
molecular photocopying (PCR) 50
Monocyte chemoattractant protein 1 (MCP-1) 38
Mo, T. 183
MPT64 secretory protein 111
mucin 16 protein 4, 261
Mucin short variant S1 (MUC1) 28, 279–80
multiplexing, of multiple signals 216
multi-walled carbon nanotubes (MWCNT) 115,
    236
MXene-enabled electrochemical aptasensors 65,
    258
Mycobacterium tuberculosis 4, 111, 181, 190, 261
myeloma 21

nanoarray aptamer-based chip assay 117
nanobiosensors 119
nanoparticles (NPs) 119
    aptamer 27–28
    fluorescent 8
    gold (*see* gold nanoparticles (AuNPs))
    magnetic 8
    silica 152
    silver 135, 257
nanotechnology 74, 118–19
nanotubes
    carbon nanotube field-effect transistors 179

material-based colorimetric biosensors
150–51
multi-walled carbon nanotubes 115, 236
nanovescicles, from human tissues/cell detection
184
N-doped carbon aerogel (NCA) 237, *238*
near-patient testing *see* point-of-care testing
(POCT) technology
Nedorezova, D.D. 189
neurodegenerative disorders 27, 187
neurological diseases 39
New, R.R.C. 187
NeXagen 2
NeXstar 2
next-generation sequencing (NGS) 57
Nguyen, N.V. 220
Ni, R. 183
noninvasive ExoPCD microfluidic chip 12
non-small-cell lung cancer (NSCLC) cells 8
nucleic acid aptamers 24, 100
SELEX 173–76
synthesis of 173–76
nucleolin 37, 193, 196
NX1838 2

ochratoxin-A (OTA) 35, 152, 155
oligonucleotide 101
oncology
aptamer 37–38
aptasensors 271–83
oncomiRs 195
optical method
aptasensors 116, 274
biosensors 82, 252
microfluidics-enabled aptasensors 214
Ovine follicle-stimulating hormone (oFSH-α)
model protein 32

Paniagua, G. 276
paper-based lateral flow immunoassays (LFIA)
114
paper microchips
microfluidics-enabled aptasensors 215
parasitic infections
point-of-care technology 112–13
pathogen detections
beacon probes 180
fluorescence biosensors 255
molecular aptamer beacon probes 189–90
surface-enhanced Raman spectroscopy 256
patterning methods, microfluidics-enabled
aptasensors
digital light processing printing 213
inkjet printing 213
lithography 213–14
plasma printing 213
wax printing 212–13

Penner, G. 35
peptide aptamers 24–25, 171, 185
applications 187–88
characterization 187
combinatorial libraries of 186
Percze, K. 190
PerkinElmer's AlphaScreen® technology 57
Pheno SELEX 175
photolithography 213–14
plasma printing 213
plasmodium lactate dehydrogenase (pLDH)
enzyme 106
plasmodium vivax 113
plastic-based microchips 215–16
platelet-derived growth factor (PDGFR) 38, 182
point-of-careology 120
point-of-care testing (POCT) technology 1, 99,
101, 103–4, 108
bacterial infections 109–12
biosensors (*see* biosensors)
cancer 282
colorimetric biosensing assay 154–56, *156*
diagnostics devices 104–9, *107*
for infectious diseases 99–101, 109–16, *110*
laboratory technique and **105**
in medical industry 107–9, **108**
protozoa parasitic infections 112–13
rapid 100
3D printing *260, 260*–61
viral infections 113–16
in vitro diagnostic methods 249
polydiacetylene (PDA) liposomes 148
polymerase chain reaction (PCR) 25, 233,
252–53
biomarkers 31–32
Systematic Evolution of Ligands by
Exponential Enrichment 51, 52
primer extension reactions (PEX) 233
prostate specific antigen (PSA) 240, 242, 278
proteinaceous antibodies 56
protein aptamer
cell surface **197**
web-based 176
protein biomarkers 72–73
aptamer-based biosensors 4–5
for cancer 276
identification 261, *262*
protein tyrosine kinase 7 (PTK7) 38
Pseudomonas aeruginosa 257
Pu, Y. 13
quantum dots (QDs) 151, 218, 264
cadmium telluride 118
graphene 115
quencher-free molecular aptamer beacon (MAB)
189

Qureshi, A. 280

Rabiee, N. 185
radiotherapy 27
Rahi, A. 278
Ramos cells 278
rapid detection
    aflatoxin B1 181
    infectious agents 40
    microfluidics-enabled aptasensors 216
Ray, J. 31
real-time polymerase chain reaction (RT-PCR)
    101, 115
reduced graphene oxide-silver nanoparticles
    (rGo-AgNPs) 240
Ren, Q. 4
resazurin dye 113
rGOSELEX 117, 118
RNA aptamers
    ligand-binding 131
    in living cells 190
    small molecules 194–95
rolling circle amplification (RCA) 8, 193, 249
Rothberg, L.J. 148
Roushani, M. 115, 257
Rous sarcoma virus detection 190

Salmonella aureus 111
    magnetic beads 180
    SELEX 111
Salmonella sp. 36
    S. enterotoxin 111
    S. typhimurium 150, 151
sandwich-like detection methods 132–33, 235
Sanger sequencing 9
SARS-CoV-2 detection *see* severe acute
    respiratory syndrome Coronavirus 2
    (SARS-CoV-2) detection
schistosomiasis 113
screen-printed carbon electrode (SPCE) 239
seasonal infectious illnesses 105
SELEX *see* Systematic Evolution of Ligands by
    Exponential Enrichment (SELEX)
self-powered FRET (SPF) flares 193
Seo, Y.J. 189
severe acute respiratory syndrome Coronavirus 2
    (SARS-CoV-2) detection 35, *36,* 113,
    115, 190, 248
    epidemic of 59
    inhibitory effect on 181
    point-of-care diagnostics 107, 155
    receptor-binding region 60
    spike protein 181, 187
Shen, H. 7, 276
Shu, D. 196
silica beads 152
silica nanoparticles (SiNPs) 152
silver nanoparticles (AgNPs) 135, 257
silver-nanowires (AgNWs) 256, *256*

Singh, V.K. 118
single-stranded oligonucleotides 101
single-stranded RNA (ssRNA) 24
slow Off-Rate Modified Aptamer (SOMAmers)
    103
small molecules 196
    aptasensing strategy **262**
    biomarkers 4, **5,** 261–63, **262**
    colorimetric aptasensor for 154
    detection of 150
    immuno-techniques of 133
    limit of detection **262**
    molecular biology tool for 29
    RNA 194–95
smallpox 113
smart phone-based aptasensor 151
sol–gel SELEX 176, *176*
SOMAmers 26
SOMAscan 25–27, 100, 103
southwestern blotting 31
Spanish flu virus 114
Spiegelmer 25, 38, 41
split-aptamer-based cytometric bead assay
    (SACBA) 178
square wave voltammetry 118
Stanton, M. 171
Staphylococcus aureus 106, 180, 236, 254, *255*
stem cell recognition 182–83
Stojanovic, M.N. 154
stonelike Au nanoparticles (SL-AuNPs) 237–38,
    238
structure-switching process 130
Sun, L. 181
surface-enhanced Raman spectroscopy/scattering
    (SERS) 8, 9, 35, 184, 214, 223, 254–57,
    256, 276
surface plasmon resonance (SPR) 117,
    177, 274
    gold nanoparticles 135
    for health care monitoring 234, 235
Systematic Evolution of Ligands by Exponential
    Enrichment (SELEX) 2, 26, *27,* 49–51,
    52, 101, 250
    advanced methods 56–57, **58**
    advantages and disadvantage **251**
    AFM-SELEX 175
    aptasensors 273, *275*
    bead-based 174
    capillary electrophoresis 52, 175–76
    capture-SELEX method 117
    cell-SELEX 53–54, *54,* 102, 174–75
    conventional 51–52, *53*
    electrochemical biosensor 232, 233
    extension 55–56
    magnetic-bead-based 53
    malaria 113
    methodology 250–51, **251**

microfluidic 55, 174
nucleic acid aptamer synthesis 173–76
optimization 265
point-of-care diagnostics 100–102, 249
Salmonella aureus 111
sol–gel 176, *176*
in solution 175–76
variants on target types 173–77
in vivo *54,* 55, 175
whole-cell SELEX technique 112
Szostak, J.W. 2, 23

Tabrizi, M.A. 276
TA6NT-AKTin-DOX 183
Tan, W. 171
targeted drug delivery 28, 39–40, 184, 195
target-induced dissociation/displacement (TID) mode 133
target-induced reassembly (TIR) mode *134,* 134–35
target-induced structure switching (TISS) mode 130–32, *131*
Tarokh, A. 151
3,3',5,5'-tetramethylbenzidine (TMB) 253
thioredoxin (trxA) 185–86
three-dimensional Cell-SELEX 175
3D printing *260,* 260–61
thrombin 4, 30, 152–53, 171, 172, 175, 177, 233, 257, 261
tissue samples, aptamer-based biosensors 13
toxins, microfluidics-enabled aptasensors (MeAS) 220
transistor-based method 214
Trypanosama sp.
    T. cruzi 36, 113
    T. evansi 112
tuberculosis (TB) 111
Tuerk, C. 23, 51
tularemia 110
tumour necrosis factor-alpha (TNF-α) 4, 219, 261, 278
two-dimensional metal nanoplates 151

Ulucan-Karnak, F. 279
unnatural base pairs (UBPs) 50, 56

Valero, J. 181
vascular epithelial growth factor (VEGF) 219
Vibrio sp.

V. cholera 111
V. parahaemolyticus 152, 216, 218
viral infections
    aptamer against *60*
    beacon probes 181
    notorious 37
    point-of-care technology 113–16
Vivekananda, J. 110
voltammetric immunosensors 90

Walter, J.G. 134
Wang, C. 181
Wang, T. 31
Wang, Y. 152
wax printing 212–13
web-based protein aptamer 176
Wei, H. 148
western blotting 34
whole-cell detection
    microfluidics-enabled aptasensors 218–19
    pathogen 7, 263
whole-cell SELEX technique 112
Wu, S. 150

xenografts 175, 196, 198
xeno-nucleic acid system 185
Xia, Y. 150
XNA-based aptamers 55–56, 61
Xu, H. 12
Xu, W. 182
Xu, Y. 7
Xu, Z. 183

Yuan, B. 13
Yüce, M. 199
Yu, X. 277

zeolite imidazole frameworks (ZIF) 192–93
zeolitic imidazolate framework-8 (ZIF-8) 192
Zhang, G. 12, 258
Zhang, J. 8, 276
Zhang, X. 258
Zhang, Z. 155
Zhao, C. 13
Zhao, Q. 181
Zhao, X. 184
Zheng, C. 192
Zika virus 187

For Product Safety Concerns and Information please contact our EU
representative GPSR@taylorandfrancis.com
Taylor & Francis Verlag GmbH, Kaufingerstraße 24, 80331 München, Germany

www.ingramcontent.com/pod-product-compliance
Lightning Source LLC
Chambersburg PA
CBHW060329220326
41598CB00023B/2652